Oxford Specialist Handbooks in Anaesthesia
Anaesthesia for Emergency Care

Edited by

Jerry Nolan

Consultant in Anaesthesia and Intensive Care Medicine
Royal United Hospital NHS Trust,
Bath, UK

Jasmeet Soar

Consultant in Anaesthesia and Intensive Care Medicine
Southmead Hospital, North Bristol NHS Trust,
Bristol, UK

D1355597

OXFORD
UNIVERSITY PRESS

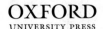

OXFORD
UNIVERSITY PRESS

Great Clarendon Street, Oxford OX2 6DP,
United Kingdom

Oxford University Press is a department of the University of Oxford.
It furthers the University's objective of excellence in research, scholarship,
and education by publishing worldwide. Oxford is a registered trade mark of
Oxford University Press in the UK and in certain other countries

British Library Cataloguing in Publication Data

Data available

Library of Congress Cataloging in Publication Data
Library of Congress Control Number: 2012933283

ISBN 978-0-19-958897-8

Printed in China by
C & C Offset Printing Co, Ltd

Preface

Anaesthetizing patients for surgical and medical emergencies can be challenging. The time critical nature of the intervention may mean proceeding with a limited medical history and only a brief assessment with minimal investigations. Ideally, these patients should be fully resuscitated, but in some circumstances (e.g. after major trauma) anaesthetizing the patient can be an essential component of the initial resuscitation.

When planning this book, we aimed to include most of procedures encountered by the 'on-call' anaesthetist, both during the day and out-of-hours. In keeping with the Oxford Handbook series, the style is concise but we have tried to include the essential information needed to anaesthetize these patients safely. The first section comprises a series of topics that are generic to many emergencies and the remaining sections cover a full range of conditions that may require anaesthesia in the operating room, emergency department, critical care unit, and radiology suite. In recognition of the increasing role of doctors in prehospital emergency medicine, we have included a section on prehospital anaesthesia and transport. Clearly, every possible scenario cannot be covered in this book. If there is any doubt about the best way to proceed in an emergency, seek expert help early.

Although aimed principally at the anaesthetic trainee, this book should be of value to consultants in anaesthesia and critical care and to trainees and consultants in emergency medicine.

We would appreciate feedback (to the e mail address below) about this book, particularly in relation to topics that we have omitted or any errors that we have missed. Finally, we thank all the authors for their high quality contributions in the face of pressing deadlines and our wives and children who now struggle to remember what we look like.

Jerry and Jasmeet
jerry.nolan@nhs.net
2012

Contents

Contributors

Anne-Marie Amphlett
Specialist Trainee
Bristol School of Anaesthesia

Monica Baird
Consultant in Anaesthesia
Royal United Hospital NHS Trust
Bath

Guy Bayley
Consultant in Paediatric
Anaesthesia,
Bristol Royal Hospital for Children

Jonathan Benger
Professor of Emergency Care,
University of the West of England,
Bristol and Consultant in
Emergency Medicine,
University Hospitals Bristol
NHS Foundation Trust

Craig Carroll
Consultant in Anaesthesia
Salford Royal Hospital NHS
Foundation Trust

Emma Clow
Specialist Trainee
Bristol School of Anaesthesia

Tim Cook
Consultant in Anaesthesia
and Intensive Care,
Royal United Hospital NHS
Trust, Bath

Jules Cranshaw
Consultant in Anaesthesia and
Intensive Care Medicine
Royal Bournemouth Hospital,
Bournemouth

Rhys Davies
Consultant in Anaesthesia
North Bristol NHS Trust, Bristol

Charles Deakin
Consultant in Cardiac Anaesthesia
and Intensive Care Medicine
University Hospital Southampton

Simon Finney
Consultant in Anaesthesia and
Intensive Care Medicine
Royal Brompton Hospital, London

Andrew Georgiou
Specialist Trainee
Bristol School of Anaesthesia

Ben Gibbison
Specialist Trainee
Bristol School of Anaesthesia

Amit Goswami
Specialist Trainee
Bristol School of Anaesthesia

Richard Griffiths
Consultant in Anaesthesia
Peterborough and Stamford
Hospitals NHS Trust

Kim J. Gupta
Consultant in Anaesthesia and
Intensive Care Medicine,
Royal United Hospital NHS Trust,
Bath

Carl Gwinnutt
Formerly Consultant in
Anaesthesia
Salford Royal Hospital NHS
Foundation Trust

Clare Hommers
Specialist Trainee
Bristol School of Anaesthesia

Tim Hooper
Specialist Trainee
Bristol School of Anaesthesia

Dom Hurford
Specialist Trainee
Bristol School of Anaesthesia

Rob Jackson
Specialist Trainee
Bristol School of Anaesthesia

Chris Johnson
Consultant in Anaesthesia
North Bristol NHS Trust, Bristol

Alistair Johnstone
Specialist Trainee
Bristol School of Anaesthesia

Rebecca Leslie
Specialist Trainee
Bristol School of Anaesthesia

David Lockey
Consultant in Anaesthesia and
Intensive Care Medicine, North
Bristol NHS Trust and London
Helicopter Emergency
Medical Service,
Royal London Hospital

Melanie McDonald
Specialist Trainee
Bristol School of Anaesthesia

Patrick Magee
Consultant in Anaesthesia
Royal United Hospital NHS Trust,
Bath

Thomas Martin
Specialist Trainee
Bristol School of Anaesthesia

Lucy Miller
Specialist Trainee
Bristol School of Anaesthesia

Ronelle Mouton
Consultant in Anaesthesia
Royal United Hospital NHS Trust,
Bath

Henry Murdoch
Specialist Trainee
Bristol School of Anaesthesia

Jerry Nolan
Consultant in Anaesthesia and
Intensive Care Medicine,
Royal United Hospital NHS Trust,
Bath

Judith Nolan
Consultant in Paediatric
Anaesthesia,
Bristol Royal Hospital for Children

Sonja Payne
Specialist Trainee
Bristol School of Anaesthesia

Carol J. Peden
Consultant in Anaesthesia and
Intensive Care Medicine,
Royal United Hospital NHS Trust,
Bath

Susanna Ritchie-McLean
Specialist Traineee in Anaesthesia,
Peterborough & Stamford
Hospitals NHS Foundation Trust

Edward Scarth
Specialist Trainee
Bristol School of Anaesthesia

Joe Sebastian
Consultant in Anaesthesia
Salford Royal Hospital NHS
Foundation Trust

Jasmeet Soar
Consultant in Anaesthesia
and Intensive Care Medicine,
North Bristol NHS Trust,
Bristol

Matt Thomas
Consultant in Anaesthesia and
Intensive Care Medicine,
University Hospitals Bristol NHS
Foundation Trust

Julian Thompson
Specialist Registrar in Prehospital
Care, London Helicopter
Emergency Medical Service,
Royal London Hospital

Jenny Tuckey
Consultant in Anaesthesia
Royal United Hospital NHS Trust,
Bath

Medha Vanarase
Consultant in Anaesthesia
John Radcliffe Hospital, Oxford

Michelle White
Consultant in Anaesthesia,
Mercy Ships, formerly Consultant
in Paediatric Anaesthesia,
Bristol Royal Hospital for Children

Andy Weale
Consultant Vascular Surgeon
North Bristol NHS Trust, Bristol

Nicola Weale
Consultant in Anaesthesia
North Bristol NHS Trust, Bristol

David Windsor
Specialist Trainee
Bristol School of Anaesthesia

Helen Wise
Consultant in Anaesthesia, Poole
Hospital NHS Foundation Trust

Symbols and Abbreviations

$\square$	cross reference
↑	increased
↓	decreased
~	approximately
→	leading to
±	plus/minus
▶	important
#	fracture
#NOF	fractured neck of femur
✍	website
A–a	alveolar–arterial
AAA	abdominal aortic aneurysm
AAGBI	Association of Anaesthetists of Great Britain and Ireland
ABCDE	airway, breathing, circulation, disability, exposure
ABG	arterial blood gas
ACEI	angiotensin converting enzyme inhibitor
ADH	anti-diuretic hormone
AKI	acute kidney injury
ALI	acute lung injury
ALS	advanced life support
APTT	activated partial thromboplastin time
ARDS	acute respiratory distress syndrome
ASA	American Society of Anesthesiologists
AV	atrioventricular
BP	blood pressure
Ca	calcium
CABG	coronary artery bypass grafting
CBF	cerebral blood flow
CDH	Congenital diaphragmatic hernia
CEA	carotid endarterectomy
CICV	can't intubate, can't ventilate'
cLMA	classic laryngeal mask airway
$CMRO_2$	cerebral metabolic rate of O_2
CNB	central neuraxial block
CNS	central nervous system

CO_2	carbon dioxide
COPD	chronic obstructive pulmonary disease
CP	cricoid pressure
CPAP	continuous positive airway pressure
CPB	cardiopulmonary bypass
CPP	cerebral perfusion pressure
CPR	cardiopulmonary resuscitation
Cr	creatinine
CS	Caesarean section
CSF	cerebrospinal fluid
CSI	cervical spine injury
CT	computed tomography
CTPA	computed tomography pulmonary angiography
CV	central venous
CVC	central venous catheter
CVP	central venous pressure
DBD	donation after brain death
DBP	diastolic blood pressure
DCD	donation after circulatory death
DI	diabetes insipidus
DIC	disseminated intravascular coagulation
DND	delayed neurological deficit
DVT	deep venous thrombosis
ECG	electrocardiogram
ED	emergency department
EDH	extradural haematoma
EEG	electroencephalogram
EMG	electromyograph
ENT	ear, nose, and throat
ET	end-tidal
ETO_2	end-tidal oxygen concentration
EVAR	endovascular aneurysm repair
EVD	external ventricular drain
FAST	focused assessment by sonography in trauma
FBC	full blood count
$F_{ET}O_2$	fraction of end-tidal oxygen
FFP	fresh frozen plasma
FiO_2	fraction of inspired oxygen
FOI	fibreoptic intubation
FRC	functional residual capacity

GA	general anaesthesia/anaesthetic
GCS	Glasgow Coma Scale
GI	gastrointestinal
h	hour/s
H^+	hydrogen ion
HAS	human albumin solution
Hb	haemoglobin
HDU	high-dependency unit
HELLP	haemolysis, elevated liver enzymes, low platelets
HFOV	high-frequency oscillatory ventilation
HIV	human immunodeficiency virus
HLA	human leucocyte antigen
HME	heat and moisture exchanger
HTLV	human T-lymphotropic virus
ICD	implantable cardioverter-defibrillator
ICH	intracerebral haematoma
ICP	intracranial pressure
ICS	Intensive Care Society
ICU	intensive care unit
Ig	immunoglobulin
ILM	intubating laryngeal mask
IM	intramuscular
INR	international normalized ratio
IO	intraosseous
IOP	intraocular pressure
IPPV	intermittent positive pressure ventilation
IVC	intravenous
IVC	inferior vena cava
K^+	potassium ion
LA	local anaesthesia/anaesthetic
LFT	liver function test
LMA	laryngeal mask airway
LMWH	low-molecular-weight heparin
LV	left ventricular
MAC	minimum alveolar concentration
MAP	mean arterial pressure
mg	milligram/s
MH	malignant hyperthermia
MI	myocardial infarction
MILS	manual in-line stabilization

min	minute/s
mL	millilitre/s
MRI	magnetic resonance imaging
Na^+	sodium ion
NICE	National Institute for Health and Clinical Excellence
NIV	non-invasive ventilation
NMBA	neuromuscular blocking agent
NSAID	non-steroidal anti-inflammatory drug
O_2	oxygen
PA	pulmonary artery
$PaCO_2$	partial pressure of arterial carbon dioxide
PCA	patient-controlled analgesia
PCC	prothrombin complex concentrate
PCI	percutaneous coronary intervention
PCO_2	partial pressure of carbon dioxide
PE	pulmonary embolism
PEA	pulseless electrical activity
PEEP	positive end-expiratory pressure
PET	pre-eclamptic toxaemia
PICU	paediatric intensive care unit
PIP	peak inspiratory pressure
PNB	peripheral nerve block
PO	orally (per os)
PO_2	partial pressure of oxygen
PONV	postoperative nausea and vomiting
PPH	postpartum haemorrhage
PR	rectally (per rectum)
PRN	as needed (pro re nata)
PT	prothrombin time
RA	regional anaesthesia/anaesthetic
RBC	red blood cell
rFVIIa	recombinant Factor VIIa
RNA	ribonucleic acid
RRT	renal replacement therapy
RSI	rapid sequence induction
RV	right ventricular
s	second/s
SAD	supraglottic airway device
SAH	subarachnoid haemorrhage
SaO_2	arterial oxygen saturation

SBP	systolic blood pressure
SC	subcutaneous
$ScvO_2$	oxygen saturation of central venous blood
SIGN	Scottish Intercollegiate Guidelines Network
SIRS	systemic inflammatory response syndrome
SSEP	somatosensory evoked potential
STEMI	ST-elevation myocardial infarction
SVC	superior vena cava
SVR	systemic vascular resistance
TAP	transversus abdominis plane
TBI	traumatic brain injury
TEG	thromboelastogram
TIA	transient ischaemic attack
TIPSS	transjugular intrahepatic portosystemic shunt
TIVA	total intravenous anaesthesia
TOF	tracheo-oesophageal fistula
TRALI	transfusion-related acute lung injury
TT	tracheal tube
U&Es	urea and electrolytes
US	ultrasound
VF	ventricular fibrillation
VP	ventriculoperitoneal
VT	ventricular tachycardia
VTE	venous thromboembolism
WFNS	World Federation of Neurological Surgeons

General Principles

Preoperative assessment

Key points

The principles of preoperative assessment for the emergency patient are the same as those that apply to the elective situation but they may need to be abbreviated in an emergency.

Background

- Thorough preoperative assessment of the emergency patient is as important as that of the patient attending for planned surgery.
- The usual principles of obtaining a history, examining the patient, and performing investigations apply, although potentially in an abbreviated form appropriate to the degree of urgency of surgery.
▶ Assessment can be made more challenging by the lack of a complete set of patient notes and investigations. Consideration must be given to which investigations are essential for safe anaesthesia to continue, and those that will cause unnecessary delays to surgical management.

History

Obtain a focused history, concentrating on those areas likely to have the greatest impact on choice of anaesthetic technique, postoperative care, and potential complications. Emergency patients may have a depressed conscious level; in this case, seek a history from all available sources such as patient notes and relatives/carers.

- Nature of the acute problem—timescale over which it has occurred and details of the surgical plan and urgency of surgery.
- Previous medical history—pay particular attention to cardiovascular and respiratory disease. Obtain an indication of exercise tolerance and frequency of angina. Orthopnoea and paroxysmal nocturnal dyspnoea imply poor cardiovascular reserve.
- Previous anaesthetic history—any known problems with previous anaesthetics? If the notes are available, scrutinize previous charts (if available) for details of airway problems or drug reactions.
- Drug history—obtain an accurate list of current medication and any changes made in hospital. Anticoagulants or antiplatelet drugs may not have been stopped in advance, precluding use of neuraxial techniques. Patients may have been nil by mouth for many days and not have received their usual medication. Check that appropriate antibiotic therapy has been given in sepsis; if not, give immediately.
- Allergies—document confirmed or suspected drug reactions.
- Fasting times should be identified carefully. Patients may be considered fasted after the following intervals:
  - 6h since solid food/formula milk.
  - 4h since breast milk.
  - 2h since clear fluids.
- Gastric emptying is prolonged in trauma (especially in children) when fasting times are considered to be the duration between last oral intake and the injury. Opioid use, poorly controlled diabetes mellitus, and renal failure may also delay gastric emptying. Patients with peritonitis should be assumed to have a full stomach.

- Social history—ensure pregnancy has been either excluded or identified in women of childbearing age. Ascertain functional level, and support required at home. This may be particularly important if an intensive care unit (ICU) admission is being considered.

Examination

- *Airway*—airway management problems are disproportionately common in emergency cases. Examine the airway carefully to identify potential difficulties and plan ahead for failed intubation or ventilation. Difficult intubation may be more likely to occur in the morbidly obese, patients with musculoskeletal disease resulting in reduced neck and jaw movement, patients with small mouths, large incisors, hypognathia, macroglossia, and short thyromental distance. Assessment should include inspection of the mouth, the Mallampati score, and assessment of range of motion of the neck. Maintain cervical spine immobilization in trauma patients until cervical spine fracture has been excluded. No simple bedside test can exclude all difficult airways. It is vital to have a well-rehearsed approach to dealing with airway management problems.
- *Respiratory*—untreated pulmonary oedema is associated with a poor outcome and should be excluded. Baseline oxygen saturation of arterial blood on air or supplemental oxygen may indicate likelihood of success of postoperative extubation. Evidence of acute lung injury may justify use of reduced tidal volume ventilation intraoperatively.
- *Cardiovascular*—identify the patient's normal blood pressure (BP): intraoperative mean arterial pressure (MAP) should be kept within 20% of this. Assess intravascular volume and extracellular fluid loss. Patients may be inadequately resuscitated; consider a period of stabilization prior to induction, this may need to occur in the anaesthetic room or ICU. Consider measuring central venous saturation and applying goal-directed therapy protocols. Arrhythmias are more common in emergency patients and may require preoperative treatment.
- *Neurological*—accurate documentation of pre-induction Glasgow Coma Scale (GCS) score can be vital for postoperative assessment and management. Pre-existing neurological deficit should be documented.

Investigations

The time available to obtain information from investigations is frequently limited; avoid unnecessary delays awaiting results. The choice of investigations is guided by the clinical situation, but generally includes the following:

- Electrocardiogram (ECG).
- Full blood count (FBC), creatinine, urea and electrolytes (U&Es), blood sugar.
- Group and screen or formal crossmatch.
- Arterial blood gas (ABG) analysis including lactate—will give valuable information about adequacy of resuscitation and severity of metabolic disturbance. The patient with severe metabolic acidosis will require extreme care on induction, and attention to ventilator settings.
- Clotting screen—especially if taking anticoagulants, or after transfusion.
- Liver function tests—if malnourished, alcoholic, or known liver disease.

- Echocardiogram—focused studies may rule out significant pathology and give useful information on ventricular function and filling status.
- Pregnancy test.
- Chest X-ray—if specifically indicated.
- Computed tomography (CT) scanning—ensure cervical spine has been cleared in trauma.

Consent

- Obtaining valid, informed consent from all patients is an ethical and professional duty. In an emergency, make reasonable efforts to obtain appropriate consent. Focus discussions on:
  - The proposed techniques.
  - The potential benefits and risk of complications (see Box 1.1).
  - Alternative treatments available.
- In life-threatening emergencies where obtaining consent would cause unacceptable delays it is acceptable to treat patients in their best interests without waiting. Consent obtained in an anaesthetic room immediately pre-induction may be later considered invalid. Where the patient is unconscious or deemed 'incompetent' the opinions of family members or close friends should be sought. If such opinions are unavailable, and time allows, the opinion of an Independent Mental Capacity Advocate (IMCA) may need to be sought to comply with the Mental Capacity Act 2005.
- A 'competent' child aged 16–18yrs may give consent for their own treatment and separate parental consent is not required. If a child aged 16–18 refuses treatment, consent may be obtained from their parents provided failure to act will result in permanent injury or death. Consent should be obtained from parents or guardians for all children below the age of 18, who are unable to give consent themselves. In life-threatening emergencies it is acceptable to treat in best interests if time does not allow for consent to occur.
- If patients are expected to be admitted to the ICU postoperatively, discuss with them the treatment they will receive there, including details of intravenous (IV) access, catheters, monitoring, and ventilation.
- Advanced directives (living wills) may impose legal restrictions on what treatment can be given. Any such directive should be examined carefully and its contents and implications discussed fully with the patient or relatives. Seek expert opinion (e.g. from hospital legal teams) if there is doubt over the application of the advance directive.
- Jehovah's Witnesses may place limits on the use of blood products. Each patient must be treated individually because attitudes toward use of cell salvage and other blood conservation strategies differ.

Box 1.1 Royal College of Anaesthetists' definitions of risk

- Very common: ~1 in 10.
- Rare: ~1 in 10,000.
- Very rare: ~1 in 100,000.

Further reading

Rivers E, Nguyen B, Havstad S, et al. Early goal-directed therapy in the treatment of severe sepsis and septic shock. N Engl J Med 2001; **345**:1368–77.

Rapid sequence induction and tracheal intubation

Key points
- The aim of raid sequence induction (RSI) and tracheal intubation is to reduce the risk of aspiration by minimizing the time between loss of protective airway reflexes and placement of a cuffed tracheal tube.
- Considerations and controversies include choice of drugs, use of an opioid, application of cricoid pressure, ventilation of the lungs during the procedure, and the choice of rescue techniques in the event of failed intubation.

Choice of anaesthetic technique
- The exact method of induction and the choice of airway will be determined by the nature of the patient's acute and chronic illness, and the operative procedure.
▶ Some emergency cases will be managed best by postponement of surgery until the patient is fasted adequately, followed by use of supraglottic airways or regional techniques. In many cases, however, tracheal intubation is the method of choice, the usual route being orotracheal.
- Inadequate fasting times, severe injury, peritonitis, pregnancy, or other causes of ↑ risk of aspiration generally require the use of RSI of anaesthesia.
- Communication with the surgical and operating room teams is essential.
- In the haemodynamically unstable patient it may be necessary to induce the patient on the operating table with the abdomen prepared and surgical team scrubbed and ready to proceed as soon as the airway is secured.
- It may also be necessary to defer some procedures performed normally before surgery (e.g. central venous pressure (CVP) lines) until after surgery commences.
- Cases where airway management is anticipated to be problematic may also require surgeons to be present and scrubbed to assist with 2nd- or 3rd-line airway plans.

Rapid sequence induction
- The aim of the RSI is to reduce the risk of aspiration by minimizing the length of time between abolition of protective airway reflexes by anaesthesia and establishment of a secure airway by tracheal intubation with a cuffed tube.
- Additional precautions to help prevent aspiration of stomach contents include application of cricoid pressure and avoidance of manual ventilation by facemask to reduce the risk of inflating the stomach with gas. A period of preoxygenation before induction prolongs the duration of apnoea before desaturation occurs.
- Use of RSI increases the incidence of intubation failure by 8–10-fold; rescue techniques will be needed in 0.3–1.0% of RSIs. Planning for failure is essential.
- The Difficult Airway Society has produced specific guidelines for the management of failed intubation following RSI (see 📖 Failed tracheal intubation, p.356). Repeated attempts at intubation may result

in desaturation of arterial blood, airway injury, and aspiration. In many cases the correct procedure is to wake the patient and use a different approach (e.g. awake fibreoptic intubation). If abandoning surgery is inappropriate, a balance must be struck between achieving an airway via other means (e.g. supraglottic airway) to facilitate surgery, and the risk of aspiration.

- All anaesthetists must be practised in failed intubation and 'can't intubate, can't ventilate' (CICV) drills and be familiar with the use of difficult airway equipment and rescue devices—specifically the ones available to them locally.
- During RSI, a precalculated dose of induction drug is given, which may cause haemodynamic compromise in the unstable patient. Consider pre-induction fluid loading and ensure appropriate vasopressor drugs are immediately available.
- Insertion of an arterial line before induction is often invaluable.
- Patients who require RSI generally remain at risk of aspiration at the end of surgery. Appropriate management of emergence and extubation (usually extubation awake in the lateral position) is as important as that of induction.

Conduct of rapid sequence induction

- Obtain informed consent from patient.
- Ensure sufficient personnel who are appropriately trained and briefed are present.
- Perform pre-induction checks (e.g. World Health Organization surgical safety checklist).
- Ensure adequate IV access and monitoring.
- Ensure availability and correct function of equipment (see Box 1.2).
- Pre-oxygenate (generally 3–5 min of 100% oxygen via tight-fitting mask and anaesthetic breathing system) until end-tidal oxygen concentration (ETO_2) is 90%. Consider head-up position and use of continuous positive airway pressure (CPAP) to optimize pre-oxygenation.
- Consider use of a short-acting opioid (e.g. alfentanil).
- Induce anaesthesia using pre-calculated dose of rapid onset IV induction drug.
- Apply cricoid pressure—10 N (1 kg) applied with injection of induction drug, increasing to 30 N (3 kg) with loss of consciousness. Avoid higher forces.
- Paralyse with rapid onset muscle relaxant (normally suxamethonium 1–2 mg kg^{-1} or rocuronium 1 mg kg^{-1}).
- Continue passive oxygenation until relaxation has occurred (about 30 s); facemask ventilation is not usually undertaken but may be essential if normal arterial oxygen saturation could not be achieved despite attempted pre-oxygenation (e.g. acute lung injury).
- Intubate the trachea, inflate the tracheal tube cuff, and secure the tube.
- Confirm tracheal intubation by presence of exhaled carbon dioxide (CO_2) trace on waveform capnography and bilateral auscultation of chest before release of cricoid pressure.
- Continue anaesthesia and controlled ventilation.
- If suxamethonium has been used, give a non-depolarizing neuromuscular blocker to maintain muscle relaxation.

Box 1.2 Equipment required for rapid sequence intubation
- Patient trolley with head-down tilt function.
- Suction (Yankauer tip) on and within reach of intubator.
- Suitable pillow for patient positioning.
- Laryngoscopes with variety of suitable blades (checked and working).
- Bougie/stylet.
- Tracheal tubes of appropriate size and smaller in reserve.
- Lubricating gel.
- Magill forceps.
- Syringe for cuff inflation.
- Waveform capnograph connected to breathing circuit.
- Breathing circuit.
- Separate reserve oxygen supply and self-inflating bag.
- Means to secure tracheal tube (tape or tie).
- Stethoscope.
- Equipment for failed intubation (supraglottic and front-of-neck devices).
- Drugs (induction agent/relaxant/vasopressors/atropine).

Additional considerations and modifications

Choice of induction agent and neuromuscular blocking drug
See also 📖 Drugs for emergency anaesthesia, p.10.
- Thiopental and propofol achieve rapid anaesthesia but cause hypotension. Consider using ketamine in septic, shocked, and trauma patients—it is cardiovascularly more stable and considered by some to be the optimal drug for critically ill patients. Etomidate is associated with ↑ mortality in septic patients.
- Suxamethonium: use a dose of 1–2 mg kg^{-1} for RSI. Higher doses produce better intubation conditions but prolong the duration of apnoea (median 5–10 min).
- Rocuronium: doses of 1.0 mg kg^{-1} will produce similar intubating conditions to suxamethonium within 1 min. Addition of a short-acting opioid improves intubation conditions. Sugammadex will reverse the neuromuscular blockade produced by rocuronium within minutes (dose dictated by scenario).
- Emergency intubation without neuromuscular blockade is associated with ↑ rates of aspiration, airway trauma, and death. It is not recommended.

Cricoid pressure
- Although regarded as standard practice, use of cricoid pressure (CP) is controversial: it lacks a robust evidence base but evidence of its harm is also absent.
- While RSI/CP does not guarantee prevention of aspiration, failure to perform CP during RSI is currently medicolegally indefensible.
- When performed well, CP is unlikely to interfere with laryngoscopy.
- CP is frequently taught poorly and performed poorly.
- Bimanual CP is not recommended for routine use.
- If laryngoscopy is difficult, change the CP to BURP (backwards, upwards, and rightward pressure).

- If laryngoscopy remains difficult, reduce the CP and if no improvement occurs, remove completely while having suction immediately available.
- If a supraglottic airway device (SAD), e.g. classic laryngeal mask airway (cLMA) or a Pro-Seal® LMA, is used to rescue failed intubation, remove the CP to enable correct placement and function of the airway device.

Use of opioids

- The addition of an opioid to RSI attenuates the sympathetic response to laryngoscopy.
- Frequency of awareness may also be decreased.
- If RSI is abandoned, the risks of prolonged apnoea can be reduced by use of short-acting drugs (e.g. alfentanil) and availability of naloxone.
- Use of opioids has not been associated with worse outcome following RSI.

Ventilation during rapid sequence induction

- The original description of CP included ventilation via facemask. Although generally avoided to reduce risk of stomach inflation it is used occasionally during RSI in small children and in those patients at high risk of developing hypoxaemia rapidly.
- Correctly applied CP will avoid gastric inflation.

Nasogastric tubes

- If a nasogastric tube is in place prior to anaesthesia it should be aspirated before induction and left on free drainage.
- It is unlikely that the presence of a nasogastric tube decreases efficacy of cricoid pressure.

Failed intubation and rescue techniques

- Poor view at laryngoscopy and failed intubation is a potentially dangerous situation. All anaesthetists should be familiar with approaches for maintaining patient safety in this scenario.
- Oxygenation is the priority. It is important to have prepared for failed intubation in advance. This includes communication and planning (equipment, roles) by the whole 'airway team'. The default management technique is to wake the patient; however, the airway usually needs to be managed actively during this period to prevent hypoxaemia.
- Facemask ventilation or insertion of a SAD is indicated in order to achieve adequate oxygenation and/or continue anaesthesia where necessary. Insertion of, and ventilation through, a SAD is impeded by CP. Insertion of a Pro-Seal® LMA by 'railroading' over an inverted bougie inserted deliberately into the oesophagus is a reliable method of achieving an effective airway with reasonable protection from aspiration in a failed intubation.
- Where rescue with facemask ventilation or a SAD fails, emergency access to the trachea (cricothyroidotomy or immediate surgical airway) is likely to be lifesaving. Those performing RSI should be trained, able, and willing to perform such techniques.
- Following airway rescue, empty the stomach.

Further reading

Difficult Airway Society Guidelines. Available at: ♙ http://www.das.uk.com.

El-Orbany M, Connolly LA. Rapid sequence induction and intubation: current controversy. *Anaesth Analg* 2010; **110**:1318–25.

Vanner RG, Asai T. Safe use of cricoid pressure. *Anaesthesia* 1999; **54**:1–3.

Drugs for emergency anaesthesia

Key points
- None of the current hypnotic drugs or neuromuscular blockers is ideal for inducing anaesthesia in an emergency.
- Despite its tendency to cause hypotension, propofol is a popular choice because of its familiarity.
- Ketamine is more cardiovascularly stable and may be the drug of choice in critically ill patients.
- Although suxamethonium remains the most commonly used neuromuscular blocking drug for RSI, more experienced anaesthetists are increasingly using rocuronium, particularly with the introduction of sugammadex, which enables rapid reversal.

General principles
- Patients undergoing emergency anaesthesia are acutely unwell, may be haemodynamically unstable, and frequently have co-morbid disease.
- The pharmacokinetic properties of drugs may be affected by intravascular volume, cardiac output, and variation in protein binding.
▶ Drugs may act in a more potent manner or have more pronounced side effects and longer duration of action in the critically ill patient.
- The ideal anaesthetic drugs would have the following properties:
  - Easily calculable doses.
  - Rapid onset and predictable duration of action.
  - Minimal impact on cardiovascular status.
  - No unwanted side effects.
  - No drug interactions.
  - Reliable metabolism despite acute or chronic illness.
- Such drugs do not exist and therefore any choice will be a compromise. Selection of drugs for use in emergencies may be based purely on pharmacological properties; however, familiarity of the anaesthetist with the drug may also have a role.
- It is possible that a frequently used drug will be used more safely than one with which the anaesthetist has limited experience.
- Emergency drugs (suxamethonium, atropine, adrenaline, dantrolene) should always be checked and available prior to commencing anaesthesia.

Induction drugs
Thiopental
- Typical dose 3–7 mg kg^{-1}.
- A barbiturate; produces reliable, rapid-onset anaesthesia with inhibition of airway reflexes and respiratory drive.
- Decreases cardiac output and systemic vascular resistance with resulting reduction in BP, especially in shocked patients.
- Reduces cerebral metabolism, cerebral blood flow, intracranial pressure, and intraocular pressure.
- Has a long history of use in RSI, but works less well when used with supraglottic airways.

- Severe anaphylactic reactions in 1:20,000.
- Metabolized in the liver with inactive products excreted by the kidneys. No effect on uterine tone.

Propofol

- Typical dose 1.5–2.5 mg kg^{-1}.
- A phenol derivative; produces rapid-onset anaesthesia, though large dose reductions are required in the shocked and unwell patient.
- Marked airway reflex inhibition, making it very suitable for use with supraglottic airways.
- Surveys suggest widespread use in RSI, though its tendency to cause profound hypotension in susceptible patients makes this controversial.
- Pharmacokinetics enable target-controlled infusion for sedation and anaesthesia. Renal and hepatic disease do not affect metabolism significantly.
- Propofol infusion syndrome may complicate use on intensive care, especially in the young, resulting in ↑ mortality.

Ketamine

- Typical dose 1–2 mg kg^{-1}.
- Produces dissociative anaesthesia and an increase in sympathetic tone resulting in a slight rise in BP.
- Airway reflexes are preserved and mild respiratory stimulation occurs.
- Considered by some to be the optimal drug for critically ill patients because of its cardiovascular stability.
- Use in traumatic brain injury is more controversial because of concerns about elevation in intracranial pressure; this may be balanced by a reduction in cerebral oxygen consumption and ↑ systemic BP.
- Prolongs duration of neuromuscular blockade achieved with muscle relaxants.

Etomidate

- Typical dose 0.3 mg kg^{-1}.
- Rapid induction of anaesthesia though frequently associated with involuntary muscle movement.
- Limited impact on the cardiovascular system with preservation of pressor response to laryngoscopy.
- Associated with marked suppression of endogenous steroid synthesis, even after a single dose, and associated with ↑ mortality in patients with sepsis. Its use in critically ill patients has diminished as a result.

Benzodiazepines

Midazolam

- Typical dose 0.07–0.1 mg kg^{-1}.
- Produces anxiolysis, amnesia, and sedation; may be used as a co-induction drug.
- Slow onset (5–7 min) limits its use in RSI.
- May reduce BP slightly; responses in the unwell and very old may be variable.
- Hepatically metabolized; inactive metabolites are renally cleared.
- Effects may be reversed by flumazenil (0.1–1 mg in titrated doses).

Non-depolarizing muscle relaxants
- Duration of block prolonged by:
  - Metabolic disturbance (dehydration, acidosis, hypercapnia).
  - Electrolyte disturbance (hypokalaemia, hypocalcaemia, hypermagnesaemia) and hypoproteinaemia).
  - Drugs (volatile agents, induction drugs, fentanyl, suxamethonium, diuretics, calcium channel blockers, alpha/beta antagonists, metronidazole, aminoglycosides, protamine).

Atracurium
- Typical dose 0.3–0.6 mg kg^{-1}.
- Produces maximal blockade after 90 s. 95% recovery within 35 min. Does not accumulate with repeated doses; metabolism occurs mainly via Hofmann degradation, which is not dependent on hepatic or renal function.
- May cause histamine release; not a trigger for malignant hyperthermia (MH).

Rocuronium
- Typical dose 0.6 mg kg^{-1} (normal intubation dose); 1–1.2 mg kg^{-1} (RSI dose).
- May be used for RSI but less likely than suxamethonium to produce excellent intubation conditions.
- Non-MH trigger and does not produce hyperkalaemia.
- Produces prolonged block (>45 min) after large doses, and should be used only in patients at low risk of airway management difficulties (unless sugammadex is available). (See 📖 Sugammadex, p.13) reverses blockade rapidly and may be useful after failed intubation. Predominantly hepatic clearance.

Vecuronium
- Typical dose 0.1 mg kg^{-1}; intubating conditions are achieved in 120 s.
- Duration prolonged in hepatic failure, though not significantly in renal failure; non-MH trigger.

Depolarizing muscle relaxant
Suxamethonium
- Typical dose 1.0–2.0 mg kg^{-1}.
- Produces excellent intubating conditions within 30 s, and is most frequently used for RSI. Higher doses produce better intubation conditions but may prolong apnoea duration (median 5–10 min).
- Duration of action may impede adequate ventilation in patients woken in failed intubation scenarios.
- May produce bradycardia (have atropine available). Resultant hyperkalaemia may be fatal in chronically immobile or burned patients; MH trigger (see 📖 Malignant hyperthermia, p.378); risk of anaphylaxis.

Neuromuscular blockade reversal drugs
Neostigmine
- Typical dose 0.05–0.07 mg kg^{-1}.
- Reversible cholinesterase inhibitor useful for assisting reversal of partial neuromuscular blockade.

- Peak effect achieved after 10 min. Normally injected with anticholinergic drug (glycopyrronium) to prevent bradycardia. Prolongs duration of action of suxamethonium.

Sugammadex

- A modified gamma-cyclodextrin that encapsulates and inactivates aminosteroid neuromuscular blockers (rocuronium and vecuronium).
- It is not active for other drugs; the drug complex is renally cleared.
- Doses: $2 \, mg \, kg^{-1}$ (reversal of moderate blockade); $4 \, mg \, kg^{-1}$ (deep blockade); $16 \, mg \, kg^{-1}$ (for immediate reversal of profound blockade, e.g. failed intubation during RSI with rocuronium).
- Neuromuscular blockade in the 24 h following administration may be achieved with non-steroidal drugs (e.g. atracurium).

Opioids

- Opioid analgesia is a mainstay of pre-, intra-, and postoperative pain control in emergency cases.
- Patients may have already received large doses of morphine or other opioid before induction.
- Opioids are classed by strength—weak (codeine) or strong (morphine, diamorphine)—or by duration of action. It may be better to use small doses of strong drugs than larger doses of weak drugs.
- The effectiveness of codeine between patients is highly variable. All opioids cause respiratory depression, nausea, vomiting, and constipation and may cause itching, confusion, and dysphoria in some. Respiratory depression can be reversed by naloxone (100–200-microgram bolus titrated to effect).

Remifentanil

- Ultra-short-acting drug. Especially useful as intraoperative infusion during major surgery ($0.01–1 \, micrograms \, kg^{-1} \, min^{-1}$).
- Bolus doses may cause severe bradycardia and difficulty with ventilation ('stiff chest').
- Context sensitive half-life is 3–5 min irrespective of duration of infusion.

Alfentanil

- Typical dose $10–25 \, micrograms \, kg^{-1}$. Short-acting drug (duration 5–10 min).
- Usefully given as a bolus for short but intensely stimulating surgical procedures. May produce bradycardia and 'stiff chest'. Given frequently by continuous infusion on ICUs.

Fentanyl

- Typical dose $1–5 \, micrograms \, kg^{-1}$; short-acting drug (duration 30–60 min).
- Useful as co-induction drug, intraoperatively, and for 'rescue' analgesia postoperatively.
- May produce bradycardia and 'stiff chest'. Also used in patient-controlled analgesia (PCA) devices and in patches for chronic pain.

Morphine
- Typical dose 5–20 mg 4-hourly via oral route; 2.5-mg IV doses should be titrated to effect.
- Peak effect after 30 min and duration of 3–4 h; dose should be reduced in renal failure due to accumulation of glucuronide conjugates.
- Used in PCA devices.

Inotropes and vasopressors
- There are few data to guide specific choices of inotropes and vasopressors in emergency surgery.
- Trials comparing different drugs given by continuous infusion on ICUs have failed to identify significant mortality differences.
- The use of non-invasive cardiac output monitoring may guide drug use, although these devices are not validated in emergency surgery.
- Ephedrine and metaraminol are convenient drugs for bolus use, with predominantly beta-1 and alpha-1 agonist effects respectively, but the use of infusions of noradrenaline and adrenaline should be considered early in emergency cases to prevent swings in BP, and prolonged periods of hypotension intraoperatively.

Antimuscarinics
Antimuscarinic drugs must be available immediately in the anaesthetic room to treat bradycardia caused by anaesthetic drugs or surgical procedures.
- Atropine—0.02 mg kg^{-1} up to 3 mg to achieve complete vagal blockade in the adult. Rapidly produces tachycardia, bronchodilation and ↓ secretions, but may also cause central excitation or depression.
- Glycopyrronium—0.2–0.4 mg; has a slower onset and prolonged duration of action compared with atropine; limited central effects due to its inability to cross the blood–brain barrier.

Dantrolene
Dantrolene is used in the treatment of MH to inhibit calcium release and therefore reduce skeletal muscle contraction. Initial dose of 2–3 mg kg^{-1} followed by 1 mg kg^{-1} as required PRN (see 📖 Malignant hyperthermia, p.378). May cause sedation. Reconstitution is hard work and requires a dedicated team member; it is made easier by using warm (40°C) diluent.

Further reading
Morris C, Perris A, Klein J, *et al*. Anaesthesia in haemodynamically compromised emergency patients. *Anaesthesia* 2009; **64**:532–9.

Perry JJ, Lee JS, Sillberg VAH, Wells GA. Rocuronium versus succinylcholine for rapid sequence induction intubation. *Cochrane Database Syst Rev* 2008; **2**:CD002788.

Smith S, Scarth E, Sasada M. *Drugs in Anaesthesia and Intensive Care* (4th edn). Oxford: Oxford University Press, 2011.

Vascular access

Key points
- The safe provision of anaesthesia for an emergency procedure depends on obtaining reliable and adequate intravenous (IV) access.
- Ultrasound (US)-directed internal jugular venous cannulation has almost replaced the landmark technique and US-guided subclavian cannulation may also be preferable to the landmark technique.
- In an emergency, if peripheral venous cannulation is not possible, the intraosseous (IO) route will provide rapid vascular access in both children and adults.

Background
- In an emergency, vascular access is achieved best by inserting at least one large-bore (14- or 16-G) peripheral IV cannula.
- The femoral vein is also very useful for urgent IV access and can be cannulated with a Seldinger technique with or without the aid of US.
- In an extreme emergency, such as cardiac arrest, if immediate IV access is not possible, the IO route will enable resuscitation drugs and fluids to be delivered.
- Relative contraindications to central venous cannulation are severe coagulopathy and local sepsis.

Ultrasound-directed vascular access
- In the UK, US-directed central venous cannulation is now the standard technique for access to the internal jugular and femoral veins.
- The advantages of using US are:
  - Direct visualization of the vessels and surrounding structures.
  - Identification of abnormal anatomy and thromboses.
  - Reduction of puncture-related complications.

Peripheral intravenous cannulation
- If rapid fluid infusion is likely to be required it is achieved most easily by inserting one or two 14- or 16-G cannula into peripheral veins in the upper limb.
- Although US can be used to aid insertion of a peripheral venous cannula, in an emergency it will be faster to cannulate the femoral vein using the landmark technique or insert an IO needle.

Femoral venous cannulation
- Cannulation of the femoral vein is relatively easy using either the US or landmark technique and avoids the risk of pneumothorax, which is associated with both the internal jugular and subclavian routes.
- The incidence of septic and thrombotic complications is 4 and 11 × higher with the femoral route than with the subclavian route.
- The femoral vein lies immediately medial to the femoral artery just below the inguinal ligament.
- A large-bore cannula can be inserted using the Seldinger technique.

- An 8.5 F introducer sheath can be inserted if rapid fluid infusion is required.
- Alternatively, a multiple lumen central venous catheter (CVC) can be placed—this will enable multiple drug infusions as well as providing a route for fluid infusion.
- The tip of a 15–20-cm catheter will lie in the common iliac vein or inferior vena cava, depending on the size of the patient and the length of the line.
- The CVP measured via the femoral route correlates well with that measured via the subclavian and internal jugular routes.

Internal jugular venous cannulation

- Right internal jugular vein cannulation is more likely to result in correct placement than subclavian cannulation; it is also less likely to cause pneumothorax.
- It is associated with a higher incidence of infection than the subclavian route, but less than the femoral route.
- It is best avoided in patients with carotid artery disease or those with raised intracranial pressure.
- Most commonly, a multilumen CVC is inserted but this route can also be used for the insertion of a dialysis catheter.
- The procedure is undertaken using a fully aseptic, Seldinger technique with the patient head-down and with the head turned slightly to the opposite side.
- There are many landmark approaches to the internal jugular vein but one of the most commonly used is just lateral to the carotid artery at the level of the cricoid cartilage and aiming at the ipsilateral nipple.
- A post-procedural check X-ray is essential: the tip of the CVC should be in the long axis of superior vena cava (SVC), level with the carina—this will be above the pericardial reflection. For a CVC placed via the right internal jugular vein, this is typically 12–15 cm from the insertion site.
- If a CVC has been placed via the left internal jugular or subclavian veins, ensure the tip is not abutting the wall of the SVC—this can cause perforation of the vein. Either advance the CVC, so that it is in the long axis of the SVC, or withdraw it into the brachiocephalic vein.

Subclavian vein cannulation

- A CVC placed in the subclavian vein is easier to keep clean and is more comfortable for the patient in the long term; however, it is associated with a higher incidence of immediate complications, particularly pneumothorax.
- It is possible to use US to guide insertion but this typically means a more lateral approach, which is more difficult.
- When using the landmark technique, the insertion point is just below the junction of the medial 1/3 and outer 2/3 of the clavicle. Aim initially to hit the clavicle; redirect the needle to aim at the suprasternal notch while staying directly behind the clavicle.

Complications of central venous cannulation

See Table 1.1.

Table 1.1 Complications of central venous cannulation

Early	Late
Arrhythmias (caused by the guidewire)	Infection—colonization and systemic sepsis
Arterial puncture	Thrombosis
Venous laceration	Embolization
Pneumothorax	Perforation of vessels
Haemothorax	Cardiac tamponade
Nerve injury (phrenic, vagus, recurrent laryngeal, brachial plexus)	
Thoracic duct laceration	
Cardiac tamponade	
Embolization	

Reproduced with the kind permission of the Resuscitation Council (UK).

Intraosseous infusion

- The IO route has been recognized for many years as a valuable means of drug and fluid delivery in children.
- Partly because of improvements in the IO devices, this route is being used increasingly in adults and has now largely replaced cutdown as a means of obtaining access rapidly to the circulation in an emergency.
- Contraindications include: fracture near or proximal to the insertion site; local infection; osteogenesis imperfecta.
- Insertion sites are the proximal tibia (most common), distal tibia, proximal humerus, distal femur, and sternum (adults only).
- The proximal tibial insertion site is 1–2 cm inferior and medial to the tibial tuberosity (on the flat surface of the tibia).
- Options for IO devices are: manual purpose-made IO needles or screws; drill-assisted devices; and spring-loaded devices.
- Proper placement is confirmed by the ability to aspirate bone marrow contents and/or absence of local swelling on careful injection of saline.
- Samples obtained from an IO device can be used for glucose, electrolyte and pH analysis, culture, and blood typing.
- Drugs and fluid can be 'syringed' in via a 3-way tap; pressure bags and infusion pumps may also be used.
- Remove the IO device as soon as more definitive access is obtained.
- The commonest complication is extravasation of fluid and drugs. Fractures and infection can occur, but these are less common.

Further reading

Duffy M, Sair M. Cannulation of central veins. *Anaesth Intensive Care Med* 2006; **8**:17–20.

Fragou M, Gravvanis A, Dimitriou V, *et al*. Real-time ultrasound-guided subclavian vein cannulation versus the landmark method in critical care patients: a prospective randomized study. *Crit Care Med* 2011; **39**:1607–12.

Nagler J, Krauss B. Intraosseous catheter placement in children. *N Engl J Med* 2011; **364**:e14.

Ortega R, Song M, Hansen CJ, *et al*. Ultrasound-guided internal jugular vein cannulation. *N Engl J Med* 2010; **362**:e57.

Tobias JD, Ross AK. Intraosseous infusions: a review for the anesthesiologist with a focus on pediatric use. *Anesth Analg* 2010; **110**:391–401.

Walsh JT, Hildick-Smith DJR, Newell SA, *et al*. Comparison of central venous and inferior vena caval pressures. *Am J Cardiol* 2000; **85**:518–20.

Transfusion

Key points
- Consider carefully the risks and benefits of transfusing blood and blood products.
- Understand the indications for blood which is fully matched versus group confirmed versus group O blood.
- Know your hospital massive transfusion protocol.
- If major blood loss anticipated before surgery, consider use of cell salvage.

Blood products
- All blood donations in the UK are tested for hepatitis B (surface antigen), human immunodeficiency virus (HIV; antibody), human T-lymphotropic virus (HTLV) (antibody), hepatitis C (antibody and ribonucleic acid, RNA), and syphilis (antibody).
- The ABO and Rhesus D (RhD) group of the donor's cells are determined and those that are group O are assessed for titres of anti-A or anti-B antibody.
- Almost all whole-blood donations in the UK are separated into red cells, platelets, and plasma. The donor's blood is collected into packs containing citrate phosphate dextrose adenine ($CPDA_1$), an anticoagulant-preservative solution. The whole blood is filtered to remove white cells.

Red cells
In the UK, a standard unit of red cells contains only 20 mL of residual plasma; the rest of the plasma is replaced with an 'optimal additive' solution of saline, adenine, glucose, and mannitol (SAGM). The final mean volume (standard deviation (SD)) of these red cell solutions is 282 mL (± 32) and the haematocrit is 57% (± 3).

Platelets
- An adult dose unit comprises the platelets from 4–6 whole-blood donations. It will include about 250 mL of plasma and 60 mL of anticoagulant.
- Platelets are best stored at 22°C and are agitated continuously. This temperature is accompanied by the risk of bacterial contamination and platelets are now cultured before being issued.

Plasma
- A single pack of fresh frozen plasma (FFP) includes a mean of 220 mL of plasma and 60 mL of anticoagulant. The usual adult dose is 12–15 mL kg^{-1}, which is typically about 4 packs.
- FFP contains significant quantities of fibrinogen (20–50 g L^{-1}) and an adult dose will typically increase the fibrinogen concentration by about 1 g L^{-1}—this is the same as would result from an adult dose of cryoprecipitate.
- The risk of microbial infectivity with FFP can be reduced with treatment with either methylene blue (single donor units) or solvent and detergent (pools of 300–5000 plasma donations).

Cryoprecipitate
A typical adult therapeutic dose (ATD) is equivalent to 10 single donor units—this contains 3–6 g fibrinogen in a volume of 200–500 mL.

Other plasma derivatives
- Factor II, VII, IX, and X concentrate (prothrombin complex concentrate, PCC) is indicated when there is life-threatening bleeding associated with warfarin overdose.
- Recombinant Factor VIIa (rFVIIa) is used when traumatic, surgical, or obstetric haemorrhage continues despite treatment with appropriate quantities of other blood products and, when indicated, attempts to control bleeding surgically.

Compatibility procedures
Group and screen
- The patient's ABO and RhD type is determined and any red cell antibodies (that could haemolyse transfused red cells) are identified.
- In the absence of antibodies, and if the sample is <7 days old, compatible blood can be issued with 15–20 min.

Red cell compatibility testing
The compatibility of the patient's blood is confirmed with each unit of red cells to be transfused (a physical crossmatch). Fully matched blood can be issued within 50 min of receipt of a sample.

Electronic issue
ABO and RhD compatible red cells can be issued safely without a physical crossmatch as long as:
- The patient's ABO and RhD type have been tested and confirmed on a second sample, retested on the first sample, or the patient is group O.
- The patient has no irregular red cell antibodies.
- The patient and the sample are identified reliably.
- The patient's previous results can be correctly identified.

Indications for transfusion of blood products in association with surgery and critical illness
Red blood cells
- Acutely bleeding patients will require blood transfusion if they have lost >30–40% of their blood volume.
- A haemoglobin concentration of $7.0\,g\,dL^{-1}$ is a reasonable transfusion threshold in the absence of evidence of ischaemic heart disease.
- For patients with evidence of ischaemic heart disease it is reasonable to maintain a haemoglobin concentration of $9.0\,g\,dL^{-1}$.

Fresh frozen plasma
- Acute disseminated intravascular coagulation (DIC)—the underlying cause should be treated. FFP may be required to correct coagulation abnormalities if bleeding or if invasive procedure is planned.
- Need for massive transfusion (see 📖 Massive blood loss, p.22).
- Thrombotic thrombocytopenic purpura (TTP).

Cryoprecipitate
- Fibrinogen supplementation (when fibrinogen concentration $<1\,g\,L^{-1}$) in fulminant DIC, advanced liver disease, massive blood transfusion, and reversal of fibrinolytic therapy.
- Von Willebrand factor replacement in renal failure where desmopressin contraindicated.

Platelets
- Platelet function disorders with bleeding or if an invasive procedure is planned. Stop antiplatelet drugs and consider other measures, e.g. desmopressin.
- Massive blood transfusion—aim to keep platelets above $75 \times 10^9\,L^{-1}$ ($100 \times 10^9/L$ if multiple trauma or neurotrauma).
- DIC.

Massive blood loss

Definition of massive blood loss
One or more of the following:
- Replacement of the blood volume within 24-h period.
- Replacement of 50% of the total blood volume within 3 h.
- Need for at least 4 units of red blood cells (RBCs) within 4 h in the setting of continued major bleeding.
- Blood loss exceeding $150\,mL\,min^{-1}$.
- Need for plasma and platelet replacement.

Management of massive blood loss
See also 📖 Coagulopathy, p.130.
- Stop the bleeding—this may mean urgent surgery, angiography, and embolization or other haemostatic techniques.
- Alert key support staff and request laboratory investigations—FBC, clotting screen, crossmatch, and biochemistry. Retesting of FBC and clotting will be required at intervals until bleeding is controlled.
- Restore circulation volume—insert two wide-bore cannulae, infuse warmed crystalloid (Hartmann's solution is generally preferred to normal saline), or blood, aiming to maintain and adequate BP and a urine output of $>30\,mL\,h^{-1}$. *Keep the patient warm.* In the presence of uncontrolled bleeding it may be appropriate to allow the BP to stay relatively low (80–100 mmHg systolic) until the bleeding is controlled. Exceptions to this strategy of 'permissive hypotension' are patients with severe head injuries, the elderly, and those with ischaemic heart disease.
- Request suitable red cells:
  - Uncrossmatched group O RhD negative may be given in extreme urgency—this can be issued immediately. Ascertain the patient's blood group and give group specific or crossmatched blood as rapidly as possible.
  - ABO group specific blood may be given when the blood group is known—this can usually be issued in 15–20 min. Full compatibility testing is undertaken retrospectively.
  - Crossmatched blood is required if antibodies are present or if time allows—a full crossmatch will take about 40 min if no atypical

antibodies are detected. A full crossmatch is not required after
10 units have been transfused in <24 h.

- Use a high-capacity blood warmer wherever possible.
- Consider red cell salvage if available and appropriate.
- To conserve stocks of O RhD negative blood, O RhD positive
  blood can be given to RhD negative men and post-menopausal RhD
  negative women.

- Ideally, use of FFP, platelets, and cryoprecipitate is guided by results of
  coagulation studies, but in massive haemorrhage the results of these
  investigations will usually lag behind the clinical condition of the patient.
  Under these circumstances, give plasma components without waiting
  for the results of the coagulation studies but use the results to confirm
  clinical impressions about the progress of the coagulopathy.
- If haemorrhage is rapid, after 4 units of RBCs and faced with continued
  blood loss, request a 'haemostatic pack'—15 mL kg^{-1} FFP and an adult
  therapeutic dose of platelets. Group compatible units will subsequently
  be used when the patient's blood group is known. Infuse tranexamic
  acid 1 g over 10 min, followed by a further 1 g infused
  over 8 h.
- Repeat the FFP and platelet administration after each 4–6 units
  (equivalent to a ratio of 1:1:1), or as guided by tests:
  - Give 15 mL kg^{-1} of FFP if prothrombin time (PT) and/or activated
    partial thromboplastin time (APTT) >1.5 × control.
  - Give two packs of cryoprecipitate (pooled) empirically or if
    fibrinogen is <1 g L^{-1}.
  - Give at least 1 'adult dose unit' of platelets if platelet count is
    <75 × 10^9/L (<100 × 10^9/L if multiple/central nervous system (CNS)
    trauma).
  - Give calcium chloride 10 mL if ionized calcium <0.9 mmol L^{-1}.
- When appropriate, consider the following specific measures:
  - Reversal of warfarin (vitamin K, PCC).
  - Reversal of heparin (protamine sulphate).
  - Desmopressin 0.3 micrograms kg^{-1} in 50 mL normal saline over
    30 min for von Willebrand's disease and patients with chronic renal
    failure.
- Consider giving rFVIIa if conventional therapy has failed to control the
  blood loss (usually 10 units of RBCs, 8 units of FFP, 2 adult dose units of
  platelets, and 2 packs of cryoprecipitate will have been given); and
  - Bleeding with coagulopathy continues; and
  - All surgical and embolization procedures have been attempted; and
  - Ideally, the following values have been achieved: platelet count
    >50 × 10^9 L^{-1}, fibrinogen concentration >1 g L^{-1}, pH >7.2,
    temperature >32°C, ionized calcium concentration >0.9 mmol L^{-1}.
  - Give rFVIIa 100 micrograms kg^{-1}. A clinical response is usually
    obvious within 20 min. If no response within 20 min, consider a
    second dose of 100 micrograms kg^{-1} rFVIIa.

Complications of transfusion

The adverse effects of transfusion fall into three domains: acute life-threatening
complications; delayed complications; and transmitted infections.

Acute life-threatening complications

- Acute haemolytic reaction:
    - The patient's anti-A or anti-B antibodies react with incompatible transfused red cells activating the complement pathway and causing haemolysis, release of cytokines, degranulation of mast cells with resulting hypotension.
    - Surprisingly, only 20–30% of ABO-incompatible transfusions cause some morbidity and 5–10% contribute to the cause of death.
    - Infusion of platelets or FFP containing high-titre anti-red cell antibodies can also cause haemolysis.
    - Treatment includes stopping the transfusion, fluid resuscitation, and vasopressors as required. Inform the blood bank and take samples for culture from the component pack.
- Infusion of blood product contaminated with bacteria:
    - Causes severe reaction with hypotension and rigors.
    - Rare, but most commonly caused by contaminated platelets because these are stored at room temperature.
    - Treat as for acute haemolytic reaction and, guided by a microbiologist, give antibiotics to cover both Gram-positive and Gram-negative.
- Transfusion-related acute lung injury (TRALI):
    - Causes hypoxaemia, dyspnoea, and relative hypovolaemia within 6 h of transfusion. Radiological appearances of acute respiratory distress syndrome (ARDS). May be accompanied by fever and rigors. There may be transient leucopenia.
    - Often caused by donor plasma antibodies that react with the patient's leucocytes. The donors are usually parous women (in the UK, only male donors are used for FFP).
    - There is no rapid clinically relevant diagnostic test.
    - Likely to require admission to the ICU for non-invasive support or tracheal intubation and positive pressure ventilation. Mortality is 5–10%.
- Transfusion-associated circulatory overload (TACO):
    - Pulmonary oedema will need treatment with a diuretic and oxygen.
- Allergic reactions:
    - Anaphylaxis may occur if there are pre-existing immunoglobulin (Ig) E antibodies although severe reactions may also occur to IgG antibodies. Some patients with severe IgA deficiency have antibodies to IgA and may develop anaphylaxis if exposed to IgA by transfusion.
    - Urticaria and itching are common during transfusion—symptoms may resolve if the transfusion rate is reduced and an antihistamine given.
    - Febrile non-haemolytic transfusion reactions involving fever and rigors occurring toward the end of the transfusion affect up to 2% of recipients; they can usually be treated by slowing the rate of transfusion and giving paracetamol.

Delayed complications of transfusion

- Delayed haemolytic transfusion reaction—occurs >24 h after transfusion in a patient sensitized by a previous transfusion or pregnancy. The Kidd and the Rh systems are the most common cause of these delayed reactions. May cause ↓ haemoglobin concentration, jaundice, fever, and, rarely, renal failure.

- Transfusion associated graft-versus-host disease—rare but serious complications (usually fatal) caused by reaction between donor lymphocytes and HLA antigens on recipient cells.
- Post-transfusion purpura—rare but very serious complication of transfusion of red cells or platelets. Profound thrombocytopenia occurring 5–9 days after transfusion.

Infections transmissible by transfusion

Every donation is tested for hepatitis B surface antigen, hepatitis C antibody and RNA, HIV antibody, HTLV antibody, and syphilis antibody. Rarely, screening fails to detect the relevant infection in the donation.

- Hepatitis B—exists in 1 in 2.2 million donations. Can cause severe infections and may progress to chronic carrier state.
- Hepatitis C—exists in 1 in 22 million donations (screening tests introduced in 1991 and 1999). Some people infected are asymptomatic but some develop chronic liver disease or hepatic carcinoma.
- Malaria—only 5 cases of transfusion-transmitted malaria reported in the UK in the last 25 years.
- Variant Creutzfeldt–Jakob disease (vCJD)—4 possible transmissions of vCJD reported in the UK but many more known recipients of components from vCJD-infected donors are being tracked. All donated blood in the UK has been leucodepleted since 1999 in an attempt to reduce the risk of vCJD transmission.

Intraoperative cell salvage

- Intraoperative cell salvage will decrease use of donor blood. It should be considered if:
  - >20% blood volume or >1000 mL anticipated blood loss.
  - A patient is difficult to crossmatch.
  - A patient does not want donor blood products.
- Red cells can be collected by suction and by washing swabs in 0.9% saline. Blood is collected into a reservoir and an anticoagulant (e.g. 0.9% saline with heparin) added. It is then washed in 0.9% saline and centrifuged to provide a bag of red cells for reinfusion.
- Contaminated blood (cement, topical clotting factors, iodine) should be avoided. The risks and benefits should be weighed up before salvaging blood potentially containing bacteria, malignant cells, or amniotic fluid.
- Use of intraoperative cell salvage needs planning in advance and specialist equipment. For emergency surgery, ideally there should be a dedicated operator for the cell salvage machine.
- In massive haemorrhage, donor blood and blood products are also likely to be needed. There is also a risk of dilutional coagulopathy.

Further reading

Association of Anaesthetists of Great Britain and Ireland. *Blood Transfusion and the Anaesthetist – Red Cell Transfusion 2*. London: AAGBI, 2008. Available at: ℜ http://www.aagbi.org/publications.

Association of Anaesthetists of Great Britain and Ireland. *Blood Transfusion and the Anaesthetist – Intra-operative Cell Salvage*. London: AAGBI, 2009. Available at: ℜ http://www.aagbi.org/publications.

Association of Anaesthetists of Great Britain and Ireland. *Blood Transfusion and the Anaesthetist – Management of Massive Haemorrhage*. London: AAGBI, 2010. Available at: ℜ http://www.aagbi.org/publications.

McClelland DBL. *United Kingdom Blood Services Handbook of Transfusion Medicine* (4th edn). Norwich: The Stationery Office, 2007.

Fluid therapy

Key points
- A crystalloid is a solution of small non-ionic or ionic particles; its distribution is determined mainly by its sodium concentration.
- Colloidal solutions are fluids containing large molecules (e.g. gelatin, dextran, and starch) that exert an oncotic pressure at the capillary membrane.
- There are very few high-quality data showing benefit for fluid resuscitation with colloid instead of, or in addition to, crystalloid.
- In most patients, in most clinical circumstances, fluid resuscitation should be undertaken with crystalloid, along with blood products as indicated.

Physiology
- Intracellular fluid (ICF) is separated from extracellular fluid (ECF) by a cell membrane (Fig. 1.1) that is highly permeable to water but not to most electrolytes.
- Intracellular volume is maintained by the membrane sodium–potassium pump, which moves sodium out of the cell (carrying water with it) in exchange for potassium. There are significant differences in the electrolytic composition of intracellular and extracellular fluid.
- The intravascular space and the interstitial fluid (ISF) are separated by the endothelial cells of the capillary wall (the capillary membrane). This wall is permeable to water and small molecules including ions. It is impermeable to larger molecules such as proteins. The higher hydrostatic pressure inside capillaries (compared with that in the ISF) tends to force fluid out of the vessel into the ISF.
- The osmotic pressure of a solution is related directly to the number of osmotically active particles it contains. The total osmolarity of each of the fluid compartments is approximately 280 mOsm L^{-1}. Oncotic pressure is that component of osmotic pressure provided by proteins. The higher osmotic pressure inside capillaries tends to pull fluid back in to the vessels.

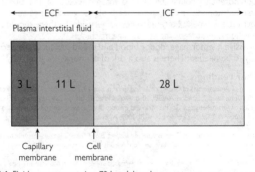

Fig. 1.1 Fluid compartments in a 70-kg adult male.

Crystalloids

The composition of some of the commonly prescribed crystalloids is given in Table 1.2.

- Distribution of a crystalloid is determined mainly by its sodium concentration. Fluids with high sodium concentrations (e.g. 0.9% saline) will be distributed in the ECF. After rapid infusion, the distribution phase lasts about 30 min and about 60% of the volume remains intravascular initially. Haemorrhage, anaesthesia, and surgery reduce clearance by 50%.
- Solutions with lower sodium concentrations (e.g. 5% glucose) will be distributed throughout both ECF and the intracellular compartment.
- In comparison with Hartmann's solution, the higher sodium content of 0.9% saline will result in slightly better intravascular volume expansion (about 10% more).
- After head injury, 0.9% saline is the preferred resuscitation fluid because Hartmann's solution is slightly hypotonic relative to plasma and may worsen cerebral oedema.
- Large volumes of 0.9% saline cause hyperchloraemic acidosis—animal data indicate that this causes renal vasoconstriction and reduces glomerular filtration rate. In clinical studies, hyperchloraemic acidosis has been associated with reduced urine production and increase in postoperative nausea and vomiting. Attempts to correct the metabolic acidosis with fluid resuscitation may be harmful.

Table 1.2 Composition of some commonly prescribed crystalloids

Crystalloid	Osmolality (mosmol kg^{-1})	pH	Na^+ (mmol L^{-1})	K^+ (mmol L^{-1})	HCO_3^- (mmol L^{-1})	Cl^- (mmol L^{-1})	Ca^{2+} (mmol L^{-1})
0.9% saline	308	5.0	154	0	0	154	0
Hartmann's solution	275	6.5	131	5.0	29[a]	111	2
Plasma-Lyte 148®	295	5.5	140	5	50[b]	98	0
5% glucose	278	4.0	0	0	0	0	0
4% glucose in 0.18% saline	283	4.5	31	0	0	31	0

[a] HCO_3^- is provided as lactate.
[b] 27 mmol L^{-1} as acetate and 23 mmol L^{-1} as gluconate.

Colloids

- Colloidal solutions are fluids containing large molecules that exert an oncotic pressure at the capillary membrane.
- Natural colloids include blood and albumin.
- Artificial colloids contain large molecules such as gelatin, dextran, and starch. IV colloids will initially expand mainly the intravascular compartment. Intravascular persistence depends on molecular size, shape, ionic charge, and capillary permeability.

Blood

Blood is an appropriate replacement fluid following severe haemorrhage. It will increase oxygen carriage and expand the intravascular compartment with little or no increase in interstitial fluid (see 📖 Transfusion, p.20).

Albumin
- Human albumin is a single polypeptide with a molecular weight of around 68 kDa. It is negatively charged and is repelled by the negatively charged endothelial glycocalyx, which extends its intravascular duration.
- Albumin has transport functions and anticoagulant properties, and it scavenges free radicals. In health, it contributes about 80% of oncotic pressure but in the critically ill, serum albumin correlates poorly with colloid oncotic pressure.
- Albumin is prepared in two concentrations (4.5% and 20%) from many thousands of pooled donors.
- The half-life of exogenous albumin in the circulating compartment is 5–10 days assuming an intact capillary wall membrane. It is expensive to prepare but has a long shelf life.
- In the critically ill patient, capillary leak limits its effectiveness. The treatment of hypoalbuminaemia with albumin does not alter outcome in the critically ill. Despite the lack of outcome data, albumin remains a mainstay of colloid therapy in paediatric intensive care.
- A randomized control comparing saline with albumin in the critically ill showed no difference in 28-day mortality but an increase in mortality with albumin in a subgroup of patients with severe head injury. A recent meta-analysis of studies involving patients with sepsis showed that survival was higher in those treated with albumin.

Gelatins
- Gelatins comprise modified bovine collagens suspended in ionic solutions. The collagen is sourced from outside the UK.
- Gelatin solutions have long shelf lives and do not transmit infection.
- Gelatin solutions contain molecules of widely varying molecular weight. Despite a quoted average molecular weight of ~35 kDa, most of the molecules are considerably smaller than this and are excreted rapidly by the kidney. Thus, gelatin solutions remain in the circulating compartment for a short period. They maintain their maximal volume effect for only 1.5 h, and only 15% remains in the intravascular space 24 h after administration. Although anaphylaxis to colloids is rare, gelatins are the most common to be implicated.

Dextrans
- Dextrans are polysaccharide products of sucrose.
- Dextran 70 (average molecular weight 70 000) has an intravascular half-life of about 12 h.
- Dextrans cause a mild alteration in platelet stickiness and function and thus have an antithrombotic effect.
- Dextran in combination with hypertonic saline (hypertonic saline dextran (HSD)) has undergone extensive investigation, particularly in trauma patients, but outcome is not improved.

Hydroxyethyl starch
- Hydroxyethyl starch (HES) is manufactured by polymerizing corn or potato starch. Several HES solutions are available, each with a different average molecular weight.
- Most HES solutions have a longer intravascular half-life than other synthetic colloids, with a significant volume effect for at least 6 h.

- The higher molecular weight starch solutions (450 kDa), particularly when combined with high substitution ratios (e.g. 0.7 or 7 hydroxyethyl groups for every 10 glucose rings), prolong clotting time by impairing factor VII and von Willebrand factor.
- The medium-weight starches (200 kDa) have less effect on coagulation but there is now good evidence that they can cause renal failure in patients with sepsis. There is some evidence that this might be related to their hyperoncotic properties (causing a reduction in glomerular filtration rate) and that other hyperoncotic fluids may cause the same problem.
- Newer low molecular weight starches (140 kDa with a substitution ratio of 0.4) are less likely to cause any of these complications but that has yet to be proven in large clinical trials.

Crystalloid versus colloid

- There are very few high-quality data showing benefit for fluid resuscitation with colloid instead of, or in addition to, crystalloid.
- In most patients, in most clinical circumstances, fluid resuscitation should be undertaken with crystalloid, along with blood products as indicated.
- Some clinicians prefer to use colloids in patients with 'leaky' capillaries, such as those with sepsis. However, the theoretical advantages associated with better retention in the intravascular have not been translated into improved outcome in clinical trials.

Controlled fluid resuscitation

- In the presence of uncontrolled bleeding, aggressive fluid resuscitation may be harmful because increasing the BP with fluid accelerates the loss of RBCs and may impair clotting.
- There is a balance between the risk of inducing organ ischaemia and the risk of accelerating haemorrhage. Older patients and those with a significant head injury require fluid resuscitation to restore vital organ perfusion.

Balanced solutions

- Plasma-Lyte 148® is a crystalloid with a balanced electrolyte content—it does not cause hyperchloraemic acidosis, even when give in high volumes.
- There are now available starch and gelatin solutions with balanced electrolyte content; they may improve renal and gastrointestinal (GI) function and reduce their impact on coagulation.

Further reading

Brunkhorst FM, Engel C, Bloos F, et al. Intensive insulin therapy and pentastarch resuscitation in severe sepsis. N Engl J Med 2008; **358**:125–39.

Delaney AP, Dan A, McCaffrey J, Finfer S. The role of albumin as a resuscitation fluid for patients with sepsis: A systematic review and meta-analysis. Crit Care Med 2011; **39**:386–91.

Finfer S, Bellomo R, Boyce N, et al. A comparison of albumin and saline for fluid resuscitation in the intensive care unit. N Engl J Med 2004; **350**:2247–56.

Hahn RG. Volume kinetics for infusion fluids. Anesthesiology 2010; **113**:470–81.

Electrolytes[1]

Key points
- Serious electrolyte abnormalities will require correction perioperatively.
- Major changes in total body K^+ can occur without significant effect on plasma K^+ concentration.
- Treatment of hyperkalaemia includes: cardiac protection by antagonizing the effects of hyperkalaemia; shifting K^+ into cells; and removing K^+ from the body.
- Hyponatraemia is associated most commonly with ↑ total body water and Na^+, but may occur with low, normal, or high total body Na^+.
- The rate of correction of the hyponatraemia depends on the underlying condition and the clinical features; if chronic, there is no indication for correction before emergency surgery.

Potassium
- A 70-kg adult has 3500 mmol potassium (K^+) of which about 60 mmol (2%) is extracellular. The normal extracellular K^+ concentration is 3.5–5.1 mmol L^{-1} and the intracellular concentration is 150 mmol L^{-1}.
- Large changes in total body K^+ can occur without significant effect on plasma K^+ concentration. The daily maintenance requirement for K^+ is ~1 mmol kg^{-1} but considerably more may be needed to replace other losses.

Hypokalaemia
Hypokalaemia is a serum K^+ <3.5 mmol L^{-1}; severe hypokalaemia is K^+ <2.5 mmol L^{-1}. Causes of hypokalaemia include: GI losses (diarrhoea); drugs (diuretics, laxatives, steroids, adrenaline, isoprenaline, etc.); renal losses (renal tubular disorders, diabetes insipidus (DI), dialysis); endocrine disorders (Cushing's syndrome, hyperaldosteronism); metabolic alkalosis; magnesium depletion; poor dietary intake.

Recognition of hypokalaemia
- As serum K^+ concentration decreases, the nerves and muscles are predominantly affected, causing fatigue, weakness, leg cramps, constipation. In severe cases, rhabdomyolysis, ascending paralysis and respiratory impairment may occur.
- ECG changes include large U waves, flattened or inverted T waves, ST-segment depression, and cardiac arrest.

Treatment of hypokalaemia
- Treatment depends on the severity, and the presence of symptoms and ECG abnormalities.
- Gradual replacement of potassium is preferable, but in an emergency, IV K^+ is required.

---

[1] Some of this topic has been adapted from: Resuscitation Council (UK) *Advanced Life Support* (6th edn), London: Resuscitation Council (UK), 2011, republished with kind permission. The section on Sodium is based on TM Craft, JP Nolan, and MJA Parr *Key Topics in Critical Care* Second edition, 2004, republished with permission from TM Craft.

- The maximum recommended IV infusion rate of K^+ is 20 mmol h^{-1}, but more rapid infusion (e.g. 2 mmol min^{-1} for 10 min, followed by 10 mmol over 5–10 min) with ECG monitoring is required if there are unstable arrhythmias.
- Adjust the dose after repeated sampling of serum K^+ values.
- Patients who are K^+ deficient can also be deficient in magnesium. Repletion of magnesium stores will facilitate more rapid correction of hypokalaemia and is recommended in severe cases of hypokalaemia.

Hyperkalaemia

Hyperkalaemia (serum K^+ >5.5 mmol L^{-1}) is caused usually by ↑ K^+ release from cells or impaired excretion by the kidneys. Severe hyperkalaemia is a serum K^+ >6.5 mmol L^{-1}.

Causes of hyperkalaemia

- The causes of hyperkalaemia include: renal failure; drugs (angiotensin converting enzyme inhibitors (ACEIs), angiotensin II receptor blockers (ARB), potassium sparing diuretics, non-steroidal anti-inflammatory drugs (NSAIDs), beta-blockers, trimethoprim); tissue breakdown (skeletal muscle (rhabdomyolysis), tumour lysis, haemolysis); metabolic acidosis; endocrine disorders (Addison's disease); hyperkalaemic periodic paralysis; diet (may be the principal cause in patients receiving chronic renal replacement therapy).
- The risk of hyperkalaemia increases when there is a combination of causative factors such as the concomitant use of ACEIs and NSAIDs or K^+ sparing diuretics.

Recognition of hyperkalaemia

- Weakness progressing to flaccid paralysis, paraesthesia, or depressed deep tendon reflexes.
- ECG effects depend on the absolute serum K^+ value as well as the rate of increase. ECG changes include: 1st-degree heart block; flattened or absent P waves; tall, peaked T waves; ST-segment depression; widened QRS; bradycardia (sinus bradycardia or AV block); ventricular tachycardia (VT); cardiac arrest (pulseless electrical activity (PEA), ventricular fibrillation (VF)/VT, asystole).
- Most patients will have ECG abnormalities at K^+ >6.7 mmol L^{-1}.

Treatment of hyperkalaemia

The five key steps in treating hyperkalaemia are:

- 1. Cardiac protection by antagonizing the effects of hyperkalaemia.
- 2. Shifting K^+ into cells.
- 3. Removing K^+ from the body.
- 4. Monitoring serum K^+ concentration for rebound hyperkalaemia.
- 5. Prevention of recurrence of hyperkalaemia.

If hypovolaemic, give fluid to enhance urinary potassium excretion. Obtain IV access, check serum K^+, and record an ECG. Treatment is determined according to severity of hyperkalaemia.

Mild elevation (5.5–5.9 mmol L^{-1}): remove potassium from the body with:

- Potassium exchange resins—calcium polystyrene sulphonate 15–30 g *or* sodium polystyrene sulphonate 15–30 g in 50–100 mL of 20 % sorbitol, given either orally or by retention enema (onset in 1–3 h; maximal effect at 6 h), or
- Diuretics: furosemide 1 mg kg^{-1} IV slowly (onset with the diuresis).

Moderate elevation (6–6.4 mmol L^{-1}) without ECG changes: use strategies as for mild elevation plus: shift K$^+$ into cells with:

- Shift potassium into cells with glucose/insulin: 10 units short-acting insulin and 25 g glucose IV over 15–30 min (onset in 15–30 min; maximal effect at 30–60 min; monitor blood glucose).
- Consider renal replacement therapy (e.g. haemodialysis) to remove potassium from the body if patient is oliguric or K$^+$ value increasing or not improving.

Severe elevation (≥6.5 mmol L^{-1}) without ECG changes: shift K$^+$ into cells with:

- Glucose/insulin (as for moderate elevation).
- Salbutamol 5 mg nebulized. Several doses (10–20 mg) may be required (onset in 15–30 min).
- Sodium bicarbonate: 50 mmol IV over 5–15 min if metabolic acidosis present (onset in 15–30 min). Bicarbonate alone is less effective than glucose plus insulin or nebulized salbutamol; it is best used in conjunction with these medications.

Remove K$^+$ from the body with multiple strategies as previously listed.

Severe elevation (≥6.5 mmol L^{-1}) with toxic ECG changes: protect the heart first with:

- Calcium chloride: 10 mL 10% calcium chloride IV over 2–5 min to antagonize the toxic effects of hyperkalaemia at the myocardial cell membrane. This protects the heart by reducing the risk of VF, but does not lower serum K$^+$ (onset in 1–3 min).
- Use K$^+$ removal and shifting strategies stated previously.
- Prompt specialist referral is essential. In hospitals without a dedicated renal unit, intensive care units can often provide emergency renal replacement therapies.

Sodium

Sodium (Na$^+$) is the principle extracellular cation. Normal plasma values are in the range 133–145 mmol L^{-1} with a requirement of 1–2 mmol kg^{-1} per day.

Hyponatraemia

- Hyponatraemia is the most common electrolyte abnormality seen in hospitalized patients.
- Although hyponatraemia is associated most commonly with ↑ total body water and Na$^+$, it may occur with low, normal, or high total body Na$^+$ and may be associated with a low, normal, or high serum osmolality.

Causes of hyponatraemia

- Shift of water out of cells secondary to osmotic shifts (hyperglycaemia, mannitol, alcohol).
- Shift of Na$^+$ into cells to maintain electrical neutrality (hypokalaemia).
- Excessive water retention (renal failure, oedematous states, syndrome of inappropriate anti-diuretic hormone (SIADH)).
- Excessive water administration.
- Excessive Na$^+$ loss (renal, bowel loss).
- Hyperglycaemia accounts for up to 15% of cases of hyponatraemia; every 5.6 mmol L^{-1} increase in serum glucose reduces the serum Na$^+$ by 1.6 mmol L^{-1}.

Causes of hyponatraemia associated with volume depletion are:
- Renal loss: diuretics, osmotic diuresis (glucose, mannitol), renal tubular acidosis, salt losing nephropathy, mineralocorticoid deficiency/antagonist.
- Non-renal loss: vomiting, diarrhoea, pancreatitis, peritonitis, burns.

Causes of hyponatraemia associated with normal or ↑ circulating volume are:
- Water intoxication: postoperative 5% glucose administration, TURP syndrome, SIADH, renal failure.
- Oedematous states (congestive heart failure, cirrhosis, nephrotic syndrome).
- Glucocorticoid deficiency, hypothyroidism.

Recognition of hyponatraemia

The rate of change of serum Na^+ is more important than the absolute concentration. Symptoms are rare with serum Na^+ >125 mmol L^{-1}.
- Mild: confusion, nausea, cramps, weakness.
- Severe (Na^+ usually <120 mmol L^{-1}): headache, ataxia, muscle twitching, convulsions, cerebral oedema, coma, and respiratory depression.

Diagnosis of hyponatraemia

- Exclude hyperglycaemia and measure urine and plasma osmolalities simultaneously.
- The urine osmolality is inappropriately high with SIADH and advanced renal failure.
- In SIADH the serum osmolality is <270 mosmol k^{-1}g and the urine osmolality is inappropriately high (>100 mosmol kg^{-1}). The urine Na^+ ↑ despite a normal salt and water intake.

Treatment of hyponatraemia

- The rate of correction of the hyponatraemia depends on the underlying condition and the clinical features.
- In chronic causes with mild or no symptoms, there will be no indication for correction before emergency surgery. The hyponatraemia is corrected slowly over a period of days with the use of fluid restriction (<1 L day^{-1}) and demeclocycline (ADH antagonist) if required; rapid correction may precipitate osmotic demyelination. There is ↑ risk of demyelination in the presence of: malnutrition, alcoholism, hypokalaemia, severe burns, and elderly females taking thiazides.
- The rate of correction of acute and symptomatic hyponatraemia is more difficult to determine; the risk of acute cerebral oedema is higher in children, females, and psychiatric patients. Acute hyponatraemia developing over less than 48 h carries a high risk of permanent neurological damage and rapid partial correction of the hyponatraemia is indicated. Depending on the underlying cause, rapid partial correction of hyponatraemia may be accomplished by: stopping all hypotonic fluids, hypertonic saline (e.g. 3% sodium chloride solution at 1 mL kg^{-1} h^{-1}), and low dose infusion of furosemide.
- For acute symptomatic hyponatraemia, aim to increase the serum Na^+ by 1–2 mmol L^{-1} h^{-1} until symptoms resolve (accompanied with frequent measurements of serum Na^+). In the acute setting an increase of serum Na^+ of 12 mmol L^{-1} day^{-1} is safe.
- The risks of rapid correction (central pontine myelinolysis) are weighed against the risk of continued symptomatic hyponatraemia.

Hypernatraemia

- Hypernatraemia results from inadequate urine concentration, loss of hypotonic fluids, or from excessive administration of Na^+.
- High-risk groups include infants and the elderly, patients on hypertonic infusions and osmotic diuretics.
- Hypernatraemia occurs in the context of low, normal, or high total body Na^+.
- Low total body Na^+ and hypernatraemia results from loss of both Na^+ and water, but the water loss is proportionately greater. It is caused by hypotonic fluid loss from the kidney or gut and is accompanied by signs of hypovolaemia.
- ↑ total body Na^+ and hypernatraemia usually follows administration of hypertonic Na^+ containing solutions.
- Normal total body Na^+ and hypernatraemia is caused by loss of water in greater proportion than Na^+. This usually results from renal losses due to central or nephrogenic DI. Initially, euvolaemia is maintained, but uncorrected water loss will lead eventually to severe dehydration and hypovolaemia.

Diabetes insipidus

- DI is caused by impaired reabsorption of water by the kidney. Water reabsorption is regulated by anti-diuretic hormone (ADH).
- Cranial DI is caused by lack of ADH production or release; nephrogenic DI results from renal insensitivity to the effects of ADH.
- Causes of cranial DI include: head injury; neurosurgery; pituitary tumour; meningitis/encephalitis; Guillain–Barré syndrome; raised intra-cranial pressure; drugs (ethanol, phenytoin).
- Causes of nephrogenic DI include: drugs (lithium, demeclocycline); congenital nephrogenic DI; chronic renal failure; sickle cell disease; hypokalaemia; hyperkalaemia.
- Polyuria (may be >$400\,mL\,h^{-1}$) in the presence of a raised serum osmolality (>$300\,mosmol\,kg^{-1}$) is suggestive of DI. The diagnosis is confirmed by measuring urine and plasma osmolalities simultaneously. In DI the urine osmolality is inappropriately low (often <$150\,mosmol\,kg^{-1}$) while serum osmolality is abnormally high.

Clinical features of hypernatraemia

Signs and symptoms of hypernatraemia are often non-specific and include lethargy, irritability, confusion, nausea and vomiting, muscle twitching, hyper-reflexia and spasticity, seizures, and coma.

Treatment of hypernatraemia

- Treat the underlying pathology and replace water (using 5% glucose IV).
- Central DI is treated with desmopressin. Nephrogenic DI is treated by removal of precipitating drugs and sometimes with thiazide diuretics or NSAIDs.
- Correct slowly at $1\,mmol\,L^{-1}\,h^{-1}$ (more slowly if hypernatraemia is chronic) to avoid the risk of cerebral oedema.

Calcium, magnesium and phosphate

The recognition and management of calcium, magnesium, and phosphate disorders is summarized in Table 1.3.

Table 1.3 Recognition and management of calcium, magnesium, and phosphate disorders[a]

Disorder	Causes	Presentation	ECG	Treatment
Hypercalcaemia Total calcium[b] >2.6 mmol L^{-1}	Primary or tertiary hyperparathyroidism Malignancy Sarcoidosis Drugs	Confusion Weakness Abdominal pain Hypotension Arrhythmias Cardiac arrest	Short QT interval Prolonged QRS Interval Flat T waves AV block Cardiac arrest	Fluid replacement IV Furosemide 1 mg kg^{-1} IV Hydrocortisone 200–300 mg IV Pamidronate 30–90 mg IV Treat underlying cause
Hypocalcaemia Total calcium[b] <2.1 mmol L^{-1}	Chronic renal failure Acute pancreatitis Calcium channel blocker overdose Toxic shock syndrome Rhabdomyolysis Tumour lysis syndrome	Paraesthesia Tetany Seizures AV block Cardiac arrest	Prolonged QT interval T-wave inversion Heart block Cardiac arrest	Calcium chloride 10% 10–40 mL Magnesium sulphate 50% 4–8 mmol (if necessary)

(continued)

Table 1.3 (continued)

Disorder	Causes	Presentation	ECG	Treatment
Hypermagnesaemia Magnesium >1.1 mmol L^{-1}	Renal failure Iatrogenic	Confusion Weakness Respiratory depression AV block Cardiac arrest	Prolonged PR and QT intervals T-wave peaking AV block Cardiac arrest	Consider treatment when magnesium >1.75 mmol L^{-1} Calcium chloride 10% 5–10 mL repeated if necessary Ventilatory support if necessary Saline diuresis—0.9% saline with furosemide 1 mg kg^{-1} IV Haemodialysis
Hypomagnesaemia Magnesium <0.6 mmol L^{-1}	GI loss Polyuria Starvation Alcoholism Malabsorption	Tremor Ataxia Nystagmus Seizures Arrhythmias—torsade de pointes Cardiac arrest	Prolonged PR and QT intervals ST-segment depression T-wave inversion Flattened P waves ↑ QRS duration Torsade de pointes	Severe or symptomatic: 2 g 50% magnesium sulphate (4 mL; 8 mmol) IV over 15 min. Torsade de pointes: 2 g 50% magnesium sulphate (4 mL; 8 mmol) IV over 1–2 min. Seizure: 2 g 50% magnesium sulphate (4 mL; 8 mmol) IV over 10 min.

Hyperphosphataemia Phosphate > 1.45 mmol l⁻¹	Reduced renal excretion:	Hypocalcaemia	Prolonged QT interval	Treat underlying cause
	• renal failure,	Tetany		Aluminium hydroxide: a binding agent.
	• hypoparathyroidism,	Ectopic calcification in		Magnesium and calcium salts
	• acromegaly,	tissues		Dialysis may be required
	• bisphosphonate therapy,	Nephrocalcinosis		
	• magnesium deficiency.	Renal stones		
	Increased exogenous load:			
	• intravenous infusion,			
	• excess oral therapy,			
	• phosphate-containing enemas.			
	Increased endogenous load:			
	• tumour-lysis syndrome,			
	• rhabdomyolysis,			
	• bowel infarction,			
	• malignant hyperthermia,			
	• haemolysis,			
	• acidosis.			

(continued)

Table 1.3 (continued)

Condition	Cause	Clinical features	ECG	Treatment
Hypophosphataemia Phosphate <0.75 mmol l⁻¹ Severe = <0.4 mmol l⁻¹	Internal redistribution of phosphate: • respiratory alkalosis, • refeeding after malnutrition, • recovery from diabetic ketoacidosis, • effects of insulin, glucagon, adrenaline, cortisol, glucose Increased urinary excretion of phosphate: • hyperparathyroidism, • vitamin-D deficiency, • malabsorption, • volume expansion, • renal tubular acidosis, • alcoholism. Decreased intestinal absorption: • antacid abuse, • vitamin-D deficiency, • chronic diarrhoea.	Seen usually when level <0.3 mmol l⁻¹ Weakness (which may contribute to respiratory failure and problems with weaning from mechanical ventilation), Cardiac dysfunction Paraesthesia Coma Seizures	Prolonged QRS AV Block	Correct underlying cause Oral phosphate 2–3 g daily Potassium phosphate 10 mmol IV over 60 minutes and repeat based on plasma levels Check and maintain adequate serum calcium levels

[a] Reproduced with the kind permission of the Resuscitation Council (UK).

[b] A normal *total calcium* is about 2.2–2.6 mmol L⁻¹. A normal *ionized calcium* is about 1.1–1.3 mmol L⁻¹. Calcium levels must be interpreted with caution. Total calcium depends on the concentration of serum albumin and will need to be corrected for low albumin values (corrected total calcium). Ionized calcium values are often measured by blood gas analysers.

Further reading

Alfonzo AVM, Isles C, Geddes C, *et al.* Potassium disorders – clinical spectrum and emergency management. *Resuscitation* 2006; **70**:10–25.

Craft TM, Nolan JP, Parr MJA (eds). *Key Topics in Critical Care* (2nd edn). London: Taylor & Francis, 2004.

Nolan J, Soar J, Lockey A, *et al.* (eds). *Advanced Life Support* (6th edn). 2011 London: Resuscitation Council UK, London.

Reynolds RM, Padfield PL, Seckl JR. Disorders of sodium balance. *BMJ* 2006; **332**:702–5.

Acute pain management

Key points

- The principles of pain management in the context of emergency anaesthesia and surgery are the same as during elective surgery, but the emergency context modifies the relative benefit and risks of several drugs.
- Physical and psychological aspects of pain should be given the same priority as drug administration.
- Paracetamol has minimal side effects and should be given regularly.
- Opioids are the mainstay but hypotension, respiratory depression, nausea/vomiting, and sedation/dysphoria may lead to more problems than normal in the emergency setting.
- Non-steroidal anti-inflammatory drugs (NSAIDs) should be considered but are often contraindicated because of the risk of complications due to effects on gastrointestinal (GI) integrity, bleeding risk and renal function.
- Other adjuncts such as gabapentin, pregabalin, clonidine and ketamine are increasingly important in the emergency setting.
- General anaesthesia (GA) may be an appropriate way to manage the patient whose pain cannot otherwise be relieved effectively and safely, and who will subsequently require surgery or management in intensive care.

General principles of pain management

- Pain relief is a human right and is a primary role of anaesthetists.
- Before considering drugs for analgesia, address other aspects of pain management (physical and psychological), e.g. immobilizing or reducing fractured limbs, patient explanation, reassurance and information, parental or partner attendance, anxiolysis, temperature control, control of fear, hunger, thirst, etc.
- Balanced analgesia (i.e. multimodal analgesia) has benefits over unimodal approaches. Balanced analgesia may include paracetamol, NSAIDs, opioids, tramadol, loco-regional analgesic techniques, physical methods and adjuncts.
- Analgesic choices should be individualized based on patient age, weight, co-morbidity, and clinical context.
▶ Regular analgesia is more effective than 'as required' analgesia partly because 'as required' drugs are generally given at more extended intervals and in lower doses than prescribed. It is rare for more than 25% of the maximum cumulative dose of an 'as required' prescription to be administered. Regular analgesia with co-prescription of adequate doses of rescue analgesia is the optimal technique.
- Self-administration of drugs (e.g. oral self-medication, IV PCA, epidural PCA) has benefits but may be complicated in emergency settings.
- Prescription of drugs to manage the side effects of analgesic drugs should be a routine part of analgesic prescription. These may include anti-emetics, gastroprotective agents and laxatives.

- The emergency setting increases the frequency of recognized side effects and complications of analgesic drugs and may lead to other less recognized ones.
- Analgesic route may need to be modified in the emergency setting.

Paracetamol

- Paracetamol is effective as a solo drug for minor pain and reduces requirements for other analgesics in moderate and severe pain.
- There are multiple possible routes of administration; the IV route increases bioavailability by 30–40%.
- There are minimal side effects in standard doses and paracetamol should be the default first analgesic prescribed.
- There is a risk of overdose if regular IV dosing not adjusted for patient size (<50 kg need <1g per dose) and age (children should have specific weight-based dosing). Use cautious dosing in patients with liver disease or malnourishment.

Opioids

- Opioids are the mainstay of pain management in the emergency setting because of ubiquitous availability, rapid onset, and lack of ceiling effect.
- The accompanying sedation is frequently beneficial in anxious patients but interferes with assessment of conscious level.
- Alternative routes (e.g. nasal, buccal, rectal, transcutaneous) may be useful in specific settings.
- Dosing should be adjusted and individualized in critical illness.
- Nausea and vomiting are both unpleasant and may have adverse physiological effects (e.g. in head injury or abdominal pathology).
- The risk of respiratory depression is increased in patients with critical injury or illness.
- There is a risk of hypotension in concealed or overt hypovolaemia.
- Dysphoria and euphoria may make critically ill patients difficult to manage or reduce safety.
- Prolonged use leads inevitably to constipation and occasional serious GI complications (ileus, perforation). Co-prescription of laxatives and monitoring of bowel activity is mandatory.

Tramadol

- Tramadol is considered separately from opioids because the differing effects of its stereo-isomers means that much of its analgesic effect is not mediated by mu (µ) opioid receptors.
- Side effects of tramadol are similar in frequency and type to opioids but patients who do not tolerate opioids may tolerate tramadol and vice versa.
- There is a ceiling effect on respiratory depression and less sedation than high dose opioids.

Non-steroidal anti-inflammatory drugs

- The major benefit of NSAIDs is the absence of opioid side effects. They are effective analgesics for minor and some moderate pain (with paracetamol) and they reduce requirements for other analgesics in severe pain.

- The side effects of NSAIDs are likely to be increased in the severely injured and critically ill and this often precludes their use.
  - Risk of GI bleeding is ↑. When NSAIDs are prescribed, co-prescribe regular protective agents (H_2 blockers or proton pump inhibitors).
  - ↑ risk of renal failure. NSAID-induced renal impairment is caused by a reduction in glomerular flow rate (GFR). This NSAID effect exacerbates any other causes of reduced GFR: hypovolaemia, hypotension, hypothermia.
  - ↑ risk of bleeding. Antiplatelet effect of NSAIDs may exacerbate bleeding particularly if critical illness has already altered coagulation. Omit NSAIDs where coagulation is impaired, bleeding is extensive, or where even minor bleeding is hazardous (e.g. head injury).
- The cyclo-oxygenase (COX)-2 antagonists are alternatives to NSAIDs and have the benefit of less risk of GI complications and of platelet-inhibited bleeding. They affect GFR similarly to NSAIDs. Their prolonged use is associated with an increase in cardiac thrombotic events, but whether this is true for short-duration use is uncertain. Several are not licensed for postoperative analgesia; parecoxib is.
- In critical illness and injury NSAIDs are frequently not appropriate until adequacy of bleeding control and renal function are confirmed. After such time NSAIDs can be used, with careful monitoring of effect.

Inhalational analgesia

Nitrous oxide has value as a rapid onset and rapid offset analgesic of moderate potency. Its use is restricted largely to obstetrics and the emergency department as Entonox® (50:50 oxygen: nitrous oxide).

There are numerous side effects described but few that limit its use in emergencies. Relevant limitations include:
- Loss of consciousness is possible.
- It should not be used in the presence of gas-filled lesions (e.g. pneumothorax, pneumomediastinum, pneumocephalus) because these will expand. For the same reason, abdominal and thoracic injuries should be fully assessed before use.
- Contraindicated if raised intracranial pressure.
- Nausea and vomiting.
- Requires specific delivery equipment and scavenging to reduce staff exposure.

Local and regional analgesia

Local and regional analgesia reduces the need for other analgesics and generally reduces the burden of analgesia-associated side effects. Its use is therefore advocated unless there are specific contraindications.
- Local anaesthesia (LA) for surgical wounds is almost never contraindicated though attention to maximum doses is always required.
- Use of elastomeric balloons and other infusion devices enable prolonged delivery of wound analgesia.
- Effective regional anaesthesia (RA) may completely eliminate the need for other analgesics (see 📖 Regional versus general anaesthesia, p.50).

- Regional anaesthesia may require additional expertise in emergency settings compared with the elective setting.
  - Integrity of coagulation should be confirmed before central neuraxial block (CNB) and major peripheral nerve block (PNB).
  - Where RA may lead to sympathetic blockade (e.g. CNB) there is a risk of hypotension with potential adverse effects. This requires careful assessment and correction of volume status before the procedure and attentive monitoring and response to hypotension following it.
  - Where RA produces profound motor or sensory blockade there should be a careful assessment of risks (e.g. secondary injury, effects of an immobile limb on mobilization and self caring, effect on pressure areas). Such effects may occasionally contraindicate RA or more often mean attentive monitoring is required after the procedure.
  - Effective relief of pain by RA may occasionally mask diagnosis of further complications (e.g. compartment syndrome in calf or forearm).

Physical methods

These may be effective alone or in combination with drugs. They should not be ignored as they have the benefit of minimal side effects when used appropriately. They include:
- Elevation (e.g. injured limbs).
- Immobilization (e.g. fractures).
- Cooling (e.g. cryocuffs, simple local cooling).
- Transcutaneous electrical nerve stimulation (TENS).
- Distraction and entertainment (especially for children).

Alternative analgesics and adjuncts

Several less commonly used drugs may have benefit in the emergency setting. This is particularly so when other drugs are contraindicated, not tolerated or ineffective; such uses are 'off-label'.

Gabapentin and pregabalin

These oral drugs have a traditional role in chronic pain management but are also effective in the acute setting. In the chronic pain setting, the dose of gabapentin is increased slowly (100 mg once daily increasing stepwise to a maximum of 300–900 mg three times daily) while pregabalin has an easier dose regimen (50–150 mg twice daily). In the acute setting, gabapentin 600–1200 mg can be given preoperatively, followed by 300 mg three times daily postoperatively. The main side effects are dizziness and sedation.

Ketamine

In low dose as bolus or infusion, this anaesthetic drug is a potent analgesic acting as a non-competitive N-methyl-D-aspartate (NMDA)-antagonist. Typical doses are 20 mg bolus or $10–20 \, mg \, h^{-1}$ infusion. Side effects include dysphoria, confusion, nausea, muscle rigidity, and hypotension, but the drug is frequently well tolerated.

Clonidine and dexmedetomidine

These alpha$_2$-adrenergic agonists may provide supplementary analgesia and sedation when administered parenterally. Hypotension and tachyphylaxis are the main side effects. When added to peripheral nerve blocks, clonidine may extend the block duration.

For more prolonged painful conditions other drugs may have a pain modifying effect and include tricyclic and serotonin re-uptake inhibitor antidepressants, and anticonvulsants.

General anaesthesia as analgesia

- GA may be an appropriate way to manage the patient whose pain cannot be relieved effectively and safely in any other way and who will subsequently require surgery.
- Continuation of intubation and sedation/anaesthesia on the ICU may in part be influenced by the ability to effectively manage pain postoperatively. The duration of such needs should be minimized by use of the principles discussed earlier in this topic.

Further reading

Macintyre PE, Schug SA, Scott DA, *et al.*; Acute Pain Management: Scientific Evidence Working Group of the Australian and New Zealand College of Anaesthetists and Faculty of Pain Medicine. *Acute Pain Management: Scientific Evidence* (3rd edn). Melbourne: ANZCA & FPM, 2010.

Monitoring

Key points

- The Association of Anaesthetists of Great Britain and Ireland (AAGBI) has published standards on monitoring during anaesthesia and recovery.
- Essential monitors for all anaesthetics are: pulse oximeter, non-invasive blood pressure (NIBP), ECG, airway gases (O_2, CO_2, and vapour), and airway pressure.
- During anaesthesia, cardiac output can be monitored non-invasively using either Doppler echocardiography or pulse contour analysis.

Monitoring the anaesthetic equipment

▶ Check carefully all equipment before providing anaesthesia for an emergency in any setting. Use the checklist published by the AAGBI—'Checking Anaesthetic Equipment'.
- Oxygen supply—monitor the breathing system using either a paramagnetic analyser, a fuel cell, or a polarographic electrode.
- Breathing systems—observation of the reservoir bag and use of capnography.
- Vapour analyser—essential whenever a volatile anaesthetic is in use.
- Infusion devices—check alarm settings and ensure infusion site is secure and visible.

Monitoring during induction and maintenance of anaesthesia

The following monitoring devices are essential:
- Pulse oximeter.
- NIBP monitor.
- ECG.
- Airway gases—O_2, CO_2, and vapour.
- Airway pressure.

Pulse oximetry

- The pulse oximeter uses plethysmography and spectroscopy to derive the oxygen saturation of arterial blood (SpO_2). The probe is placed on either a digit or an ear lobe. Its two light-emitting diodes (LEDs) emit light at 660 nm (red) and 940 nm (infrared), which passes through the tissue to a photocell.
- Oxygenated haemoglobin (Hb) and deoxygenated Hb have different spectra, but absorb differently at 660 nm and similarly at 940 nm. Other haemoglobin species, such as carboxyhaemoglobin (COHb), methaemoglobin (MetHb) and SulphHb are not accounted for.
- Software is used to eliminate the entire non-pulsatile components of absorbences and assesses only the pulsatile component. This is compared to a calibration curve in the device, and a value for SpO_2 calculated. The calibration curve is valid only between 80–100%.
- Inaccuracy may occur with an irregular pulse, low capillary pressures, or peripheral vasoconstriction. Jaundice, skin colour, and fetal

haemoglobin do not affect accuracy. COHb has a similar absorption spectrum to oxyhaemoglobin in the red range, so the pulse oximeter may not be reliable in heavy smokers and in smoke inhalation victims.

Non-invasive blood pressure

- In haemodynamically stable patients, in whom arterial blood sampling is not needed, it is acceptable to measure BP with a cuff.
- A cuff that is too small will overestimate BP, and a cuff that is too large will underestimate. The width of the inflatable part of the cuff should be 40% of the limb circumference, and its length should be twice its width.
- Oscillometry is used with a single cuff, both to compress the underlying artery, and to detect pulsations. The cuff is inflated above systolic pressure and; it is then deflated and pulsations are detected by the cuff as systolic pressure is reached. Further deflation maximizes pulsations at MAP. Further deflation towards pulsation diminishment occurs at diastolic pressure. As diastolic measurement is the least accurate, some devices calculate it.
- Prolonged use may damage skin and underlying nerves. Inaccuracy can occur when cuff deflation is too rapid, when the pulsations are irregular (e.g. atrial fibrillation), and at low BPs.

Electrocardiogram

- The surface electrocardiographic voltage is low magnitude (1–2 mV), which may be prone to interference. It is therefore important to have good quality silver/silver chloride (Ag/AgCl) gel electrodes attached properly to clean, smooth skin.
- Using the standard right arm, left arm, left leg electrode configuration, it is possible to confirm rate and rhythm, the presence of the individual components of electrical depolarization and their intervals, and the heart axis.
- By using different viewing lead configurations and signal filtering, most arrhythmias and other abnormalities can be identified. For a formal diagnosis, record a full 12-lead ECG.

Capnography

- Most methods of CO_2 analysis use infrared spectroscopy with an infrared light source and a photodetector, either in line with the airway device, or delivered to a distant monitor via a sampling line.
- Expired CO_2 monitoring confirms airway patency, and indicates ventilation adequacy. The end tidal (ET) CO_2 approximates to the partial pressure of arterial CO_2 ($PaCO_2$) unless there is pulmonary disease and/ or reduced cardiac output. In health, the normal value of $PaCO_2$ (5.3 kPa (40 mm Hg)) is controlled tightly by the respiratory centre.
- A low $ETCO_2$ value may reflect reduced CO_2 delivery to the lungs (e.g. with a reduced cardiac output or a pulmonary embolus) or hyperventilation.
- A high $ETCO_2$ value may indicate inadequate minute ventilation, ↑ dead space, ↑ generation of CO_2, (e.g. malignant hyperthermia) or surgical use of CO_2 such as in laparoscopy.
- The shape of the capnograph is informative: it is normally a square wave—a slope on either the upstroke or the plateau suggests chronic

obstructive pulmonary disease or asthma. A non-zero inspired CO_2 value or an abnormal shape suggests a problem with the breathing system or ventilator, and spontaneous respiratory effort can be observed superimposed on the square waveform.

Additional monitoring

Invasive arterial and venous pressures

- If greater accuracy or a continuous measure of arterial pressure is required, insert a 20-G arterial line in a peripheral artery. A hydraulic connection is made from the arterial cannula to a strain gauge transducer connected to a signal processor, which converts the hydraulic signal into a pulsatile waveform on a screen. The transducer must be levelled with the right atrium; it must be zeroed before use and periodically calibrated.
- Central venous pressure (CVP) monitoring requires a catheter in a central vein, to give an estimate of right atrial pressure. A 15–20-cm catheter placed in the femoral vein provides a reasonable approximation of the CVP (see 📖 Vascular access, p.16). It uses the same system as the arterial pressure measurement system, using an appropriate scale for venous pressure, which is low and relatively non-pulsatile. Therefore accurate zeroing is important.
- Pulmonary artery catheter (PAC) monitoring is no longer used commonly because of its perceived risks and lack of proven benefit. It is introduced into a central vein, advanced through the right heart, into the pulmonary artery (PA), where it is wedged with an inflatable balloon. PA occlusion pressure provides an estimate of left ventricular filling pressure. A proximal port in the catheter enables delivery of a cold fluid bolus and a thermistor at its tip enables cardiac output to be measured by the thermodilution technique, applying the Fick principle. Complications include arrhythmias, perforation of the right ventricle, and rupture of the PA.

Blood gas analysis

- Frequent blood gas analysis is essential when anaesthetizing any critically ill patient. Many hospitals will have a blood gas analyser in the operating suite.
- Many blood gas analysers include modules for measuring electrolytes and lactate—these are also very useful when anaesthetizing for emergency surgery.
- A blood gas analyser has electrodes to measure pH, PCO_2 and PO_2 in blood and it calculates oxygen saturation and bicarbonate.
  - The PO_2 electrode is a fuel cell.
  - The tip of the pH electrode is made of H^+ sensitive glass and the remainder of the Ag/AgCl electrode is filled with buffer solution to keep its internal $[H^+]$ constant. The opposite Ag/AgCl electrode, suspended in a saturated KCl solution, acts as a reference. The blood sample generates a potential difference proportional to blood $[H^+]$ or pH. Thermostatic control of the machine to 37°C is important, or a correction must be made.
  - The CO_2 electrode is a pH sensitive glass electrode in a bicarbonate solution.

Non-invasive cardiac output monitoring

Cardiac output can be monitored non-invasively using either Doppler echocardiography, pulse contour analysis, impedance plethysmography, or Fick partial rebreathing. Only the first two of these are used commonly during anaesthesia.

Doppler echocardiography

- An ultrasound wave is directed at the aorta from a probe placed in the oesophagus, in the suprasternal notch, or integrated in the tip of a tracheal tube. This wave is reflected off boundary surfaces, including red blood cells (RBCs) in the aorta.
- Doppler shift is the change in frequency of a reflected wave from that of the transmitted wave, the magnitude of which is proportional to the velocity of the RBCs, detected by the transducer. When the probe is aligned with the descending aorta a characteristic triangular waveform is produced, with a peak velocity at its apex and the flow time (systole) along its base, which is corrected to a standard heart rate.
- Cardiac output is obtained by multiplying average velocity by aortic cross sectional area; preload and afterload can also be deduced. The measurement is adequate to follow trends, and the velocity triangle provides information to enable optimization of fluid and vasoactive drugs.

Pulse contour analysis

Mathematical algorithms analyse the arterial pressure waveform to assess aortic compliance to deduce stroke volume, and hence cardiac output. Two of the existing systems (PiCCO (Pulsion Medical Systems, Germany) and LiDCO (LiDCO Ltd, UK)) must be calibrated intermittently, by using transpulmonary dilution techniques, with arterial and central venous lines. In patients receiving positive pressure ventilation, potential fluid responsiveness (indicating the need for more fluid) can be assessed from stroke volume variation (SVV) or pulse pressure variation (PPV). Values above 10% for SVV or 13% for PPV imply that the patient's haemodynamics will improve with fluid.

- PiCCO uses thermodilution to calibrate its pulse contour algorithm; the special arterial line includes a thermistor; a bolus of cold fluid is injected via the central line and a temperature curve is plotted to give a value for cardiac output.
- LiDCO uses lithium dilution for calibration; a bolus of lithium solution is injected via a central or peripheral venous line; a lithium electrode is attached to an arterial line—lithium concentration is plotted and a value for the cardiac output is derived. The more recent 'LiDCOrapid' system does not need calibration and has been designed specifically for use in the operating room.
- The Vigileo system (Edwards Lifesciences, USA) does not require calibration but there are conflicting data on the accuracy of this device.

Further reading

Association of Anaesthetists of Great Britain and Ireland. Recommendations for standards of monitoring during an-aesthesia and recovery (4th edn). London: AAGBI, 2007. Available at: ℅ http://www.aagbi.org/publications.

Davey AJ, Diba A (eds). *Ward's Anaesthetic Equipment* (5th ed). Oxford: Elsevier Saunders 2005.

Magee P, Tooley M (eds). *The Physics, Clinical Measurement, and Equipment of Anaesthetic Practice for the FRCA* (2nd ed). Oxford: Oxford University Press, 2011.

Regional versus general anaesthesia

Key points
- RA is suitable only for a minority of emergency cases but should be actively considered.
- Airway protection is paramount for both GA and RA.
- RA with poorly managed sedation may be the 'worst of both worlds'.
- Correct hypovolaemia before both RA and GA.
- Exclude coagulopathy before RA.

Background
For a subset of emergency operations there may be an option to perform surgery exclusively under RA. GA is often the default. There is little evidence to support the choice of anaesthetic techniques although Caesarean section and surgery for fractured neck of femur (#NOF) are two areas where evidence does exist.

- Urgent surgery for Caesarean section should be performed under RA where possible as there is evidence of better maternal satisfaction and fetal outcome (see 🕮 Emergency Caesarean section, p.262). For genuine emergencies (Category 1) a fine balance exists between the potential for better fetal outcome from RA and the delay required to perform it. The concept of rapid sequence spinal was introduced recently but remains controversial.
- For surgery for #NOF evidence supports the use of spinal anaesthesia because short-term outcome is improved (see 🕮 Fractured neck of femur, p.92). Evidence of long-term benefit (>6 months) is lacking.
- The large GALA study comparing GA versus RA in largely elective carotid surgery found no differences in outcome between the two anaesthetic techniques.

Pros and cons of general versus regional anaesthesia
Generally, RA is not considered as often as it might be for emergency surgery. However, there are specific pitfalls to use of RA in emergency surgery. These are discussed as pros and cons. RA is divided into CNB and PNB. Of note, the increasing reliability of ultrasound guided RA techniques make them more of a viable prospect than previously in the emergency setting.

General anaesthesia—pros and cons
Pros
- 100% effective.
- Fast—can be achieved in only a few minutes.
- Few absolute contraindications.
- Once established, airway is protected.
- Less stressful for anxious patient.
- Unconscious patient enables open communication between anaesthetist, surgeon, and other team members.
- In trauma, enables secondary survey without distress to patient.
- Consent for GA is currently tacitly assumed as part of a surgical procedure (although whether this view will persist is debatable).

Cons

- Risk of aspiration at time of induction requires rapid sequence induction and tracheal intubation.
- Risk of airway complications or failure during emergency intubation considerably higher than for elective surgery.
- Overt or concealed hypovolaemia risks profound cardiovascular instability.
- Provides minimal postoperative analgesia.
- Minimal effect on surgical stress response.

Regional anaesthesia—pros and cons
Central neuraxial block—pros

- Avoids risk of airway complications as patient maintains own airway.
- Reduces stress response.
- Minimizes postoperative opioid/sedative analgesic needs.
- Enables communication with patient during and after surgery.
- Less postoperative confusion.
- Less respiratory and potentially cardiac complications.
- Potentially less postoperative cognitive dysfunction in the elderly.
- In trauma enables secondary survey with patient cooperation.

Central neuraxial block—cons

- Taking informed consent is often challenging.
- Overt or concealed hypovolaemia risks profound cardiovascular instability.
- ↑ risk of coagulopathy and must be excluded before CNB.
- Patient cooperation may be difficult in emergency situation.
- Heavy sedation not appropriate (risk of aspiration).
- Less than 100% reliability.
- Unpredictable time to onset and finite duration of action.
- Injuries outside the area of blockade may cause symptomatic distress during surgery.
- Equipment and sterility issues make CNB generally inappropriate outside operating room.

Peripheral nerve block—pros

- Many—as for CNB.
- Role for early analgesia (e.g. femoral nerve block for #NOF).
- Potential for prolonged postoperative analgesia (particularly catheter techniques).
- May facilitate surgery as day case.

Peripheral nerve block—cons
As for CNB.

In general, RA should at least be considered for all emergencies; however, for the most major emergencies RA will be less appropriate than GA as a solo technique. When RA is chosen, it requires considerable skill to ensure performance is prompt, effective and with the minimal risk of complications.

Regional anaesthesia in combination with general anaesthesia

A combination of GA and RA enables the benefits of CNB and PNB to be achieved without many of the negative aspects listed previously. RA undoubtedly improves analgesia compared with no RA and there is conclusive evidence that CNB achieves better analgesia than parenteral opioids after major surgery. The long-standing debate over whether RA (in particular CNB) improves outcome is unresolved but, as emergency cases have an up to 2–10 fold increase in morbidity/mortality compared with elective surgery, the potential benefits of RA are likely greatest in emergency cases. Unfortunately the risks of RA in emergencies are also likely to be increased. Careful judgement of case-specific risks and benefits will remain the mainstay that guides practice for individual patients.

Further reading

Cook TM. Potential benefits of central neuraxial block. In NAP3. *The Third National Audit Project of the Royal College of Anaesthetists, Major Complications of Central Neuraxial blockade in the United Kingdom. Report and Findings.* London: Royal College of Anaesthetists, 2009, Chapter 2 pp. 17–26. Available at: http://www.rcoa.ac.uk/index.asp?PageID=717.

Macintyre PE, Schug SA, Scott DA, et al.; Acute Pain Management: Scientific Evidence Working Group of the Australian and New Zealand College of Anaesthetists and Faculty of Pain Medicine. *Acute Pain Management: Scientific Evidence* (3rd ed). Melbourne: ANZCA & FPM, 2010.

Wijeysundera DN, Beattie WS, Austin PC, et al. Epidural anaesthesia and survival after intermediate-to-high risk non-cardiac surgery: a population-based cohort study. *Lancet* 2008; **372**:562–9.

Prehospital

Prehospital anaesthesia

Key points
- The need for prehospital anaesthesia is rare.
- Prehospital anaesthesia should be undertaken by well-trained, competent practitioners using appropriate equipment and monitoring.
- Prehospital organizations require a well-defined clinical governance structure to regulate and monitor prehospital anaesthesia with the aim of preventing ↑ morbidity and mortality in this difficult setting.

Background

The prehospital setting is usually a more challenging place to perform anaesthesia than hospital. The clinician will often have other management decisions and interventions to make. The lack of trained assistance and 'bedside' senior support makes it more difficult.

Although intubation has not been shown to improve outcome in medical cardiac arrests, early intubation in those few trauma and medical patients who need it optimizes ventilation, reduces hypoxia and secondary insults, and reduces delay to definitive procedures. Robust systems are needed to ensure that high standards are achieved and patient safety is not compromised.

Indications

The decision to anaesthetize a patient is made on a patient-by-patient basis aided by an on-scene risk:benefit analysis, i.e. in this situation, do the benefits of an anaesthetic outweigh the risks? It is based on who is available to anaesthetize the patient—are they competent, current and proficient to perform this intervention in the prehospital setting? Potential indications include:
- Actual or impending airway compromise—trauma, burns, anaphylaxis.
- Ventilatory failure—trauma (pneumothorax, haemothorax, #ribs, circumferential burns), severe pulmonary oedema.
- Unconsciousness—leading to an unprotected airway (traumatic brain injury, drug overdose).
- Humanitarian indications—polytrauma or severe burns (pain), long transfer time.
- Unmanageable or agitated patient post head injury—facilitates safe transfer.
- Anticipated clinical course—need for scanning, urgent surgery.

Anaesthetic drugs

- The choice of anaesthetic drugs varies between different prehospital organizations. In general, they are chosen for their relative haemodynamic stability and reasonably wide therapeutic range.
- These are often drawn up in advance for immediate use. Predrawn syringes should be labelled clearly with drug name and date/time of drawing up.

Equipment

Equipment used in the prehospital setting should match that used in hospital. It needs to be robust, portable, able to withstand adverse conditions and have appropriate battery capacity. Like hospital equipment, it must be appropriately maintained and serviced. Equipment varies with each prehospital set up but includes that shown in the algorithm in Fig. 2.1.

Preparation

* Address scene safety before anaesthesia is considered. Personal protective equipment (PPE) should be worn as appropriate.
* If possible, move the patient to establish 360° access and, if available, place on an ambulance trolley at kneeling height.
* Connect monitoring and set it so that readings are taken at regular (2 min) intervals.
* Establish IV access and secure carefully. Ideally, two forms of access (IV, central, or IO) should be available in the event that one fails.
* Concurrent activity, including treatment of immediate needs (splintage, haemorrhage control), is essential.
* Prepare a standard 'kit dump' with all drugs and equipment needed for intubation according to local protocol (see Fig. 2.1). The prehospital team should be fully conversant with all drugs and equipment.
* Brief the assistants. Ideally, four people are required: intubator, assistant to intubation, in-line cervical spine immobilization provider, and cricoid pressure/larynx manipulator.
* Using a challenge and response strategy, the intubator and assistant run through a checklist to check the equipment and allow time for adequate pre-oxygenation before inducing anaesthesia.
* Anticipation of patient needs is important to keep scene time to a minimum. Delay to definitive care because of protracted on scene management may be harmful.

Intubation

Preinduction

* Effective pre-oxygenation will denitrogenate the lungs and increase the time from the onset of apnoea to arterial oxygen desaturation. In the spontaneously breathing patient this can be achieved using high-flow oxygen through a close fitting non-rebreathing mask with reservoir attached.
* A patent airway is essential. Consider use of nasopharyngeal and oropharyngeal airways with manual airway manoeuvres.
* If breathing is inadequate, use a bag–mask technique to achieve pre-oxygenation.
* Pre-anaesthetic sedation may be needed to facilitate control and pre-oxygenation of the agitated or combative patient. Titrate to effect small doses of midazolam (1–2 mg) but do this very carefully in the haemodynamically unstable patient.

With manual in-line cervical spine stabilization in place, remove the front of the cervical collar and head blocks to facilitate laryngoscopy.

Induction

- With the checklist complete, induction is undertaken using the same consideration for drugs and dosages as would occur in hospital, i.e. reduced doses for the haemodynamically unstable patient.
- A poor view on laryngoscopy is often caused by badly applied cricoid pressure. It may need to be adjusted or released altogether to facilitate a better view.
- Prehospital airways are often challenging because of the patient and testing environment: difficult intubations should be anticipated. Use a bougie routinely. Ensure that suction and difficult airway equipment are readily at hand.
- Once the tracheal tube has passed between the cords, confirm correct placement with both a colorimetric device and side or mainstream CO_2 detector. Also auscultate over the axillae and stomach.
- If there is an inadequate view on laryngoscopy, carry out optimization drills to improve the view:
  - Backward, upward, rightward pressure (BURP).
  - Release cricoid pressure.
  - Insert blade to maximum and slowly withdraw.
  - Suction.
  - Adjust operator position.
  - Adjust patient position.
  - Change operator.
  - Change blade—long or McCoy.
- If desaturation to below 92% occurs during attempted intubation, reoxygenate using a bag–mask before making a second attempt.
- Do not attempt tracheal intubation more than 3 times. If unsuccessful, initiate the failed intubation plan.

Failed intubation

- Every prehospital organization should have a failed intubation plan (further information can be obtained from the Difficult Airway Society and UK Training in Emergency Airway Management (TEAM) course manual).
- Consider a supraglottic airway as a rescue device in this setting.
- A surgical airway may also be considered and may be the preferred primary option if a difficult airway is anticipated (e.g. burns).
- Other options include bag–mask ventilation or waking the patient (not always feasible), although a supraglottic or surgical airway are usually preferable.

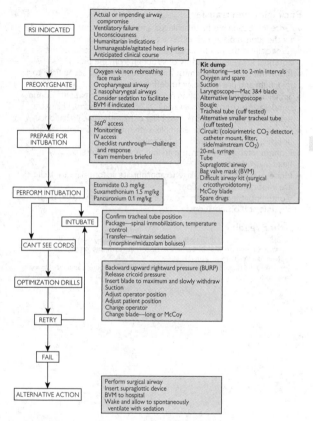

Fig. 2.1 Algorithm for prehospital anaesthesia. Adapted from Tim Nutbeam, Figure 4. *Pre-hospital RSI overview, The ABC of prehospital emergency medicine*, 2012, with permission from Wiley/Blackwell.

Packaging and transfer

- Once intubation has been achieved and tube placement confirmed, fix the tube in place with either a tie, tube holder, or adhesive tape (especially in the head-injured patient because this reduces the potential for venous outflow obstruction from the brain).
- Momentum at this stage must be continued to keep scene time to a minimum and prevent delay to definitive care.
- Spinal immobilization is often needed in the trauma patient. Consider temperature-controlled packaging (bubble wrap, thermal blankets, heaters etc.) to reduce the possibility of hypothermic coagulopathy.
- Continue anaesthesia, for example, with morphine and midazolam boluses, or with an infusion of propofol.
- Monitor vital signs and ensure adequate ventilation (especially in the head-injured patient).
- Mode of transport and triage to appropriate secondary care facilities are important considerations.
- Contemporaneous patient notes are vital, including written or printed physiological observations.

Further reading

Association of Anaesthetists of Great Britain and Ireland. *AAGBI Safety Guideline: Pre-hospital Anaesthesia*. London: AAGBI, 2009. Available at: ℘ http://www.aagbi.org/publications/guidelines/docs/prehospital_glossy09.pdf.

Benger J, Nolan J, Clancy M. *Emergency Airway Management*. Cambridge: Cambridge University Press, 2008.

Transport and transfer

Key points
- In the UK, critically ill patients are frequently transferred between hospitals. Most of these transfers are to enable access to specialist services.
- Understanding of the reasons for transfer and the principles involved will maximize safety.
- Several organizations, including the Association of Anaesthetists of Great Britain and Ireland (AAGBI) and the Intensive Care Society (ICS), have produced guidelines for transfers.
- Careful preparation is the most important factor in a safe transfer.

Reason for and speed of transfer
- The most common reason for transfer is to access specialist services, most often neurosurgery.
- The decision to transfer a patient must not be taken lightly and is usually made at consultant level. It must involve the critical care teams at the transferring and receiving hospitals.
- The urgency of the transfer is determined by the patient's medical condition. An expanding intracranial haematoma is a time-critical emergency, a diffuse axonal injury, whilst serious, has no remediable treatment that must be provided immediately in a neurosurgery centre.
- There is no indication for a 'scoop and run' immediate transfer if the patient is in a hospital with critical care facilities. Immediate life-saving treatments to stabilize a patient are undertaken first.

Who should go?
- The team at the referring hospital decides who accompanies the patient and whether any interventions are needed before transfer.
- There are no specific recommendations about seniority of doctor undertaking a transfer, but it is recommended that they should have undertaken a transfer course and these should be available in each region.
- As competency-based training increases, competencies in interhospital transfer will be developed.
- The healthcare personnel who accompany the patient on the transfer must be adequately insured for personal injury. Such insurance is included as a benefit of membership of the AAGBI and ICS.

Mode of transfer
The majority of transfers will occur in standard land ambulances. There are occasions when longer-distance transfers are undertaken in specialist ambulances or fixed or rotary wing aircraft. These longer distance transfers should be undertaken by specialist teams with experience and knowledge of that mode of transfer.

Equipment

- The equipment required for transfer should be provided by the referring hospital. It should be familiar to the doctor using it and if possible should be similar throughout a region.
- The equipment should be portable but sturdy, and have an extensive battery life. Many ambulances have only a 12-volt supply so the battery must be able to last the entire journey.
- Gravity-fed drip systems will be unreliable in an ambulance, so infusion pumps are a priority.
- Invasive BP monitoring is useful as non-invasive systems are both unreliable in a moving vehicle and deplete batteries rapidly.

The setup within the ambulance should enable the transferring doctor to see the patient, the monitors and all the equipment. Minimal monitoring comprises:

- Continuous presence of appropriately trained staff.
- ECG.
- NIBP (although frequently unreliable).
- Arterial oxygen saturation (SaO_2).
- $ETCO_2$ in ventilated patients.
- Temperature (preferably core and peripheral).

Problems

Most problems are related to the confined space and the movement and noise of the vehicle. Careful preparation should minimize these risks:

- Disconnection of equipment especially ventilator tubing.
- Inability to monitor accurately because of movement and vibration.
- Inability to examine patient because of noise.
- Equipment damaged by sudden movement.

Preparation

This is the most important part of any transfer and involves an appropriate mix of efficiency and speed whilst maintaining patient safety. An ABC approach may help to prepare:

A. Ensure the airway is adequate, this will usually mean the patient is intubated and ventilated; confirm the position of the tracheal tube, preferably radiologically. Secure the tube so it will not move, but ensure that venous drainage is unobstructed.

B. Establish the patient on the transfer ventilator and, if time allows, obtain an ABG sample to ensure the ventilator settings are correct. It is the transferring doctor's responsibility to ensure there is adequate oxygen available for the transfer. Drain any pneumothorax before transfer. Monitor $ETCO_2$ throughout the transfer.

C. Do not transfer a patient who is bleeding actively. Patients who are under resuscitated will be less stable during transfer. Ensure that there are two patent IV lines.

Take precautions to minimize any increase in intracranial pressure. Document the preintubation Glasgow Coma Scale score.

Communication

Communicate adequately with the receiving hospital and obtain details on where to go and who will be taking over. Ensure that the driver knows precisely where to go! Carry a mobile phone to ensure constant contact.

Documentation

- Take a complete copy of the patient's medical notes.
- A copy of any imaging should be available at the receiving hospital. With modern Picture Archiving and Communications Systems (PACS) this is usually possible over the Internet.
- Documentation of the transfer is also important and should include details similar to that contained on an anaesthetic chart. Regions have been encouraged to develop transfer forms.

Checklist

The pre-departure checklist produced by the AAGBI is invaluable.

Predeparture checklist

- Do attendants have adequate competencies, experience, knowledge of case, clothing, and insurance?
- Appropriate equipment and drugs?
- Batteries checked?
- Sufficient O_2?
- Trolley available?
- Ambulance service aware or ready?
- Bed confirmed? Exact location?
- Case notes, X-ray films, results, blood collected?
- Transfer chart prepared?
- Portable phone charged?
- Contact numbers known?
- Money or cards for emergencies?
- Estimated time of arrival notified?
- Return arrangements checked?
- Relatives informed?
- Patient stable, fully investigated?
- Monitoring attached and working?
- Drugs, pumps, lines rationalized and secured?
- Adequate sedation?
- Still stable after transfer to mobile equipment?
- Anything missed?

Further reading

Association of Anaesthetists of Great Britain and Ireland. *AAGBI Safety Guideline: Interhospital Transfer*. London: AAGBI, 2009. Available at: ℘ http://www.aagbi.org/publications/guidelines/docs/interhospital09.pdf.

Intensive Care Society. *ICS Guidelines on Transfer of the Critically ill Adult*. London: ICS, 2002. Available at: ℘ http://www.ics.ac.uk/intensive_care_professional/standards_and_guidelines/transport_of_the_critically_ill_2002.

The Injured Patient

Pathophysiology of trauma and hypovolaemia

Key points

- Several mechanisms are involved in the development of cellular injury after severe trauma. Haemorrhage, causing circulatory failure with poor tissue perfusion and generalized hypoxia (hypovolaemic shock) are common.
- Severe trauma is a potent cause of the systemic inflammatory response syndrome (SIRS) and this may progress to multiple organ failure.

Background

An understanding of the pathophysiology of the response to trauma and haemorrhage is essential if haemorrhagic shock is to be diagnosed and treated efficiently and effectively. A table of standardized vital signs associated with varying degrees of haemorrhage is central to trauma life support but there is wide variation from these 'typical' values.

Physiological responses to haemorrhage

Trauma compromises tissue oxygenation because haemorrhage reduces oxygen delivery and tissue injury and inflammation increase oxygen consumption. Compensatory responses to haemorrhage are categorized into immediate, early, and late:

- Immediate—the loss of blood volume is detected by low-pressure stretch receptors in the atria and arterial baroreceptors in the aorta and carotid artery. Efferent responses from the vasomotor centre trigger an increase in catecholamines, which causes arteriolar constriction, venoconstriction, and tachycardia.
- Early compensatory mechanisms (5–60 min) include movement of fluid from the interstitium to the intravascular space and mobilization of intracellular fluid.
- Long-term compensation to haemorrhage includes: reduced glomerular filtration rate, salt and water reabsorption (aldosterone and vasopressin), thirst, and ↑ erythropoiesis.

Hypovolaemic shock is divided into four classes (Table 3.1).

- Blood loss of 15–30% of the total blood volume will typically be associated with a tachycardia >100 min^{-1} and reduced pulse pressure; the increase in diastolic pressure reflects peripheral vasoconstriction.
- A decrease in systolic pressure implies a loss of >30% of total blood volume (approximately 1500 mL in a 70-kg adult).
- Pure haemorrhage without significant tissue injury may not cause this typical pattern of a stepwise increase in heart rate. Occasionally, the heart rate may remain relatively low until the onset of cardiovascular collapse.

Haemorrhagic shock causes a significant lactic acidosis:

- Once the mitochondrial PO_2 is less than 2 mmHg, oxidative phosphorylation is inhibited and pyruvate is unable to enter the Krebs cycle. Instead, pyruvate undergoes anaerobic metabolism in the cytoplasm—a process that is relatively inefficient for adenosine triphosphate (ATP) generation.
- ATP depletion causes cell membrane pump failure and cell death.
▶Resuscitation must restore oxygen delivery rapidly if irreversible haemorrhagic shock and death of the patient is to be prevented.

Table 3.1 Classification of hypovolaemic shock according to blood loss (adult)

	Class I	Class II	Class III	Class IV
Blood loss (%)	<15	15–30	30–40	>40
Blood loss (mL)	<750	750–1500	1500–2000	>2000
Systolic BP	Unchanged	Normal	Reduced	Very low
Diastolic BP	Unchanged	Raised	Reduced	Unrecordable
Pulse (beats/min)	Slight tachycardia	100–120	120 (thready)	>120 (very thready)
Capillary refill	Normal	Slow (>2 s)	Slow (>2 s)	Undetectable
Respiratory rate	Normal	Tachypnoea	Tachypnoea (>20/min)	Tachypnoea (>20/min)
Urine output (mL/h)	>30	20–30	10–20	0–10
Extremities	Normal	Pale	Pale	Pale, cold, clammy
Complexion	Normal	Pale	Pale	Ashen
Mental state	Alert	Anxious or aggressive	Anxious, aggressive or drowsy	Drowsy, confused or unconscious

Systemic inflammatory response syndrome

Severe trauma is a potent trigger of SIRS (Box 3.1).
- Crushed and wounded tissues activate complement which in turn triggers a cascade of inflammatory mediators (C3a, C5a, tumour necrosis factor-a (TNF-a), interleukin (IL)-1, IL-6, and IL-8).
- The extent of the inflammatory response to trauma in individuals is influenced significantly by genetic polymorphisms.
- Polymorphonuclear neutrophils (PMNs) are released from human bone marrow and adhere tightly to endothelium and migrate into the surrounding parenchyma where they are activated to release superoxide anion (O^{2-}) and elastase.
- The classic metabolic response to severe trauma is biphasic and multiple organ failure can occur during either of these of these phases:
  - SIRS occurs during the initial 3–5 days; during this phase, a second insult (or hit), such as surgery, may provoke an exaggerated inflammatory response.
  - Up to 50% of the patients developing organ failure early after trauma do so in the absence of bacterial infection.
  - The initial phase is followed by a period (perhaps 10–14 days) of immunosuppression when the patient is prone to infection.
- This temporal response is probably overly simplistic. Recent data suggest that there is a balance between inflammation and anti-inflammation—local inflammation is accompanied by systemic anti-inflammation. The anti-inflammatory response dominates outside the local area of inflammation—this enables phagocytes to be concentrated at the site of injury. But sometimes these protective systemic responses can become immunosuppressive.

Box 3.1 The systemic inflammatory response syndrome (SIRS)

Manifested by two or more of the following conditions:
- Temperature >38°C or <36°C.
- Heart rate >90 beats min^{-1}.
- Respiratory rate >20 breaths min^{-1} or $PaCO_2$ <4.3 kPa.
- WBC >12 000 cells mm^{-3}, <4000 cells mm^{-3}, or >10% immature (band) forms.

Further reading

American College of Surgeons Committee on Trauma. *Advanced Trauma Life Support Program For Doctors: Student Course Manual* (8th edn). Chicago, IL: American College of Surgeons, 2008.

Benger J, Nolan J, Clancy M. *Emergency Airway Management*. Cambridge: Cambridge University Press, 2008.

Foëx BA. Systemic response to trauma. *Brit Med Bull* 1999; **55**:726–43.

Giannoudis PV. Current concepts of the inflammatory response after major trauma: an update. *Injury* 2003; **34**:397–404.

Huber-Wagner SR, Lefering R, Qvick LM, *et al.* Effect of whole-body CT during trauma resuscitation on survival: a retrospective, multicentre study. *Lancet* 2009; **373**:1455–61.

The primary survey

Key points

- The primary survey has undergone important changes including the prioritization of life-threatening haemorrhage, a revised fluid resuscitation strategy, and ↑ use of modern imaging techniques.
- The primary survey should be led by an experienced clinician with clearly articulated goals and subject to regular audit and review.

Background

The primary survey is a systematic, initial assessment that identifies and addresses immediately life-threatening problems. First developed in trauma care, it has subsequently been adapted to a broader range of ill and injured patients. The underlying principle is a widely recognized 'ABC' approach, in which the:

- Airway is established first, *then immediate*
- Breathing problems are addressed, *before*
- Circulation is assessed and managed.

This system still has much to offer as a starting point, particularly for novice clinicians, locations where resources are very limited, and situations in which healthcare demand significantly exceeds supply.

The modern approach to the primary survey

The primary survey has been adapted and refined in developed countries because:

- The initial hospital management of severely-injured patients is now conducted by trauma teams—the components of the primary survey are completed simultaneously, not in sequence.
- Recent military experience has identified catastrophic external haemorrhage as an important cause of death in the first few minutes following trauma—its treatment comes before airway.
- Where there is a formal system of prehospital care much of the primary survey will have been addressed before hospital arrival. The average time between trauma and hospital arrival for non-trapped patients in the UK is 60 min. If a patient with truly life-threatening injuries has survived this time they are unlikely to arrive in hospital with a problem that must be immediately addressed to prevent death in the next few minutes.

Assessment and intervention follows the priorities listed in the modern primary survey—in a hospital emergency department these are likely to be undertaken simultaneously:

- Control of catastrophic external haemorrhage.
- Airway (with cervical spine control).
- Breathing.
- Circulation.
- Disability.
- Exposure and environment.

Control of catastrophic external haemorrhage

Catastrophic external haemorrhage is of such severity that it threatens the patient's life within minutes, and cannot be controlled by pressure, elevation, and conventional wound dressings. It is usually caused by severe vascular injury in the limbs, groin, axilla, or neck. In the civilian setting, patients with true catastrophic external haemorrhage will either have had this controlled or will have died before they reach hospital. Where direct pressure and elevation are not effective the following two techniques are available:

Tourniquets
- Suitable for control of catastrophic limb haemorrhage when they can be placed proximal to the point of injury.
- Once control of haemorrhage has been achieved, effective wound dressing, sometimes using specialist pressure dressings, may enable the tourniquet to be fully loosened prior to formal surgical intervention.
- Minimize limb ischaemia: communicate the presence of a tourniquet and document the application and removal time.

Haemostatic dressings
- Wide range available: packing, gauze, and bandages.
- Use physical and/or chemical methods to promote rapid haemostasis in sites where tourniquets cannot be applied (e.g. the groin, axilla, or neck); suitable for packing large tissue defects associated with catastrophic external haemorrhage.
- Require removal of excess blood followed by application of the product and direct pressure.
- Initial problems with heat generation (exothermic reactions) now resolved.
- Remove dressings under controlled conditions in an operating room.

Airway (with cervical spine control)

- Establish airway patency and apply high-flow oxygen and monitoring at the earliest opportunity. Use adjuncts only when needed to maintain airway patency: oropharyngeal airways may precipitate vomiting (particularly if too long) and nasopharyngeal airways may cause bleeding (particularly if too large). Where adjuncts are required, particularly if effective oxygenation proves challenging, use bilateral nasopharyngeal airways and an oral airway: concerns about the use of nasopharyngeal airways in head injury are unfounded provided these are inserted correctly.
- The airway in a trauma patient may prove exceptionally difficult to manage: blood in the airway, the risk of neck injury requiring cervical spine immobilization, injuries involving the upper airway and physiological compromise are factors that may contribute to the difficulty.
- Very few patients require tracheal intubation immediately on hospital arrival; the vast majority will benefit from airway and physiological optimization.
- Tracheal intubation is considerably more challenging in trauma patients, and a senior airway clinician should therefore be present with a clear plan and preparation for failed intubation.

Intubation and cervical spine immobilization in trauma patients

A failed airway may occur at least 10 times more frequently in the trauma patient compared with elective surgical patients: in the USA, 0.5% of intubations recorded in the National Emergency Airway Registry (NEAR) required a surgical airway. Immobilization of the cervical spine reduces the laryngeal view by, on average, one Cormack and Lehane grade.

During the primary survey, the cervical spine is immobilized if there is a risk of cervical spine injury, but this must not compromise effective airway management. Effective oxygenation takes precedence over small movements of the cervical spine because:

- Most injured patients do not have an unstable neck injury: about 10% of unconscious polytrauma patients (the highest risk group) will have a cervical spine injury and most of these are stable.
- Any associated spinal cord injury is most likely to occur at the point of initial injury: subsequent controlled movements of the spine are very unlikely to cause further damage.
- Direct laryngoscopy and intubation is unlikely to cause clinically significant movements of the neck—in this context manual inline stabilization probably contributes little additional value.

Breathing

Careful assessment of the patient's chest is an essential component of the primary survey. In a crowded and noisy resuscitation room, auscultation is of limited value; inspection and palpation of the chest can reveal important information.

Inspection

- Expose the chest and observe the patient's breathing from the end of the bed.
- Small ↑ in respiratory rate and/or minute volume may be caused by early hypovolaemia or direct chest trauma; anxiety is also a possibility but only if the former causes have been excluded.
- ↑ work of breathing, especially with external signs of injury, implies chest trauma; hyperventilation caused by haemorrhagic shock tends not to be associated with ↑ respiratory effort or patient distress.
- Chest asymmetry during respiration may indicate a flail segment or pneumothorax.

Palpation

- Allows asymmetry to be further assessed and may reveal tenderness, rib crepitus, and/or surgical emphysema.
- Failure to palpate the chest may delay the detection of significant chest injury.
- ABG analysis should occur as soon as the primary survey is completed, or earlier if there are adequate personnel. Treat immediately life-threatening problems (see 📖 Thoracic injury, p.74). Tracheal intubation and positive pressure ventilation may convert a simple pneumothorax into a tension pneumothorax—this will require immediate decompression.

Circulation

- Measure the pulse and BP; assess the capillary refill, colour, and autonomic state. A patient who is anxious, pale, and sweaty is likely to have both significant hypovolaemia and a 'normal' pulse and BP.
- Pulse rate and haemoglobin concentration are not reliable indicators of circulatory status.
- A metabolic acidosis and/or an ↑ plasma lactate value implies significant blood loss.
- Control external haemorrhage, secure IV access and obtain venous blood for routine testing including crossmatch and coagulation studies.
- It is much better to conserve the patient's blood volume than to replace it; any internal bleeding must be controlled rapidly; this may mean laparotomy, pelvic fixation (preceded by application of an external pelvic binder), and long-bone stabilization (e.g. by the application of a femoral traction splint—see ⬚ Pelvic fractures, p.88).

Fluid resuscitation in trauma

Previous guidance advocating the use of rapidly infused crystalloids is being revised in the favour of two alternative strategies:

- *Permissive hypotension.* The use of minimal or no IV fluids and the acceptance of temporary hypoperfusion/hypotension until haemorrhage is controlled. This strategy is most applicable to penetrating trauma, particularly in previously healthy patients where definitive haemorrhage control can be achieved rapidly. This strategy avoids both the dilution of clotting factors and transient increases in BP that may precipitate further haemorrhage. It may be applicable in some blunt trauma cases, particularly where there is an early end point at which definitive haemorrhage control will be achieved, but there are few data in these patients.
- *Early use of blood and blood products.* Recent military experience suggests that blood loss is best replaced by blood, with particular attention to the provision of clotting factors and platelets (see ⬚ Coagulopathy, p.130). The optimal approach, and ratio of blood product administration, has yet to be determined; data from observational studies supports the early and liberal use of blood products. The effectiveness of this strategy has not been proven in prospective studies.

Disability

- The Glasgow Coma Scale (GCS) score and pupillary response remains the mainstay of trauma disability assessment. The best response is documented with particular attention to the motor component since this has the greatest prognostic value.
- Assess motor function in all four limbs and the pattern of respiration (to seek diaphragmatic breathing) to rule out spinal cord injury (see ⬚ Spinal injury, p.104). Practitioners responsible for airway management and trauma intubation may be accused of causing neurological deficit in patients subsequently shown to have unstable cervical spine injuries, unless such deficit was clearly documented at the outset.

Exposure and environment

- Examine the patient's entire skin surface including the back and buttocks (by log-rolling). The log roll is done once only—all clothes, wet and soiled sheets, and injury debris removed at the same time. Rectal examination is not required routinely in the conscious and alert trauma patient without neurological deficit.
- Avoid hypothermia: exposure should be brief, with heat conservation and warming methods applied from the outset. Monitor the temperature continuously.

Complete at this stage any other simple adjunctive investigations (venous and arterial blood sampling, blood glucose measurement, ECG).

Trauma imaging

- Ideally, the CT scanner is co-located with the emergency department resuscitation facilities—the patient can then be comprehensively scanned immediately following the primary survey, reducing the need for the three 'trauma radiographs' (cervical spine, chest, and pelvis) that have been emphasized in traditional teaching.
- Cervical spine X-rays have now been replaced by CT scanning in all patients with significant head injury and/or multisystem trauma. Chest and pelvic X-rays remain routine in many centres, but selected patients are increasingly undergoing CT as their initial imaging modality.
- Ultrasound is also being used increasingly in the initial assessment of trauma, with FAST (focused assessment by sonography in trauma) scanning used as an adjunct to the primary survey or even in the pre-hospital phase of care (see Intra-abdominal trauma, p.80).

Team leadership

- Ideally, an experienced consultant should lead the trauma team.
- The effective team leader stands back, coordinates the team, directs care, and does not get involved in delivering the required interventions.
- The team leader provides clear, calm, and consistent direction, prioritizes the patient's requirements and maintains momentum. This requires the non-technical skills of communication, leadership, situational awareness, and task management; factors that influence outcome as much as the clinical skills of the team.

Goals and endpoints

- The aim of the primary survey is to rapidly assess the trauma patient, identifying and addressing life-threatening pathology whilst quantifying the degree of physiological derangement and likely injuries.
- The primary survey is not an end in itself—it is just part of the patient's journey towards definitive care (usually the operating room or ICU).
- Maintain a forward momentum and set clear goals.
- Set and audit key standards such as the time between arrival and transfer for CT scan or surgery.

Further reading

Benger J, Nolan J, Clancy M (eds). *Emergency Airway Management*. Cambridge: Cambridge University Press, 2008.

Graham CA, Beard D, Oglesby AJ, *et al*. Rapid sequence intubation in Scottish urban emergency departments. *Emerg Med J* 2003; **20**:3–5.

Holcomb JB, Wade CE, Michalek JE, *et al*. Increased plasma and platelet to red blood cell ratios improves outcome in 466 massively transfused civilian trauma patients. *Ann Surg* 2008; **248**:447–58.

Manoach S, Paladino L. Manual in-line stabilization for acute airway management of suspected cervical spine injury: Historical review and current questions. *Ann Emerg Med*. 2007; **50**:236–45.

Shlamovitz GZ, Mower WR, Bergman J, *et al*. Poor test characteristics for the digital rectal examination in trauma patients. *Ann Emerg Med* 2007; **50**:25–33.

Thoracic injury

Key points
- Most thoracic injuries can be treated effectively with relatively simple interventions.
- All patients with suspected thoracic injury should receive high-flow oxygen.
- Immediately life-threatening injuries are treated during the primary survey.

Background
Thoracic injuries are grouped into two: (a) those that are immediately life threatening should be detected and treated in the primary survey; (b) potentially life-threatening injuries are detected later, usually after imaging or other investigations that form part of the secondary survey.

Life-threatening thoracic injuries
These injuries may be identified during the primary survey and must be treated immediately.
- Tension pneumothorax
- Open pneumothorax
- Massive haemothorax
- Flail chest
- Cardiac tamponade.

Tension pneumothorax
Tension pneumothorax develops if gas progressively enters the pleural space though a 'one-way valve' air leak but is unable to leave. This process increases the pressure in the pleural space, collapsing the lung on the affected side, pushing the mediastinum to the opposite side, compressing great vessels and preventing venous return. Life-threatening deterioration may be rapid, particularly during positive pressure ventilation.

Symptoms and signs (often unreliable and late)
- Absent breath sounds, hyperinflation, and hyper-resonance to percussion on the affected side.
- Tachycardia and hypotension.
- Visibly distended neck veins (unless concomitant hypovolaemia).
- Trachea deviated away from the affected side.

Management
- Immediate needle thoracocentesis: insert a wide-bore cannula (14 G) into the 2nd intercostal space in the midclavicular line of the affected hemithorax. This intervention may convert a tension into a simple pneumothorax. It does not allow lung reinflation and may fail due to insufficient cannula depth to penetrate the pleural space and subsequent cannula displacement or kinking; in this case, decompression is achieved with immediate thoracostomy.
- Definitive management requires intercostal chest drain insertion.

Open pneumothorax

When a chest wall defect is more than 2/3 the diameter of the trachea, air enters the pleural cavity preferentially through the wound and prevents alveolar ventilation.

Symptoms and signs
- Absent breath sounds on the affected side.
- Hypoxia and hypercapnia.

Management
- Immediate wound closure with an occlusive three-sided dressing or manufactured one-way valve. This creates a flutter valve, preventing both air entry via the wound during inspiration and air trapping within the pleural cavity causing tension physiology. Such dressings are prone to blocking or failing to remain attached to the chest wall.
- Definitive management requires sealing the wound with an occlusive dressing or surgical repair and inserting an intercostal chest drain remote from the wound.

Massive haemothorax

Rapid accumulation of >1500 mL or >30% blood volume in the hemithorax can cause life-threatening respiratory and circulatory compromise. Hypovolaemia will compound ventilatory failure and increase tissue hypoxia.

Symptoms and signs
- Reduced breath sounds and dullness to percussion on the affected side.
- Haemorrhagic shock.

Management
- Once IV access has been obtained, insert a large chest drain (32 FG) in the 5th intercostal space (anterior axillary) line and connect to an underwater seal drain. Restore blood volume and consider autotransfusion.
- Consider early thoracotomy.
- Incomplete drainage may cause complications such as an empyema.

Flail chest

When more than one consecutive rib is fractured in more than one place, an unstable segment is created, which disrupts normal chest wall movement. The degree of underlying pulmonary contusion and subsequent hypoxia determines the severity of the injury.

Symptoms and signs
- Paradoxical, asymmetrical, or uncoordinated chest wall movement—the diagnosis of a flail chest is based on the clinical observation of these signs.
- Palpable crepitus.
- Pain.
- Signs of underlying lung injury.

Management
- Systemic analgesia while watching for opioid-induced respiratory depression.
- LA: intercostal, intrapleural, or epidural blocks may provide excellent analgesia and avoid the need for intubation.
- Assess ABGs and ventilate if respiratory failure develops.

Cardiac tamponade

Blood in the pericardial space that increases the pressure in the pericardial sac will constrict cardiac filling and eventually lead to pulseless electrical activity (PEA). Penetrating injury is the most common cause of cardiac tamponade. Entry wounds may be remote from the pericardium and wounds between the nipple lines, in the epigastrium and between the shoulder blades should give a high index of suspicion.

Symptoms and signs
- Distended neck veins in the presence of hypotension are suggestive of cardiac tamponade, although after rapid volume resuscitation myocardial contusion may also present in this way. Tension pneumothorax may also mimic tamponade.
- Normal breath sounds unless concurrent lung injury.
- Pulsus paradoxus (a reduction in the volume of the peripheral pulse during inspiration).
- FAST is sensitive and specific for the evaluation of the pericardium for cardiac tamponade in penetrating trauma.
- Muffled heart sounds are meaningless in the midst of a busy resuscitation room.

Management
- Thoracotomy is the definitive management of cardiac tamponade.
- In the absence of the surgical capability for thoracotomy, needle pericardiocentesis has been advocated but is only rarely effective.
- Emergency thoracotomy for cardiac tamponade has been performed with successful outcome following traumatic cardiac arrest by appropriately trained non-surgical physicians.

Potentially life-threatening thoracic injuries

There are six potentially life-threatening injuries (two contusions and four 'ruptures'):
- Pulmonary contusion.
- Cardiac contusion.
- Aortic rupture—blunt aortic injury.
- Ruptured diaphragm.
- Oesophageal rupture.
- Rupture of the tracheobronchial tree.

Pulmonary contusion
- Inspection of the chest may reveal signs indicating considerable decelerating forces, such as seatbelt bruising.
- Pulmonary contusion is the commonest potentially lethal chest injury.
- Young adults and children have particularly compliant ribs and considerable energy can be transmitted to the lungs in the absence of rib fractures.
- The earliest indication of pulmonary contusion is hypoxaemia (reduced PaO_2/FiO_2 ratio).
- The chest radiograph shows patchy infiltrates over the affected area, but may be normal initially.

- Increasing the FiO_2 may provide sufficient oxygenation, if not, the patient may require mask CPAP or tracheal intubation and positive pressure ventilation.
- Use small tidal volumes (6 mL kg^{-1}—based on ideal body weight) to minimize volutrauma. Try to keep the peak inspiratory pressure <30 cmH$_2$O.
- The patient with chest trauma requires appropriate fluid resuscitation but fluid overload will compound the lung contusion.

Myocardial contusion
- Cardiac contusion must be considered in any patient with severe blunt chest trauma, particularly those with sternal fractures.
- Cardiac arrhythmias, ST changes on the ECG, and elevated serum concentrations of cardiac troponin suggest cardiac contusion.
- Elevated CVP in the presence of hypotension is the earliest indication of myocardial dysfunction secondary to severe cardiac contusion, but cardiac tamponade must be excluded.
- Echocardiography is the best method of confirming a cardiac contusion.
- The severely contused myocardium will require inotropic support (e.g. dobutamine).

Aortic disruption
- The thoracic aorta is at risk in any patient sustaining a significant decelerating force (e.g. fall from a height or high-speed road traffic crash). Only 10–15% of these patients will reach hospital alive.
- The commonest site for aortic injury is at the aortic isthmus, just distal to the origin of the left subclavian artery at the level of the ligamentum arteriosum. Deceleration produces large shear forces at this site because the relatively mobile aortic arch travels forward relative to the fixed descending aorta.
- The tear in the intima and media may involve either part of or the whole circumference of the aorta, and in survivors the haematoma is contained by an intact aortic adventitia and mediastinal pleura.
- Patients sustaining blunt aortic injury usually have multiple injuries and may be hypotensive at presentation. However, upper extremity hypertension is present in 40% of cases as the haematoma compresses the true lumen causing a 'pseudocoarctation'.
- The supine chest radiograph will show a widened mediastinum in the vast majority of cases. Although this is a sensitive sign of blunt aortic injury, it is not very specific—90% of cases of widened mediastinum are due to venous bleeding.
- Contrast-enhanced CT is the standard investigation for the diagnosis of blunt aortic injury.
- If blunt aortic injury is suspected, the patient's BP should be maintained at 80–100 mmHg systolic (using a beta blocker such as esmolol), in an effort to reduce the risk of further dissection or rupture. The use of pure vasodilators increases the pulse pressure and will not reduce the shear forces on the aortic wall.
- Once stable, the patient must be transferred immediately to the nearest cardiothoracic unit. In many cases these aortic injuries are now treated by endovascular stenting (see 📖 Cardiac tamponade, p.202).

Diaphragmatic rupture

- Injury to the diaphragm can occur following either blunt or penetrating chest trauma and is often a late diagnosis.
- Blunt diaphragmatic injury usually occurs on the left (75%), as the liver is relatively 'protective' of the right diaphragm. The stomach or colon commonly herniate into the chest and may strangulate.
- Diminished breath sounds on the affected side and respiratory distress may be associated with severe chest and abdominal pain in the awake patient.
- The chest radiograph may show an elevated hemidiaphragm, gas bubbles above the diaphragm, shift of the mediastinum to the opposite side, and nasogastric tube in the chest. Injecting contrast media via the nasogastric tube will confirm the diagnosis. CT is diagnostic.
- Laparotomy to repair the diaphragm is required.

Oesophageal rupture

- A severe blow to the upper abdomen may tear the lower oesophagus as gastric contents are ejected forcefully.
- The conscious patient will complain of severe chest and abdominal pain, and mediastinal air may be visible on the chest radiograph.
- Gastric contents may appear in the chest drain.
- The diagnosis is confirmed by contrast study of the oesophagus or endoscopy.
- Urgent surgery is essential—mediastinitis carries a high mortality.

Tracheobronchial injury

- Laryngeal fractures are rare.
- Signs of laryngeal injury include hoarseness, subcutaneous emphysema, and palpable fracture crepitus.
- Total airway obstruction or severe respiratory distress is managed by intubation or a surgical airway—tracheostomy is indicated rather than cricothyroidotomy.
- Less severe laryngeal injuries may be assessed by CT before any appropriate surgery.
- Transections of the trachea or bronchi proximal to the pleural reflection cause massive mediastinal and cervical emphysema.
- Injuries distal to the pleural sheath lead to pneumothoraces—these will not resolve after chest drainage, since the bronchopleural fistula allows a large air leak.
- Most bronchial injuries occur within 2.5 cm of the carina and the diagnosis is confirmed by bronchoscopy.
- Tracheobronchial injuries require urgent repair through a thoracotomy.

Simple pneumothorax

- Small simple pneumothoraces may be missed on clinical examination and chest radiograph but may develop rapidly into a tension pneumothorax if positive pressure ventilation is applied.
- Intercostal chest drain insertion provides definitive management but conservative treatment of an asymptomatic pneumothorax in a self-ventilating patient may be appropriate with close clinical observation.

Further reading

American College of Surgeons Committee on Trauma. *Advanced Trauma Life Support Program For Doctors: Student Course Manual* (8th edn). Chicago, IL: American College of Surgeons, 2008.

Intra-abdominal trauma

Key points
- Life-threatening intra-abdominal haemorrhage requires rapid haemorrhage control, usually by immediate laparotomy, although interventional radiologists are increasingly successful at stopping solid organ bleeding with use of embolization.
- Induction of anaesthesia in the presence of hypovolaemia is challenging but will be necessary if a strategy of controlled fluid resuscitation has been adopted.
- Consider damage control surgery to enable the patient to be fully resuscitated once haemorrhage is controlled.

Background
- Injuries within the abdomen can be difficult to diagnose and potentially catastrophic. The primary concern is haemorrhage, particularly from the liver, spleen, and kidneys, which may require immediate surgery to control. Subsequently, however, it is important to consider the risk of more subtle injuries to the bowel and renal tract: these are harder to diagnose and may take several days to become apparent.
- All trauma patients are at risk of abdominal injury, but those with injuries above and below the abdomen (e.g. flail segment and femoral fracture) are at particular risk and need very careful assessment.

Indicators of intra-abdominal trauma
- Suggestive mechanism of injury: high velocity trauma with multisystem injury, history of direct abdominal trauma.
- External signs of abdominal injury: bruising, abrasions, swelling.
- Penetrating injury with potential involvement of the abdomen (this includes penetrating injuries to the lower chest, pelvis, and buttocks). Unless clearly very superficial, all such injuries should be formally explored in the operating room: it is notoriously difficult to assess wound depth or the involvement of intra-abdominal organs.
- Abdominal tenderness: blood within the peritoneal cavity usually causes significant pain and localized peritonitis, becoming progressively more generalized. It is important to distinguish true abdominal tenderness from pain related to the chest wall (ribs) or pelvis, though both chest and pelvic injury are associated with intra-abdominal trauma. Bowel perforation tends to present later with progressive peritonitis. The presence or absence of bowel sounds is initially unreliable.
- Trauma around the abdomen: low rib fractures, pelvic injury, and lumbar spine injury are all associated with intra-abdominal injury.
- Shock in the absence of external haemorrhage: this is usually due to blood loss within the chest, abdomen, pelvis, or retroperitoneal space. Early hypovolaemia is more difficult to identify and must be sought actively: if present, urgent abdominal imaging is indicated. Pulse rate is an unreliable indicator of circulatory status (see 📖 Pathophysiology of trauma and hypovolaemia, p.64).

Assessing the abdomen in trauma

- Careful inspection of the abdomen (front, flanks, and back) should be followed by thorough palpation. Percussion is of limited value and, as noted previously, bowel sounds are initially unreliable.
- Serial examination over time remains a useful tool in conscious and alert patients, particularly children where the relatively high radiation dose of CT scanning should be avoided if possible. However, in patients with more extensive trauma, and particularly those who are intubated, abdominal examination is unreliable and imaging preferred.

Imaging the abdomen in trauma

Previous invasive techniques, such as diagnostic peritoneal lavage, have been abandoned in favour of FAST scanning and CT.

FAST scanning

The FAST scan is a four-view ultrasound that seeks to detect fluid within the pericardium and the dependent zones of the peritoneal cavity in a supine trauma patient. In experienced hands it is a rapid and sensitive test for free fluid volumes in excess of 100–200 mL.

CT scanning

CT scanning with IV contrast provides the 'gold standard' imaging for intra-abdominal trauma. In selected and more stable patients oral (or nasogastric) contrast may be added to seek bowel injury. Modern scanners obtain very detailed images rapidly, and in selected cases this may be followed by radiological intervention such as embolization of a bleeding vessel.

CT or operating room?

Traditional trauma teaching emphasizes the need for some patients to go directly to the operating room for laparotomy in order to control intra-abdominal haemorrhage. In practice this is a very rare event, and is most strongly indicated in the presence of penetrating trauma and haemorrhagic shock. In blunt trauma, CT scanning is more often used, reflecting the increasing use of conservative or radiological approaches. In all cases there should be early consultation between the trauma team leader and an experienced surgeon.

Late complications

Signs of intra-abdominal trauma may develop over hours or days, particularly when there is localized upper GI perforation or subtle injury to the renal tract. For this reason patients suspected of significant intra-abdominal injury should be admitted for a period of observation and serial examinations.

Anaesthesia for the patient with intra-abdominal trauma

- Patients with significant intra-abdominal injuries are typically haemodynamically unstable and in many cases a strategy of controlled fluid resuscitation will have been adopted appropriately. This makes RSI particularly challenging—an arterial line before induction is invaluable.
- Fear of inducing profound hypotension may make the anaesthetist reluctant to anaesthetize the patient in the ED, but in many cases this will enable all necessary interventions, including CT scan—if appropriate—to be undertaken much faster; it will generally get the laparotomy underway much quicker.

- The counter view is that the patient with intra-abdominal trauma should be treated in the same way as a patient with ruptured abdominal aneurysm (see 📖 Emergency abdominal aortic aneurysm repair, p.180): in these cases, fear that the loss of abdominal tone will exacerbate bleeding means that anaesthesia is usually not induced until the patient is in the operating room and the surgeons are scrubbed.
- The priority is haemorrhage control. In the patient with multiple intra-abdominal injuries, who is cold, acidotic, and coagulopathic, it may be best to adopt a strategy of 'damage control' surgery, e.g. packing a bleeding liver, preventing ongoing intra-abdominal contamination from bowel lacerations by creating stomas and using a temporary closure (e.g. Bogota bag) enabling the patient to be transferred to the ICU for further fluid resuscitation, haemodynamic optimization, and rewarming. Once stabilization has been achieved, the patient is transferred back to the operating room for definitive surgical correction of the intra-abdominal injuries.
- The decision to undertake damage control surgery is undertaken jointly by the surgeon and the anaesthetist.

Postoperative

- The patient with major intra-abdominal injuries will need postoperative care on an ICU.
- Most of these patients will remain intubated until full resuscitation has been achieved, including rewarming, and correction of acidaemia and coagulopathy.
- Once coagulopathy has been corrected and spinal injury has been excluded, it may be appropriate to insert an epidural catheter to enable pain control before the patient is extubated.

Further reading

American College of Surgeons Committee on Trauma. *Advanced Trauma Life Support Program For Doctors: Student Course Manual* (8th edn). Chicago, IL: American College of Surgeons, 2008.

Multiple long-bone fractures

Key points
- Multiple long-bone fracture may be associated with major haemorrhage.
- Fracture immobilization will reduce blood loss and help to reduce pain.
- Consider damage control orthopaedics in the patient with multiple injuries including long-bone fractures.

Background

Musculoskeletal injuries occur in 85% of patients who sustain blunt trauma and may be life or limb threatening. Massive blood loss may complicate multiple long-bone fractures and must be addressed during the circulation phase of the primary survey. These injuries imply high-energy trauma and are often associated with spinal or other life-threatening pathology. Dramatic distal limb injuries should not distract from the management of other life-threatening injuries.

Initial management of long-bone fractures

Primary survey
- The priority remains the airway, breathing, circulation—treat the most time critical injuries first.
- Control external haemorrhage by direct pressure and consider tourniquet application in early catastrophic extremity haemorrhage.
- Blood loss from femoral shaft fracture can be significant (up to 1500 mL) and haemorrhage control can be improved by restoration of normal anatomy with traction and splinting.

Secondary survey
- Examine the limbs for fractures, deformity, wounds, or discoloration.
- Systematic assessment of vascular and neurological status of limbs.
- Reduce fractures that compromise circulation to prevent distal ischaemia by restoration of normal alignment, traction, and splintage.

Fracture immobilization
- Restores normal alignment with traction and immobilization.
- Reduces ongoing blood loss, reduces pain from movement of bone ends, and prevents further soft tissue damage.
- Requires procedural sedation and analgesia in conscious patients.
- RA may provide excellent analgesia if appropriate.

Open fractures
- Irrigate with saline and remove obvious contaminants.
- Photograph to prevent need for multiple examinations.
- Prevent dessication with saline soaked gauze and impermeable dressing.
- Early broad-spectrum IV antibiotics.
- Tetanus prophylaxis.
- Debride uncomplicated injuries within 24 h.

Complications

Vascular compromise

A cold, pale, painful, pulseless extremity indicates disruption of arterial blood flow. Partial disruption or injuries with collateral circulation may present with prolonged capillary refill and coolness. Vascular compromise requires immediate surgery and restoration of distal circulation (delay of 6h of warm ischaemia is likely to be irreversible).

Neurological compromise

Early recognition and treatment of nerve injury optimizes functional outcome. Reduction of fractures or dislocations may improve nerve compression and neurological function should be re-evaluated and documented after reduction.

Compartment syndrome

- Occurs with trauma to a site where muscle is contained within a closed fascial space (common areas include lower leg, thigh, gluteal region, forearm, foot, and hand).
- Increasing pressure in the osteofascial compartment results in tissue ischaemia and ultimately infarction. If untreated, causes neurological deficit, muscle necrosis, and may require amputation.
- Early recognition is critically important: signs include disproportionate pain, tenderness, and swelling and may be masked by RA. Neurological deficit and loss of arterial pulse are late signs. Diagnosis is confirmed if the difference between the diastolic BP and measured compartment pressure is <30mmHg.
- Urgent decompression by surgical fasciotomy is required. Late intervention increases the risk of muscle death and rhabdomyolysis.
- IV fluid to maintain good urine output may reduce the impact of myoglobulinaemia on renal function.

Fat embolism

- Pulmonary and systemic embolization of bone marrow fat globules occurs in up to 90% of traumatic bone injuries but is usually asymptomatic.
- Fat embolism syndrome (FES) develops in 1–5% of cases, typically at 24–72h post injury. Clinical manifestations involve the lungs, brain, and skin, presenting with hypoxaemia, neurological deficit, and a petechial rash.
- Diagnosis is clinical but laboratory findings may include thrombocytopenia, fat macroglobulinaemia, or sudden decrease in haemoglobin concentration.
- Treatment is supportive with early oxygen and ventilation if required.
- Mortality is up to 20% but long-term sequelae are uncommon in survivors.

Pulmonary embolism

- Pulmonary embolism is a common late cause of death in trauma patients. Patients with lower limb fractures are at high risk.
- Preventative measures include early mobilization, mechanical prophylaxis (external compression devices and inferior vena cava filters), and avoidance of dehydration.
- Pharmacological prophylaxis is essential in the polytrauma patient unless there are compelling contraindications.

Timing of surgical fixation

- The optimal timing for the fixation of long-bone fractures in polytrauma patients is controversial.
- Early fixation may reduce the incidence of fat embolism syndrome, pulmonary emboli, ARDS, and mortality. However, early fixation using intramedullary nails, particularly if reaming is included, generates fat emboli and may exacerbate secondary brain injury and the pulmonary complications of thoracic trauma.
- Timing should be individualized to each patient, with the treatment and stabilization of life-threatening injuries taking priority over limb-threatening injuries.

Intraoperative

- Fixation of multiple long-bone fractures may involve prolonged anaesthesia with risk of major haemorrhage. An arterial cannula will enable continuous BP monitoring and convenient blood sampling.
- Reaming and intramedullary nailing of femoral fractures will cause a decrease in PaO_2 (this may or may not be enough to decrease the SpO_2) as a result of microembolization of the lung. If this results in a significant reduction in SpO_2 during intramedullary nailing of the first of bilateral femoral fractures, discuss with the surgeon the option of temporary external fixation of the second side.
- If the patient has multiple injuries, including multiple long-bone fractures, discuss with the surgeon the possibility of damage control orthopaedics—temporary external fixation of fractures and a return to the operating room when stable for definitive fixation.

Postoperative

- The patient with multiple long-bone fractures is likely to need admission to the ICU postoperatively.
- Consider PCA, in combination with regular paracetamol and NSAIDs (if not contraindicated), to provide optimal pain relief.

Further reading

Dunham CM, Bosse MJ, Clancy TV, *et al.* Optimal timing of long-bone fracture stabilisation in polytrauma patients. *J Trauma* 2001; **50**:958–67.

Husebye EE, Lyberg T, Roise O. Bone marrow fat in the circulation: clinical entities and pathophysiological mechanisms. *Injury* 2006; **37S**:S8–S18.

Pelvic fractures

Key points
- Pelvic fractures are associated frequently with massive haemorrhage that may be undisclosed initially.
- The combination of massive pelvic injury and coagulopathy is frequently lethal.
- GA may be required as part of the resuscitation phase and/or to enable application of an external fixator.
- Definitive repair of major pelvic fractures requires relatively prolonged anaesthesia but is generally delayed for several days.

Background
A pelvic fracture can cause rapid exsanguination that is notoriously difficult to control. Even with optimal treatment up to 50% of open pelvic fractures will be fatal. Recent recognition that any extraneous movement in a patient with an unstable pelvic injury can lead to profound blood loss has encouraged an approach emphasizing pelvic immobilization and limited patient movement in combination with coordinated strategies to achieve haemorrhage control and aggressive replacement of blood and clotting factors.

Types of pelvic injury
Three main mechanisms of pelvic injury are recognized:
- Anteroposterior (AP) disruption, including the 'open-book' pattern.
- Lateral compression injuries, often from a side impact.
- Vertical shear, most commonly caused by a fall onto an out-stretched leg.

The Young–Burgess classification system, which has been shown to have substantial intra-observer agreement and moderate inter-observer agreement, describes seven types of fracture: three AP, three lateral compression, and one vertical shear.

The pelvis is a complete ring—major disruption usually, but not universally, occurs in at least two places. The mechanism of injury has some bearing on the most likely underlying fracture pattern, but detailed CT scanning is required to fully determine the type and extent of injury.

Assessment of the pelvis
- Do not 'spring' the pelvis to assess for instability—this test has limited diagnostic value and, in the presence of pelvic disruption, it may precipitate additional haemorrhage and clot dislodgement.
- If the mechanism of injury suggests possible pelvic trauma, apply a pelvic binder—this remains in place until definitive imaging has been obtained.
- This approach is similar to that for cervical spine management.

Pelvic binders
- These are applied to all patients with potential pelvic fracture, usually during the primary survey prehospital or in-hospital; it will stabilize any underlying injury and reduce bleeding.

- The traditional draw sheet has been replaced by a range of commercial devices that enable the pelvic ring to be closed.
- The value of these devices in different fracture patterns is debated, but the underlying injury cannot be known before imaging; apply a pelvic binder in all cases.
- Apply directly to the patient's skin to reduce the risk of pressure necrosis and do not remove until definitive imaging has been obtained (pelvic binders are specifically designed to be used during both plain radiography and CT scanning).
- A properly applied pelvic binder causes no harm and may greatly reduce the visibility of some pelvic fractures by minimizing fracture site distraction: if there is high clinical suspicion, keep the binder in place until CT scanning has been completed, even if the initial pelvic X-ray appears normal.

Treatment of pelvic fractures

The treatment of pelvic fractures is increasingly multidisciplinary, requiring close cooperation between specialist pelvic surgeons, interventional radiologists, intensivists, and anaesthetists. The main options are:

- External fixation—this is usually undertaken in the operating room, but in exceptional cases may occur in the emergency department resuscitation room.
- Internal fixation—this is rarely applied in the initial stages because of the risk of worsening profound and potentially uncontrollable haemorrhage. However, it is appropriate for some fracture types, and may be combined with internal packing. Selective radiological embolization is increasingly used.
- Conservative—if a pelvic binder is effective then it may be most appropriate to manage the patient with minimal handling on an intensive care unit, with delayed intervention at a later stage or if the patient deteriorates.

In practice a combination of these is often used. In all cases it is essential to pay close attention to the replacement of blood, clotting factors and platelets, along with the correction of acidosis and hypothermia. The combination of massive pelvic injury and coagulopathy is frequently lethal.

Associated injuries

Pelvic injuries are often associated with disruption to the lower GI and urinary tracts: urethral, bladder, and rectal injuries are particularly common and should be actively sought. Faecal and/or urinary diversion may be required at an early stage. Open pelvic injuries are particularly problematic with a very high risk of uncontrollable haemorrhage and infection.

Anaesthesia for patients with pelvic fractures

- In the resuscitation phase, pain control can be a problem. Once it is clear that the patient requires surgical intervention, induction of GA provides definitive pain relief.
- These patients are likely to be hypovolaemic: at induction, be prepared to support the BP with fluid (blood products) and/or vasopressors.

- Providing anaesthesia for embolization in the radiology suite is accompanied by all the challenges typical of providing anaesthesia outside the operating room (access to the patient, limited space, obtaining appropriate monitoring, temperature control, etc.).
- Definitive surgery is usually undertaken after about a week—these are long procedures and can be associated with considerable blood loss.

Further reading

Lee C, Porter K. The prehospital management of pelvic fractures. *Emerg Med J* 2007; **24**:130–3.

Fractured neck of femur

Key points

- Anaesthetists may be involved at all stages of care of fractured neck of femur (#NOF) patients.
- The American Society of Anesthesiologists (ASA) physical status of hip fracture patients is 3 in 52%, 4 in 10%, and 1 in <3%.
- The 30-day mortality is 5–10%, and 1-year mortality is 25–30%. Delays to definitive surgery can increase morbidity and mortality. The maximum waiting time between admission and surgery should be no more than 36 h.
- The three important anaesthetic considerations are analgesia, resuscitation, and optimization of pre-existing medical conditions.
- The Scottish Intercollegiate Guidelines Network (SIGN) recommends spinal anaesthesia over GA but there is not universal agreement with this recommendation.

Background

- The term 'neck of femur' includes fractures of the femoral neck, femoral head, trochanters, and the inter- and subtrochanteric regions, but excludes fractures of the femoral shaft and acetabulum.
- The surgery itself is relatively straightforward; it is the multitude of co-morbidities (largely cardiac, respiratory, and cognitive) that makes these patients complex for the anaesthetist.
- Many different anaesthetic techniques are used, including GA and RA, nerve blocks, and invasive monitoring.
- Despite many advances since the advent of the National Health Service (NHS), the outcome for many of these patients remains poor. In the series of deaths investigated by National Confidential Enquiry into Patient Outcome and Death (NCEPOD), 38% of the operations were for #NOF. The 30-day mortality is 5–10%, and 1-year mortality is 25–30%. These figures have changed little in the past 20 years.
- Approximately 90 000 patients with hip fracture are admitted to acute hospitals each year in the UK. 74 % of patients are female, with an average age of 84 years. The total cost of treatment plus rehabilitation is estimated at nearly £2 billion per year. These numbers are likely to increase over the next 50 years as the population ages.

Preoperative

▶ Delays in #NOF repair may increase morbidity and mortality and the aim is to optimize and operate. The maximum waiting time between admission and surgery should be no more than 36 h.

- Only 3% of patients do not receive operative treatment. Some of these patients may present late with a fracture that is already healing well. <1% of patients are too unwell for surgery. Surgery is the best form of analgesia and should be considered for palliation for even the most frail, unwell patients.

- The three important anaesthetic considerations for patients who have sustained a hip fracture are analgesia, resuscitation, and optimization of pre-existing medical conditions. Early analgesia and fluid management influences not only on survival but also future rehabilitation.

Analgesia

- Hip fractures are painful and analgesia will be needed. IV paracetamol is particularly useful because it lacks significant side effects.
- Some patients may be on regular NSAIDs before the fracture but these are rarely used acutely because of potential side effects.
- Opioids are prescribed often, but be careful in older patients because side effects such as delirium are common.
- A fascia iliaca block reduces the need for parenteral analgesia.
- Although there is some evidence that epidurals may reduce cardiac complications, they are not used routinely in the UK.

Resuscitation

- Start resuscitation immediately. All acute hospitals should have a protocol for resuscitating patients with hip fractures.
- Long-term dehydration is common in older people because of reduced fluid intake and use of diuretics. Periods of immobility or starvation before admission and bleeding from the fracture site exacerbate volume depletion. Signs of mild or moderate dehydration can be difficult to recognize clinically. Patients with chronic cardiac and/or renal failure, and vascular disease, are particularly vulnerable to the effects of hypoperfusion, which can cause organ failure. Hypovolaemia must be corrected.
- Fluid overload can be equally harmful to tissue oxygenation. Pulmonary oedema can occur with few clinical warning signs and cardiac arrest can be the first mode of presentation.
- Objective assessment of fluid status, such as non-invasive cardiac output measurement, may be helpful to guide fluid resuscitation in this population. Goal-directed fluid resuscitation is beneficial.
- Measure the haemoglobin concentration preoperatively, intraoperatively, and postoperatively. The admission haemoglobin concentration is likely to be an overestimate. Extracapsular and subtrochanteric fractures tend to bleed more than intracapsular fractures. Bleeding from extracapsular fractures may continue between the time of admission and surgery.

Medical optimization

- Most hip fracture patients have significant co-morbidities and will therefore need some degree of optimization before surgery. The reason for their fall will also need investigation. Approximately 52% of all hip fracture patients are ASA physical status 3, 10% are ASA 4, and <3% are ASA 1.
- Hip fracture patients should be prioritized particularly when other investigations are required before surgery. Close cooperation between specialities will minimize delays.

Box 3.2 lists those conditions that may delay surgery, although some of these are amenable to prompt treatment.

Box 3.2 **Acceptable reasons for delaying hip fracture surgery**

- Anaemia (haemoglobin <9.0 g dL^{-1}).
- Dehydration or acute uraemia.
- Severe electrolyte imbalance (sodium <120 or >150 mmol L^{-1}, potassium <2.8 or >6.0 mmol L^{-1}).
- Uncontrolled diabetes.
- Uncontrolled heart failure.
- Correctable cardiac arrhythmia.

Specific issues include:

Electrolyte disturbances
Electrolyte abnormalities are common; however, almost all that are serious enough to delay surgery can be corrected within 36 h.

The heart murmur
- An asymptomatic cardiac murmur may indicate significant cardiac disease and should be investigated preoperatively by echocardiography. ~20% of hip fracture patients have a heart murmur and 1/3 of these may have undiagnosed aortic stenosis. The investigation should not delay the planned surgery.
- Moderate or severe cardiac disease may alter the surgical management towards a less invasive procedure.
- The choice of anaesthetic technique for patients with known aortic stenosis should be left to the individual consultant. GA may be preferable if the aortic valve gradient is high. Invasive arterial monitoring may be helpful whichever anaesthetic technique is used.

Antiplatelet drugs
- Aspirin and clopidogrel are irreversible inhibitors of platelet activity and there will be an ↑ bleeding tendency until the inhibited platelets are replaced.
- The risks associated with stopping clopidogrel and/or aspirin should be balanced against the risks of bleeding. Patients with drug-eluting coronary stents are at high risk of coronary artery thrombosis if clopidogrel is stopped within 1 year of insertion. Although continued use of aspirin increases bleeding, it may reduce mortality. In general, aspirin should be continued perioperatively. In general clopidogrel should not be stopped and surgery should not be delayed.
- For patients on clopidogrel, GA is preferred. Spinal anaesthesia is safe in patients on low-dose aspirin.

Intraoperative
The preferred anaesthetic technique is controversial but, based on available evidence, SIGN recommends spinal anaesthesia over GA. A Cochrane systematic review found marginal benefit of RA over GA; however, this review has been criticized:
- Although there was a reduction in thromboembolic complications in the spinal group, most of the studies were conducted before thromboprophylaxis was used routinely.

- There was a significant decrease in the incidence of postoperative confusion in patients undergoing RA, but there were only 120 patients in each group.
- Some of the studies comparing general with spinal anaesthesia included the use of high doses of sedating drugs such as benzodiazepines. With prolonged elimination half-lives in older people, any perceived benefit from RA over GA could have been lost.
- Older studies may not reflect modern practice.

Intrathecal opioids
Inclusion of intrathecal opioids may enable a lower dose of LA to be used, which may reduce the risk of hypotension.

Blood transfusion
- Intraoperative blood loss is higher with intramedullary nails and hip screws than with hemi-arthroplasties.
- Measure the haemoglobin concentration in the postanaesthetic care unit (PACU) using a point-of-care technique and then in the laboratory the following day.
- There is evidence that low haemoglobin is an independent risk factor for not being able to walk after surgery. The transfusion trigger in this population is probably higher than in young adults, but the evidence is limited.

Postoperative
- Rehabilitation of patients with #NOF should start as soon as possible. Maintain oxygenation, fluid status, and BP within normal limits, avoid psychotropic and sedating drugs, and control pain.
- Avoidance of postoperative dehydration may reduce the incidence of pressure sores, decrease postoperative malaise, enhance rehabilitation, enable earlier mobilization and discharge, reduce the incidence of delirium, and reduce the need for long-term institutional care.
- Remove cannulae and catheters at the earliest opportunity to minimize the risk of infection.
- Older people frequently become confused by the experience of an acute injury and hospital stay. Simple measures such as returning hearing aids and spectacles, and ensuring adequate nutrition, can reduce confusion and greatly improves the patient's experience.

Analgesia
Hemiarthroplasty and total hip replacement for hip fracture are less painful than dynamic hip screws and nails. Adequate analgesia is essential for physiotherapy. Paracetamol 2 g intravenously may be as effective as a continuous femoral nerve block or morphine postoperatively.

National Health Service Hip Fracture Anaesthesia Network
The NHS Networks Hip Fracture Anaesthesia website provides discussion and resources for all health professional involved in the care of this group of patients: see ℘ http://www.networks.nhs.uk/nhs-networks/hip-fracture-anaesthesia.

Further reading

Foss NB, Kristensen BB, Bundgaard M, et al. Fascia iliaca compartment blockade for acute pain control in hip fracture patients: a randomized, placebo controlled trial. *Anesthesiology* 2007; **106**:773–8.

Matot I, Oppenheim-Eden A, Ratrot R, et al. Preoperative cardiac events in elderly patients with hip fracture randomized to epidural or conventional analgesia. *Anesthesiology* 2003; **98**:156–63.

McBrien ME, Heyburn G, Stevenson M, et al. Previously undiagnosed aortic stenosis revealed by auscultation in the hip fracture population – echocardiographic findings, management and outcome. *Anaesthesia* 2009; **64**:863–70.

National Hip Fracture Database. *National Report 2010*. Available at: ℘ http://www.nhfd.co.uk.

NCEPOD – Elective & Emergency Surgery in the Elderly: An Age Old Problem (2010) Available at: ℘ http://www.ncepod.org.uk/2010report3/downloads/EESE_fullReport.pdf.

Parker MJ, Handoll HHG, Griffiths R. Anaesthesia for hip fracture surgery in adults. *Cochrane Database Syst Rev* 2004; **18**(4):CD000521.

Price JD, Sear JJW, Venn RRM. Perioperative fluid volume optimisation following proximal femoral fracture (Review). *Cochrane Database Syst Rev* 2004; **1**:CD003004.

Simunovic N, Devereaux PJ, Sprague S, et al. Effect of early surgery after hip fracture on mortality and complications: Systematic review and meta-analysis. *CMAJ* 2010; **182**:1609–16.

White SM, Griffiths R, Holloway J, et al. Anaesthesia for proximal femoral fracture in the UK: first report from the NHS Hip Fracture Anaesthesia Network. *Anaesthesia* 2010; **65**:243–8.

Traumatic brain injury

Key points
- The main objective of treatment is prevention of secondary injury.
- Thorough assessment and treatment of airway, breathing, and circulation should optimize cerebral blood flow and oxygenation.

Background
Head injury is a significant cause of death, disability and cost to society with over 1 million hospital presentations per year in the UK. Not all neurological damage occurs at the moment of primary injury but develops over subsequent minutes, hours, and days. Prevention of this 'secondary' brain injury is the principal focus of management and the focus of standard 'Airway, Breathing, Circulation' treatment guidelines described in the ATLS® and European Trauma Courses.

Classification of severity of traumatic brain injury—the Glasgow Coma Scale
Traumatic brain injury (TBI) ranges from trivial to unsurvivable and a well-established classification is based on the Glasgow Coma Scale (GCS) score (Table 3.2).
- Minor: GCS 13–15.
- Moderate: GCS 9–12.
- Severe: GCS 8 or less.

Morphological classification of head injuries
Skull fractures
- Linear or stellate, open or closed, cranial vault or skull base.
- Presence of a skull fracture significantly increases the risk of intracranial injury.
- Clinical signs of basal skull fractures include periorbital or retro-auricular (Battle's sign) ecchymosis, cerebrospinal fluid (CSF) leak from nose or ears, and VIIth or VIIIth cranial nerve palsy.

Diffuse brain injury
- Ranges from mild concussion to severe hypoxic ischaemic brain injury with poor outcome.
- CT scan appearances vary from normal to diffuse cerebral oedema with loss of grey–white matter differentiation or multiple punctate haemorrhages.

Extradural haematoma
- Haemorrhage between the inner table of the skull and the adherent dura produces the CT appearance of biconvex haematoma.
- Usually arterial in origin and often located in the temporal or temporo-parietal region due to tears in the middle meningeal artery.
- Classically there is loss of consciousness, followed by a lucid interval and then neurological deterioration.
- Urgent neurosurgical intervention is required to evacuate the haematoma and prevent death.

Table 3.2 Glasgow Coma Scale score

	Response	Score
Best motor response	Obeys commands	6
	Localizes pain	5
	Normal flexion withdrawal (stimulus to supraorbital notch)	4
	Abnormal flexion to pain	3
	Extension to pain	2
	Nothing	1
Best verbal response	Orientated	5
	Confused	4
	Inappropriate words	3
	Inarticulate sounds	2
	Nothing	1
Eye opening	Eyes open	4
	Eyes open to speech	3
	Eyes open to pain	2
	No eye opening	1

Reprinted from Teasdale G, Jennett B. Assessment of coma and impaired consciousness. A practical scale. *Lancet* 1974: **304**(7872), 81–4, with permission from Elsevier.

Subdural haematoma
- Shearing of surface or bridging veins of the cerebral cortex causes haematoma over the surface of the cerebral hemisphere.
- Can be acute or chronic and often require urgent neurosurgical evacuation.

Contusions and intracerebral haematoma
- Commonly occur in the frontal and temporal lobes following trauma.
- May evolve to form intracerebral haematoma with mass effect requiring neurosurgical intervention.

Subarachnoid bleed
- Common in severe head injury and associated with poor prognosis.

Management of traumatic brain injury
Meticulous management of airway, breathing, and circulation provides the optimal immediate care for the brain following traumatic injury.

Airway
- 15 L min^{-1} oxygen via a non-rebreathing mask.
- Basic airway manoeuvres/adjuncts and suction as required.
- Low threshold for cervical spine immobilization.
- RSI as indicated by the following criteria:

Criteria for immediate intubation and ventilation
- GCS <9.
- Loss of protective laryngeal reflexes.
- Ventilatory insufficiency (PaO_2 <13 kPa (100 mmHg) on oxygen, $PaCO_2$ >6.0 kPa (45 mmHg)).
- Spontaneous hyperventilation causing $PaCO_2$ <4.0 kPa (30 mmHg).
- Respiratory arrhythmia.
- To enable CT scanning.

Criteria for intubation prior to interhospital transfer
- Significantly deteriorating conscious level (≥1 point on motor score), even if not in coma.
- Unstable fractures of the facial skeleton.
- Copious bleeding into mouth (e.g. skull base fracture).
- Seizures.

Management of intubation in the head-injured patient
- Requires a RSI with cricoid pressure and manual in-line stabilization of the head and neck (remove cervical collar, blocks, and tapes).
- Give thiopental 3–5 mg kg^{-1} or propofol 1–3 mg kg^{-1} with suxamethonium 1–2 mg kg^{-1} and fentanyl 2–5 micrograms kg^{-1} or alfentanil 15–30 micrograms kg^{-1}.
- Ventilate to a $PaCO_2$ of 4.5–5.0 kPa (34–38 mmHg)—hyperventilation can cause myocardial depression and cerebral vasoconstriction and ischaemia.
- Maintain oxygenation (SaO_2 >95%).
- Secure the tracheal tube with adhesive tape or loosely tied tape to avoid compromising venous return from the brain.
- Maintain sedation with a propofol infusion (1–3 mg kg^{-1} h^{-1}).
- Insert an orogastric tube—nasogastric tubes are contraindicated until a fractured base of skull has been excluded.
- Restore normovolaemia (0.9% saline) and give vasopressors to maintain a mean arterial BP of 90 mmHg.

Circulation
- Maintain or restore normovolaemia with 0.9% saline or blood as required to maintain Hb ≥10 g dL^{-1} (avoid hypotonic fluids).
- Maintain MAP ≥90 mmHg with infusion of fluids or vasopressors.
- Shock is almost never due to head injury and other causes must be identified.

Disability
- Serial assessment of GCS noting trends is vital.
- Record lateralizing signs and pupillary response.
- Prompt CT imaging, as indicated by the following criteria, unless physiological instability precludes safe transfer.

Criteria for CT scan of the head within 1 hour:
- GCS <13 on initial assessment in ED.
- GCS <15 at 2 h after the injury.
- Suspected open or depressed skull fracture.
- Any sign of base of skull fracture.
- Post-traumatic seizure.

- Focal neurological deficit.
- >1 episode of vomiting.
- Amnesia for events >30 min before impact.

Risk factors requiring CT scan of the head within 8 h of an injury causing loss of consciousness or amnesia include age ≥65 years, coagulopathy, or dangerous mechanism of injury.

Minimizing delay to neurosurgical assessment for evacuation of intracranial haematomas is critical to good outcome. Even in cases where no immediate intervention is required, morbidity and mortality are reduced when patients are managed in a neurosurgical centre.

Criteria for discussing patient's care with neurosurgeon
- Persisting coma (GCS <8).
- >4 h of unexplained confusion.
- Deterioration in GCS.
- Progressive focal neurological signs.
- Seizure without full recovery.
- Definite or suspected penetrating injury.

Cerebral physiology in traumatic brain injury

The maintenance of adequate cerebral blood flow and oxygenation is central to the management of TBI. Several factors determine whether this is achieved:

Munro Kelly Doctrine
- The rigid, non-expansile skull keeps the total volume of the intracranial contents constant.
- Arterial and venous blood, brain tissue, and CSF form the contents under normal conditions.
- The pressure effect of a space-occupying haematoma is initially compensated for by displacement of venous blood and CSF.
- Once the limit of this displacement is reached, the intracranial pressure (ICP) rises rapidly.

Cerebral blood flow
- Adult cerebral blood flow (CBF) is approximately 50 mL per 100 g of brain tissue per minute and in the healthy adult brain CBF is autoregulated at this value across a range of MAPs from 50–150 mmHg.
- Cerebral vasculature constricts and dilates in response to changes in $PaCO_2$ and PaO_2. Hypercapnia-induced cerebral vasodilation increases ICP.
- Autoregulation may be lost in the injured brain.

Cerebral perfusion pressure
- Cerebral perfusion pressure (CPP) = [MAP—Venous pressure (usually zero)]—ICP
- Adequate blood flow to the brain can therefore be achieved by increasing MAP or reducing ICP.

Initial treatment of traumatic brain injury on the critical care unit

Critical care with ICP monitoring and neuroprotective measures:
- 10–15° head up; avoid venous obstruction.
- CPP of 50–70 mmHg.
- PaO_2 >13 kPa and $PaCO_2$ 4.5–5 kPa.
- Temperature ≤37°C.
- Adequate sedation, analgesia, and neuromuscular blockade.
- Phenytoin 15 mg kg^{-1} if seizures.

If ICP >20 mmHg or CPP <50 mmHg then exclude neurosurgical lesion with repeat CT. If no surgical lesion consider:
- Fluid and/or vasopressor or inotrope to increase MAP.
- 20% mannitol (0.25 g kg^{-1}) until plasma osmolarity 320 mosm L^{-1}.
- Exclude seizure on electroencephalogram (EEG); institute antiepileptic therapy if required.
- Seek neurosurgical opinion about surgical decompression/CSF drainage.
- 5% NaCl 2 mL kg^{-1} (repeat as required if Na <150 mmol L^{-1}).
- Temporary mild hyperventilation to $PaCO_2$ 4.0 kPa may help reduce elevated ICP but should not be instituted until 24 h after injury.
- High-dose barbiturate may control elevated ICP refractory to maximal therapy.
- See 📖 Evacuation of traumatic intracranial haematoma, p.218, for detailed guidance on intraoperative and postoperative treatment.

Further reading

American College of Surgeons Committee on Trauma. *Advanced Trauma Life Support*® *for Doctors*, 8th *Edition*. Chicago, IL: ACS, 2008.

Brain Trauma Foundation. *Guidelines for the management of severe traumatic brain injury* (3rd edn). *J Neurotrauma* 2007; **24**, Suppl 1, S1–S106.

National Institute for Health and Clinical Excellence. *Clinical Guideline 56 Head injury: NICE guideline*. London: NICE, 2007.

Spinal injury

Key points
- Spinal injury occurs in 2–6% of blunt trauma cases and more than half involve the cervical spine.
- An unstable spinal injury is assumed in all patients with significant blunt trauma, and particularly those with head injury, and the patient's spine is initially immobilized to prevent any deterioration.
- Injury at multiple spinal levels is common: the whole spine is imaged whenever a spinal injury is identified.
- Following multitrauma, a CT of the head, cervical spine, chest, abdomen, and pelvis is normally obtained. This 'whole body' CT will provide good views of the whole spine and, if no spinal injury is detected, will normally allow spinal immobilization to be discontinued.
- A high spinal cord injury will cause bradycardia, hypotension, and profound neurological deficit but this is easy to overlook in an unconscious trauma patient with hypotension resistant to fluid resuscitation.
- In the acute setting, intubation of the patient with confirmed or potential cervical spine injury (CSI) is achieved with a RSI and manual in-line stabilization (MILS). Patients presenting later for surgical stabilization of their cervical spine may be intubated awake using a fibreoptic intubating bronchoscope.

Background
Spinal injury is relatively rare, even in multisystem trauma, but where present can have profound implications for future recovery and quality of life. Previous policies of strict and prolonged immobilization are being re-evaluated because it is now recognized that both vertebral and spinal cord injuries are most likely to occur at the time of the initial trauma; further small movements are unlikely to cause any additional harm.

How common is spinal injury?
- Spinal injury occurs in 2–6% of blunt trauma cases. The incidence in the USA is 25–50 per million people, with 10 000 new cases per year.
- More than half of these involve the cervical spine. Persons older than 65 years are at a significantly higher risk of CSI than younger patients.
- The most common causes are:
  - Motor vehicle collision (36–48%).
  - Interpersonal violence (5–29%).
  - Falls (17–21%).
  - Sports injuries (7–16%).
- The majority of CSIs (70% of cases) are fractures without associated spinal cord injury. Data from a survey of trauma centres showed:
  - 4.3% incidence of all types of CSI.
  - 3.0% incidence of CSI without spinal cord injury.
  - 0.7% incidence of spinal cord injury without fracture.
  - Delayed diagnosis of CSI in only 0.01%.

Spinal immobilization
- Assume an unstable spinal injury in all patients with significant blunt trauma, and particularly those with head injury, and immobilize the patient's spine to prevent any deterioration.
- Patients with penetrating trauma to the neck do not require immobilization in the absence of neurological deficit, and even those with neurological deficit should be immobilized cautiously because of the risk of airway compromise.
- Before immobilization, place the patient's spine in a neutral position, which may require elevation of the shoulders in children under 1 year or elevation of the head in adults, particularly those with obesity or muscular shoulders. There is a strong tendency to extend the neck when an adult patient lies on a flat surface in a semi-rigid collar.
- Prolonged immobilization can cause pressure area necrosis (which is exacerbated by spinal cord injury), respiratory compromise and raised jugular venous pressure, which will be harmful in head injury. Thus, hard spinal boards (extrication boards) have been replaced by vacuum and pressure relieving mattresses combined with policies that encourage early clearance of the spine.
- Injury at multiple spinal levels is common: image the whole spine whenever a spinal injury is identified.

Initial assessment
The initial assessment for spinal injury includes an examination of motor function, tone, and reflexes in all four limbs and an assessment of respiratory pattern, seeking evidence of diaphragmatic breathing. Assess sensation whenever possible.

The conscious trauma patient
Two clinical decision rules (the NEXUS criteria and Canadian C-Spine rule) have been extensively evaluated in conscious and cooperative trauma patients and have excellent sensitivities for detecting clinically important CSI. These have been used to formulate the recommendations of the National Institute for Health and Clinical Excellence (NICE), which are summarized as follows.

Cervical spine imaging in the conscious trauma patient (adults and children >10 years)
Request immediate three-view plain radiography of the cervical spine if any of the following are present:
- Patient cannot actively rotate neck to 45° to left and right (if safe to assess the range of movement in the neck).[*]
- Not safe to assess range of movement in the neck.[*]
- Neck pain or midline tenderness plus:
  - Age ≥65 years, or
  - Dangerous mechanism of injury.[**]
- Definitive diagnosis of CSI required urgently (e.g. before surgery).

[*]Safe assessment can be carried out if patient:
- Was involved in a simple rear-end motor vehicle collision.
- Is comfortable in a sitting position in the ED.

- Has been ambulatory at any time since injury and there is no midline cervical spine tenderness.
- Or if the patient presents with delayed onset of neck pain.

**Dangerous mechanism of injury:
- Fall from >1 m or 5 stairs.
- Axial load to head, e.g., diving; high-speed motor vehicle collision.
- Rollover motor accident.
- Ejection from a motor vehicle.
- Accident involving motorized recreational vehicles.
- Bicycle collision.

The unconscious trauma patient

It is now common to CT the cervical spine in patients with significant head injury and the whole spine in patients with multisystem trauma. This should be achieved during the patient's first trip to the CT scanner. Ensure that any radiological report specifically considers the spine, particularly in the thoracolumbar region, where injuries may be overlooked. The NICE recommendations for CT scanning of the cervical spine are summarized as follows.

Indications for CT scanning of the cervical spine in trauma patients (adults and children >10 years)
- GCS <13 on initial assessment.
- Has been intubated.
- Plain film series technically inadequate, suspicious, or definitely abnormal.
- Continued clinical suspicion of injury despite normal X-ray.
- Patient is being scanned for multiregion trauma.

A normal CT scan does not rule out ligamentous injury but still enables spinal immobilization to be discontinued unless there is clear neurological deficit or a very high suspicion of spinal cord/ligamentous injury. If the latter, try to obtain a MRI scan—this may be difficult. Where a patient's spinal immobilization is discontinued on CT findings alone, reassess spinal pain and peripheral neurology when awake.

Airway versus cervical spine
- Whilst cervical spine immobilization is important in the initial stages of trauma management, effective airway management is even more so.
- Small, controlled movements of the cervical spine are acceptable if required to establish and maintain effective oxygenation, or to achieve tracheal intubation (see 📖 The primary survey, p.68).

Neurogenic shock

Spinal cord injury may be associated with neurogenic shock, in which interruption to sympathetic outflow may lead to peripheral vasodilatation and, for some cervical and high thoracic injuries, bradycardia. The combination of bradycardia, hypotension, and profound neurological deficit is relatively easy to spot, but neurogenic causes are easy to overlook in an unconscious trauma patient with hypotension resistant to fluid resuscitation. Whilst hypovolaemia is a much more common cause of shock in trauma, and may also coexist with neurogenic shock, it is important to bear this possibility in mind, particularly when other causes have been excluded.

Septic shock

Key points
- Septic shock comprises fluid-resistant cardiovascular abnormaliti and organ dysfunction caused by infection.
- 'Early' (~first 6h) use of effective antibiotics and goal-directed resuscitation can prevent organ failure.
- Established organ failure is not improved by supranormal physiological targets, which could be harmful.
- Provide emergency tracheal intubation for a vulnerable airway an respiratory failure.
- Liaise closely with the ICU team.
- Plan urgent anaesthesia for imaging and surgical or radiological 'source control' of infection around physiological stabilization.
- Optimize and maintain the patient's physiology while responding acute exacerbations caused by interventions.
- Interventions should be the minimum essential to avert otherwise inevitable morbidity or death—mortality is high.

Background
Surgical/radiological removal of infection or emergency surgery in a pa with an unrelated cause of sepsis (e.g. pneumonia) is relatively com and carries a high mortality, especially in the elderly. Guidance for treatment of sepsis should be followed before, during, and after sur rather than waiting until transfer to an ICU.

Preoperative
- Arrange timing of procedures with operating room and radiology departments.
- Liaise with ICU about admission, optimization, current state, drugs equipment required, and the best time for transfer to and from the operating room.
- Ensure the appropriate antibiotics have been given—discuss with a microbiologist if necessary.
- Carefully manage hypovolaemia and acute electrolyte abnormalities.
- Informed consent may be impossible. Follow appropriate processes.
- If you are unfamiliar or overwhelmed with equipment (e.g. monitors, pumps, ventilators) when transferring, get senior help.
- Check all recent investigations and that blood products are available.
- Treat coagulopathy and thrombocytopenia before and during the procedu
- Continuous, reliable invasive cardiovascular monitoring is essential.
- An arterial line gives effective heart rate, BP, pulse pressure variation and contour-derived cardiac output and acute responses to fluid, leg raise and positive end-expiratory pressure (PEEP) challenges, as well inotropes and vasopressors.
- A central venous (CV) catheter shows CV pressure and allows reliabl inotrope, vasopressor and fluid administration. A well-placed SVC line in adults (inferior vena cava (IVC) in children) allows 'early' goal-directed therapy targeted to the O_2 saturation of CV blood ($ScvO_2$).

See 📖 Cervical spine fractures, p.238 for detailed guidance on anaesthesia for patients with cervical spine injury.

Further reading

Benger J, Blackham J. Why do we put cervical collars on conscious trauma patients? *Scand J Trauma Resusc Emerg Med* 2009; **17**:44.

Blackham J, Benger J. "Clearing" the cervical spine in conscious trauma patients. *Trauma* 2009; **11**:93–109.

Blackham J, Benger J. "Clearing" the cervical spine in the unconscious trauma patient. *Trauma* 2011; **13**:65–79.

Grossman MD, Reilly PM, Gillett T, et al. National survey of the incidence of cervical spine injury and approach to cervical spine clearance in U.S. trauma centers. *J Trauma* 1999; **47**(4):684–90.

McDonald JW, Sadowsky C. Spinal-cord injury. *Lancet* 2002; **359**(9304):417–25.

National Institute for Health and Clinical Excellence. *Clinical guideline 56: triage, assessment, investigation and early management of head injury in infants, children and adults.* London; NICE, 2007. Available at: 🔗 http://guidance.nice.org.uk/CG56.

Chapter 4

Anaesthesia for the Critically Ill Patient

- Cardiac output monitoring is valuable because simply targeting arterial pressure can result in undesirable vasoconstriction and hypovolaemia.
- Oesophageal Doppler-derived flow time is a potential fluid therapy guide. Transoesophageal echocardiogram-guided therapy in this dynamic setting is a rare skill.
- Point-of-care pH, PaO_2, $PaCO_2$, lactate, glucose, Hb, and Ca^{2+} as well as bicarbonate/base excess calculations are essential guides.
- Do not fluid challenge for oliguria alone. Urine output is an unreliable marker of successful resuscitation. Unnecessary fluid causes pulmonary, wound and generalized oedema increasing tissue fragility.
- In patients with severe respiratory failure, prepare for acute severe hypoxaemia and hypercarbia after induction and muscle relaxation. Spontaneous breathing, CPAP, and assisted ventilation often provide better oxygenation and minute ventilation than full positive pressure ventilation.
- A checked, preset ICU ventilator may be life-saving. Most provide better ventilation and PEEP than operating room machines. Recruitment manoeuvres and ↑ PEEP can increase PaO_2 but decrease BP and cardiac output. Support the cardiovascular system to match perfusion to recruited ventilation. Set sufficient minute ventilation to maintain acceptable pH. Relative under ventilation with an acute decrease in pH can cause cardiovascular instability. Gradual hypercarbia may not be harmful and possibly beneficial. If possible, set tidal volumes <6 mL kg^{-1} (expected weight derived from height and sex) and a plateau pressure <30 cmH$_2$O. With lung inflammation, higher values increase the risk of developing acute lung injury (ALI) or acute respiratory distress syndrome (ARDS), and increase mortality. An FiO_2 >0.8 causes atelectasis that is difficult to treat, even with recruitment manoeuvres, and recurs despite PEEP. Ventilatory requirements may delay postoperative extubation.

Intraoperative

- RSI with cricoid pressure is often indicated but be careful with rate and dose of induction drug. Anticipate a decrease in BP and reduced response to fluid and vasoconstrictors. Test bolus vasoconstrictor response pre-induction. Etomidate may be associated with ↑ mortality (adrenal suppression); therefore, consider using ketamine.
- Maintenance with a volatile anaesthetic is as appropriate as total intravenous anaesthesia (TIVA) but if transferring, TIVA/sedation may already be in use and could conveniently continue.
- Opioid-dominant balanced anaesthesia may be more cardiovascularly stable. Remifentanil avoids impaired organ-dependent metabolism.
- Monitor neuromuscular blocker action (altered kinetics). Cisatracurium and atracurium avoid impaired organ-dependent metabolism.
- Take time and seek assistance to set ventilator for optimal lung mechanics, PaO_2, $PaCO_2$, and lung protection. Physiology is altered (sometimes favourably) by thoraco/abdominal incisions and drainage e.g. nasogastric.
- Monitor blood glucose and adjust insulin infusions regularly. Patients are typically hyperglycaemic but severe shock, liver, and adrenal failure

cause hypoglycaemia. Reasonable targets are >4.0 mmol L^{-1} (~75 mg dL^{-1}) and <10 mmol L^{-1} (180 mg dL^{-1}) but carefully avoid hypoglycaemia.

- Monitor ABGs and other relevant problems (e.g. disseminated intravascular coagulopathy (DIC)) at appropriate intervals. Lactate clearance is an indicator of successful resuscitation.
- In the 'early phase', manage fluid and Hb concentration according to goal-directed guidelines. With established organ failure, ↑ O$_2$ carriage by blood transfusion and inotropes may not help and may be harmful. A Hb concentration of 7–9 g dL^{-1} may be safe if there is no coronary artery insufficiency.
- Whether to use crystalloid or colloid is uncertain (see 📖 Fluid therapy, p.26). The intravascular volume achieved matters more. Colloids achieve effects more quickly because the effective volume can be given more rapidly. But they have dose limits and more side effects—coagulopathy, renal dysfunction, and anaphylaxis.

Postoperative

Return patient to ICU/HDU for further management. Consider early extubation in patients with normal lung function. Good analgesia is essential for rapid recovery. The analgesic choice will depend on local practice. The use of epidural catheters in septic patients is controversial.

Further reading

Eissa D, Carton EG, Buggy DJ. Anaesthetic management of patients with severe sepsis. *Br J Anaesth* 2010; **105**:734–43.

Jabre P, Combes X, Lapostolle F, *et al.* KETASED Collaborative Study Group. Etomidate versus ketamine for rapid sequence intubation in acutely ill patients: a multicentre randomised controlled trial. *Lancet* 2009; **374**:293–300.

Surviving Sepsis Campaign guidelines. Available at: 🔗 http://www.survivingsepsis.org.

Cardiogenic shock

Key points
- Patients with cardiogenic shock have high perioperative morbidity and mortality.
- Cardiovascular instability should be anticipated and detected early by invasive monitoring irrespective of the anaesthetic technique.
- Maintaining coronary perfusion is critically important and often requires vasoconstrictors. Intraoperative cardiac output monitoring may be useful.
- Postoperatively, patients should be cared for in a HDU/ICU.

Background
- Cardiogenic shock occurs if the cardiac pump is acutely inadequate for organ perfusion. Patients can require anaesthesia for emergency cardiac interventions in the operating room or catheter laboratory (e.g. emergency drainage of pericardial tamponade). Causes also include acute ischaemic heart disease (common); decompensated valvular disease; congenital heart disease; cardiomyopathy and vascular obstruction (e.g. acute pulmonary embolism).
- The left ventricle receives coronary blood flow during diastole. Low diastolic BP reduces flow, function and cardiac output. Unless there is pulmonary hypertension, the right ventricle is perfused throughout the cardiac cycle.
- Cardiac output is also dependent upon heart rhythm, heart rate, appropriate filling, intrinsic myocardial function, and the vascular tone of the pulmonary and systemic circulation.

Preoperative
- Safe anaesthesia requires an understanding of the cause of cardiogenic shock. Obtain a relevant history including drug therapy and previous cardiac procedures. Biventricular pacing and implanted defibrillators often imply poor ventricular function. Serial ECGs may provide evidence of (re-)current cardiac ischaemia. Rapid echocardiography can define valve disease, pericardial effusions, regional wall abnormalities, and ventricular systolic and diastolic function.
- Coronary stents require antiplatelet therapy, e.g. aspirin and a thienopyridine. Stopping these early risks stent thrombosis and perioperative myocardial infarction with a 20% mortality. These important risks must be balanced against ↑ perioperative bleeding risk.
- Congenital heart disease is challenging, especially univentricular systems and anatomy involving a morphological right ventricle that ejects into the aorta, e.g. after Mustard or hypoplastic left-heart corrections. Seek advice from specialists in congenital heart disease management, imaging and electrophysiology and critical care. If feasible, transfer the patient to a specialist centre.
- Invasive arterial BP monitoring is mandatory before induction. Early central venous access enables reliable vasopressor administration.
- Prepare all required vasoactive agents for bolus and infusion.

- Consider monitoring cardiac output. Arterial acid–base balance, lactate, SVC oxygen saturation and urine output are influenced by factors other than cardiac output. Intra-aortic balloon pumps interfere with oesophageal Doppler measurements and pulse contour analysis.
- Consider intraoperative transoesophageal echocardiography, which can monitor cardiac output and function dynamically. Beware over-interpretation of images and distraction if solo. Arrange skilled assistance.
- Liaise closely with the skilled surgeon/cardiologist. The minimal effective intervention may be prudent to aid stabilization. Their experience must facilitate expedient surgery and minimize complications. Depending on the specialty, they may also be able to assist with arrhythmia control, AV sequential pacing to a higher heart rate, and inserting an intra-aortic balloon pump.

Intraoperative

- An anaesthetic technique may be suggested by the nature of the procedure. LA/RA (± sedation) is often preferred but this is not without risk and is not proven safer than GA.
- All induction drugs reduce BP and vascular tone so give vasoconstrictors pre-emptively. Severe hypotension that reduces coronary flow and cardiac output can be very difficult to reverse. Drug circulation time is increased so be patient. No data supports the use of a specific induction drug. Large doses of opioids, e.g. fentanyl, will not provide cardiovascular stability in cardiogenic shock: massive sympathetic activity maintains perfusion and reducing this with an opioid can cause profound hypotension.
- The importance of maintaining coronary flow with vasoconstrictors should outweigh concern of a moderately ↑ afterload.
- Thoracic epidurals increase venous capacitance, decrease cardiac preload, and decrease cardiac accelerator response, which and can all cause a large decrease in BP.
- Avoid nitrous oxide: it is a cardiodepressant. Inotrope and vasoconstrictor infusions may be necessary. Experience and local preference often dictate choice. Phosphodiesterase inhibitors, e.g. milrinone or enoximone, or levosimendan (a calcium sensitizer) may incur relatively less myocardial oxygen consumption per increase in cardiac output but both can produce considerable vasodilation.

Postoperative

- Patients should be admitted to an ICU/HDU.
- Despite correction, periods of inadequate organ perfusion may still produce organ failure.
- The use of inotropes and vasoconstrictors does not preclude allowing a patient to emerge from anaesthesia. Indeed, right ventricular function often improves in spontaneously ventilating patients and vasoconstrictor requirements are less in those not receiving sedation.

Further reading

Gatzoulis MA, Webb GD, Daubeney PEF (eds). *Diagnosis and management of adult congenital heart disease* (2nd edn). Edinburgh: Churchill Livingstone, 2010.

Howard-Alpe GM, de Bono J, Hudsmith L, *et al.* Coronary artery stents and non-cardiac surgery. *Br J Anaesth* 2007; **98**:560–74.

Chronic obstructive pulmonary disease

Key points
- In a patient with chronic obstructive pulmonary disease (COPD) and limited ventilatory function, the pulmonary complications of anaesthesia, and surgery (especially thoracic, upper abdominal, aortic, head, neck, and neuro-surgery) as well as procedures >3h can cause respiratory failure.
- Current smoking, chest malignancy, infection, cough, body mass index (BMI) >27 or <20 kg m^{-2}, age and weakness increase the risk of respiratory failure.
- Pulmonary complications are more frequent after emergency surgery.
- Chronic hypercapnia predisposes respiratory failure and cor pulmonale.
- Plan postoperative treatment carefully, including safe oxygen therapy and support for expectoration.
- Lung function tests usually add little to acute risk prediction and should not alone guide management.

Background
- COPD variably combines excessive sputum, emphysema, and partially reversible airflow limitation.
- Emphysema causes airway closure in expiration and at functional residual capacity (FRC). There is gas trapping, ↓ respiratory reserve, and ↑ dead space.
- Gas trapping and hypovolaemia can decrease pulmonary artery pressure (PAP), which is often chronically elevated and can increase dead space and ventilatory demand.
- Anaesthesia and abdominothoracic pathology can decrease FRC for 7–10 days, decrease cough efficacy, and cause sputum retention, airway closure, and atelectasis.
- Patients may have ↑ perioperative CO_2 production while effective alveolar ventilation, ventilatory capacity, and mechanical advantage are impaired.
- COPD is linked to cardiovascular disease: congestive cardiac failure is a bigger risk for pulmonary complications but is hard to diagnose in these patients.
- IV fluid and cardiac support can be difficult to titrate without invasive monitoring.

Preoperative
- Liaise with the ICU team for all high-risk cases.
- Review previous anaesthetic, surgical, and medical history for respiratory complications and polycythaemia caused by chronic hypoxaemia.
- Measure $PaCO_2$ and PaO_2. In acute/chronic hypercapnia/cor pulmonale, consider close monitoring and assisted ventilation (non-invasive ventilation (NIV) if airway safe/intermittent positive pressure ventilation (IPPV)) to cover peak CO_2 production period and recovery.

Routine postoperative IPPV does not prevent pulmonary complications and may cause nosocomial pneumonia.

- Analyse ABG values to determine the normal $PaCO_2$ and PaO_2 values for the patient and target appropriate values in the perioperative period.
- Look at previous peak flow/spirometry. Even without surgery, hospital mortality with exacerbation of COPD is approximately 7.5%. A forced vital capacity exhaled in the first second (FEV_1) of <50 mL is associated with a mortality of 10% per year.
- A chest X-ray will show coexistent pathology and provide a baseline.
- Review drugs especially corticosteroid dependence. Ensure medications or substitutes are given or increased as needed.
- Ensure adequate fluid resuscitation without overload. A 'dry' fluid strategy to avoid oedema risks a fall in PAP and ↑ dead space.
- Plan secretion management. Consider tracheostomy if copious secretions and a poor cough.
- Plan postoperative nutritional support. Poor nutritional status decreases ventilatory reserve. Feed enterally with a nasogastric tube if necessary. Nasogastric tubes can increase the risk of pulmonary complications and their need should be reviewed frequently.
- Avoid GA if possible by using effective peripheral nerve blocks with or without catheters.
- Neuraxial anaesthesia may be surgically appropriate but can cause abdominothoracic muscle weakness and impair breathing and cough.
- Beware interscalene block/deep cervical block which may paralyse the diaphragm. The patient may not be able to increase respiratory rate and thoracic cage movement and therefore may fail to compensate.
- Plan on GA for patient preference, intolerance of position, or control of coughing during surgery.
- In comparison with IV opioids, postoperative epidural analgesia helps decrease $PaCO_2$ and increase PaO_2. Diaphragm efficiency improves if the abdominal wall relaxes but lung volume maintenance is not guaranteed. Consider multimodal pain control.

Intraoperative

- Try to achieve the usual lung volumes, along with control of secretions, oxygenation, and CO_2 elimination.
- An arterial line enables $PaCO_2$ measurement to assess ventilation and shows BP swings with intrathoracic pressure changes in spontaneous ventilation (SV) or IPPV. Spontaneous ventilation under GA causes active exhalation with ↑ collapse and gas trapping.
- If using IPPV, limit the tidal volume. Set a long inspiratory-expiratory (I:E) ratio to avoid gas trapping. Beware pneumothorax: the presence of bullae increase the risk of pneumothorax but may make the chest X-ray hard to interpret.
- Oxygen administration can increase $PaCO_2$ without a decrease in minute volume by decreasing hypoxic pulmonary vasoconstriction and increasing the ventilation–perfusion (V/Q) mismatch.
- Use anaesthetic/narcotic/sedative/inhalational agents that are eliminated rapidly, but beware of desflurane, which can increase airway reflexes and cause bronchoconstriction. Residual inhalational

anaesthetic equivalent to 0.1 minimum alveolar concentration (MAC) blunts the response to hypoxaemia and hypercarbia.
- Propofol suppresses airway reflexes > etomidate > thiopental. Tolerance of supraglottic airway devices is reduced in smokers with cough, and these airways can get blocked with sputum.
- Intubation can reduce dead space and enable sputum suction.
- Maintain oxygen delivery with fluid/transfusion and monitor carefully.
- Maintaining systemic BP (as a surrogate of PAP) may improve V/Q matching.
- A stable respiratory pattern without tachypnoea is required for extubation. In the presence of chronic hypercapnia, aim for an appropriately low PaO_2.
- If blood gas values or respiratory pattern preclude extubation, transfer to the ICU.

Postoperative
- Ensure good pain control to enable physiotherapy for lung expansion (exercises, positioning, and early mobilization) and secretion management.
- Use hydration, humidification, mucolytics, bronchoscopy, and tracheostomy if required. Beware surgical contraindications to NIV.
- Prescribe titrated oxygen to decrease episodic desaturation and cardiovascular stress. A SpO_2 of 88–92% may be sufficient and decrease pulmonary hypertension.
- Admit to ICU/HDU if respiratory function declines or respiratory failure occurs.
- Treat exacerbation with guidelines, antibiotics, and expert help.
- Distinguish physiological inadequacy, pulmonary complications, and surgical complications.

Further reading
Smetana G, Conde M. Pre-operative pulmonary update. *Clin Geriatr Med* 2008; **24**:607–24.

Liver failure

Key points
- Emergency surgery with liver failure has a high perioperative morbidity and mortality.
- Risks relate to severity of liver dysfunction and surgical type.
- Cardiac surgery, laparotomies, and procedures with significant blood loss carry the greatest risks.
- Haemodynamic disturbance with anaesthesia and surgery exacerbate pre-existing multisystem dysfunction.
- Pharmacodynamic and pharmacokinetic profiles of anaesthetic agents are altered.
- Perioperative challenges are cardiovascular stability, hepatorenal protection, preventing encephalopathy, minimizing blood loss and infection risk.

Background
Obesity-related hepatic disease and improved treatment of cirrhosis mean more patients with liver failure present for emergency surgery. Anaesthesia may be required to manage specific complications (e.g. variceal bleeding, transjugular intrahepatic portosystemic shunt (TIPSS)) or for coincidental emergency surgery. Caesarean section for hepatic diseases of pregnancy (haemolysis, elevated liver enzymes, low platelets (HELLP), acute fatty liver, cholestasis) often requires urgent anaesthesia.

Risk assessment
- Obstructive jaundice, acute hepatitis of any cause, and coexistent systemic compromise are associated with poor postoperative outcome.
- Portal hypertension increases bleeding risk of abdominal procedures.
- Child–Turcotte–Pugh (CTP, Table 4.1) and Modified End-Stage Liver Disease (MELD, Box 4.1) scoring systems help quantify perioperative mortality risk.

Table 4.1 Child–Turcotte–Pugh score

	1 point	2 points	3 points
Ascites	Absent	Slight-moderate	Refractory/severe
Encephalopathy	Absent	Grade I–II	Grade III–IV
Albumin (g L^{-1})	>35	28–35	<28
Bilirubin (µmol L^{-1})	<34	34–50	>50
INR	<1.7	1.7–2.3	>2.3

Class A: 5–6 points—low risk; 4% 3-month mortality.

Class B: 7–9 points—intermediate risk; 14% 3-month mortality.

Class C: 10–15 points—high risk; 51% 3-month mortality.

Box 4.1 MELD score formula

MELD score = {[0.957 × $\log_e$ (serum creatinine mg dL^{-1})] + [0.378
× $\log_e$(total serum bilirubin mg dL^{-1})] + [1.120 ×
$\log_e$(INR)] + 0.643} × 10

- MELD <10 low risk.
- MELD 10–15 intermediate risk.
- MELD >15 high risk.

Preoperative risk assessment

Establish the cause of liver failure and assess the degree of multisystem compromise.

Cardiovascular examination

- Look for related cardiovascular risks: alcoholic cardiomyopathy, pericardial effusion, and coronary artery disease.
- 30% of cirrhotics have hyperdynamic cardiovascular systems (↑ heart rate, ↑ cardiac output, ↑ blood volume, ↓ BP, warm peripheries).
- Echocardiography may show right atrial and right ventricular dilatation and right-sided diastolic dysfunction.
- Porto-pulmonary hypertension (PAP 35–45 mmHg) causes dyspnoea, chest pain, right-sided heart failure, hypoxaemia, and syncope if severe. It significantly increases mortality but may be amenable to pharmacological treatment.
- Cirrhosis can be associated with a prolonged QT interval.

Respiratory system examination

- 50% of cirrhotics have respiratory compromise.
- Ascites and pleural effusions increase intrathoracic pressure and decrease FRC.
- End-stage liver failure can cause hepato-pulmonary syndrome—intrapulmonary shunt, V/Q mismatch, and hypoxaemia refractory to increasing FiO$_2$ and pharmacological treatment.
- Smoking or rarely, α-1 antitrypsin deficiency, causes coexistent emphysema.

Porto-systemic (hepatic) encephalopathy

- Grade I—inattention; II—disorientation; III—somnolence; IV—coma.
- Impairs mental capacity and the ability to consent.
- Intracranial haemorrhage can complicate this assessment.

Haematological tests

- A variable and complex coagulopathy develops.
- Acute liver failure without cirrhosis causes a decrease in pro- and anticoagulant factors, platelets, and dysfunctional fibrinogen and platelets.
- Excessive bleeding is usually mucosal and from punctures.
- Cirrhosis and portal hypertension cause a similar pattern but with spontaneous GI bleeding (varices, gastropathy).
- Malnutrition and cholestasis cause a decrease in vitamin K-dependent factor synthesis.
- Malnutrition, bleeding, and fluid retention cause anaemia.

Renal function tests
- Renal dysfunction is common in advanced disease. Splanchnic vasodilation, abnormal renal autoregulation, and activation of the renin–angiotensin system → renal hypoperfusion → renal failure (hepatorenal syndrome).
- This can be difficult to distinguish from relative hypovolaemia and, or low cardiac output in a previously hyperdynamic patient.
- Urea is often low (↓ hepatic production).
- Chronic hyponatraemia and hypokalaemia are common (water retention, inhibition of Na/K ATPase, diuretic therapy).

Preoperative

- Discuss optimization strategies with haematologists, hepatologists, surgeons, and ICU staff.
- Preoperative drainage of ascites and pleural effusions may improve ventilation but can cause haemodynamic instability. Albumin transfusion to compensate for related extravascular fluid shifts is usual.
- Rapid correction of severe hypokalaemia may be possible via a central venous catheter and monitored in an HDU. Chronic hyponatraemia is less important.
- Haematology—preoperative correction of coagulopathy with FFP (but there is no evidence that achieving specific targets reduces complications), cryoprecipitate, desmopressin, and platelet transfusions (vitamin K is slow) may reduce blood loss and bleeding complications (e.g. during ICP monitor insertion) but complete correction is often difficult and brief. Patients receiving large blood product volumes may require haemofiltration to prevent fluid overload. Diuretics often fail to reduce or prevent volume overload.
- Consider cell salvage for abdominal procedures or predicted heavy blood loss. Cross match appropriate volumes of blood and arrange for other products to be immediately available. Warn haematology technicians that clotting function tests may be sent in quick succession. Ask for assistance if running multiple point-of-care assays, e.g. thromboelastography.
- Consider prophylactic antifibrinolytics, e.g. tranexamic acid.
- Universal precautions must be taken by all staff for patients with infectious causes of hepatic failure.
- Perioperative supplementation may be needed for patients with autoimmune hepatitis treated with long-term steroids.
- If anxiolytic premedicant is absolutely necessary, lorazepam may be the least harmful.

Intraoperative

- Have a low threshold for using invasive haemodynamic monitoring. Transoesophageal monitoring is contraindicated in the presence of varices and use with extreme caution in coagulopathy. Neurohormonal reflexes to anaesthesia and hypovolaemia are often blunt and alterations in BPs and volume that are normally acceptable may cause hepatic and renal decompensation. Basal haemodynamic values may be highly abnormal. Cardiac contractility may worsen with the surgical problem and anaesthesia. For major surgery use cardiac

output monitoring to guide combined fluid replacement and inotropic/
vasopressor support.

- LA carries least risk of instability. Amide LAs are hepatically eliminated
  and may require dose adjustment. Neuraxial blocks are typically
  contraindicated by coagulopathy and may be complicated by epidural
  varices. As with GA, haemodynamic changes associated with neuraxial
  blocks can be sufficient to cause postoperative hepatic and renal
  decompensation.
- Cautious induction of GA avoiding hypotension is more important
  than the choice of drug. Patients often have delayed gastric emptying.
  Suxamethonium can be used safely for RSI but ↓ serum pseudo-
  cholinesterase may increase the duration of action). Use atracurium/
  cisatracurium as non-depolarizing neuromuscular blockers (hepatically
  independent metabolism). Avoid vecuronium, rocuronium, and
  pancuronium (hepatobiliary excretion). Volatile agents or TIVA are
  both reasonable choices for maintenance. Isoflurane, desflurane, or
  sevoflurane are safe. Avoid enflurane and halothane.
- Fentanyl may be the opioid of choice for perioperative analgesia.
  Remifentanil can provide intraoperative analgesia with organ-
  independent metabolism. Use opioids requiring hepatic metabolism
  with care. Avoid morphine and oxycodone in cirrhosis/severe hepatic
  impairment. Doses should generally be reduced by 50%. NSAIDs
  are contraindicated (nephrotoxic; upper GI bleeding and antiplatelet
  action). Paracetamol is safe except in severe liver failure.
- Antiemetics: reduce ondansetron dose to 8mg in 24h (↓ clearance).
  The sedative effect of cyclizine is enhanced. Avoid prochlorperazine.
- Liaise with microbiologist for loading, maintenance, and intervals of
  appropriate antibiotics and antifungals.
- Check blood glucose values frequently.
- Provide careful positioning padding, and protection. Oedematous
  tissues are more prone to blistering, pressure damage, and delayed
  healing. Heavy alcohol consumption is associated with higher risk of
  pressure damage to peripheral nerves.

Postoperative

- Patients may require postoperative ICU/HDU.
- Postoperative complications include bleeding, renal failure, infection,
  hypoglycaemia, and wound dehiscence.
- Analgesia following major or abdominal procedures is challenging.
- Encephalopathy may be exacerbated by GI bleeding, electrolyte or
  metabolic disturbance, infection, diuretics, constipation, opioids,
  benzodiazepines, and hypoxaemia.

Further reading

Hemprich U, Papadakos PJ, Lachmann B. Respiratory failure and hypoxemia in the cirrhotic patient
including hepatopulmonary syndrome. *Curr Opin Anaesthesiol* 2010; **23**(2):133–8.

Renal failure

Key points

- Optimizing airway, breathing, and circulation and treating any underlying cause may prevent the progression of acute renal failure in critically ill patients requiring surgery.
- Acute kidney injury (AKI) is associated with ↑ morbidity and mortality.
- Urgently treat AKI caused by urinary tract obstruction or intra-abdominal compartment syndrome.
- Avoid nephrotoxic drugs and drugs that accumulate in renal failure.
- Consider and plan for the need for renal replacement therapy early.

Background

- Critically ill patients requiring surgery may either have developed renal failure acutely as a consequence of their current illness or may have had longer-standing chronic kidney disease complicating their current illness.
- Patients with kidney transplants or on renal replacement therapy (RRT) may need emergency surgery outside specialist centres but need not be at greater risk of complications.
- Emergency surgical problems typically causes an inadequately filled and dilated circulation. Urine should be generated first by correcting renal perfusion and not by giving diuretics even if they are normally prescribed.

Acute renal failure definitions

AKI is common in critically ill patients and is an independent marker of ↑ mortality.

- The Acute Kidney Injury Network (AKIN) criteria for AKI are: rapid time course (<48h), a rise in serum creatinine (absolute increase ≥26.4 µmol L^{-1}, or percentage increase of ≥ 50%), and a reduction in urine output, defined as <0.5 mL kg^{-1} h^{-1} for >6 h.
- The RIFLE system is increasingly used to classify AKI (Table 4.2).

ICU mortality by RIFLE criteria:
- No kidney injury: 5.5%.
- Risk group: 8.8%.
- Injury group: 11.4%.
- Failure group: 26.3%.

Causes of acute renal failure

- Prerenal—hypovolaemia (severe, haemorrhage, nephrotic syndrome), ↓ perfusion (shock, cardiac failure, severe sepsis), ACEIs.
- Intrinsic renal—acute tubular necrosis: toxic (aminoglycosides, NSAIDS, severe rhabdomyolysis), or ischaemic; glomerulonephritis or interstitial disease.
- Post-renal (obstructive)—blocked urinary catheter or stent, renal stones, tumours, strictures, enlarged prostate, intra-abdominal hypertension.

Table 4.2 RIFLE classification of renal failure

RIFLE category	Serum creatinine/estimated glomerular filtration rate (eGFR)	Urine output
R—Risk	Serum creatinine ↑ × 1.5 or GFR ↓ by >25%	<0.5 mL kg^{-1} h^{-1} for 6 h
I—Injury	Serum creatinine ↑ × 2 or GFR ↓ by >50%	<0.5 mL kg^{-1} h^{-1} for 12 h
F—Failure	Serum creatinine ↑ × 3 or GFR ↓ by 75%	<0.3 mL kg^{-1} h^{-1} for 24 h or anuria for 12 h
L—Loss	Failure for >4 weeks	
E—End stage	Renal failure for >3 months	

Renal replacement therapy

- There are several different RRT modes (e.g. intermittent haemodialysis, continuous veno-veno haemofiltration (CVVH)). The best mode is not known.
- Indications for urgent renal replacement in the critically ill patient include: fluid overload causing respiratory failure, electrolyte (especially potassium) imbalance, severe renal metabolic acidosis, severe uraemia, severe rhabdomyolysis, and removal of certain toxins/drugs.
- The patient will require a specific central venous catheter for RRT ('vascath').
- RRT usually requires anticoagulation (unless peritoneal dialysis). The use of isolated circuit anticoagulation with citrate and calcium may prevent the need to anticoagulate the patient, but using this technique requires experience. Ensure coagulation is 'normal' at the time of surgery in patients who have had RRT.

Anaesthesia for acute renal failure (RIFLE criteria 'R' and 'I')

Aim to minimize further damage to the kidney and prevent morbidity from the potential complications.

Preoperative

- Consider transfer to ICU for optimization if time allows.
- Aim to correct any fluid or electrolyte deficit before surgery.
- Check recent blood results including blood gases.
- If not already in place, consider insertion of invasive monitoring to guide fluid resuscitation and allow frequent blood sampling intraoperatively.

Intraoperative

- Certain drugs (e.g. vecuronium, rocuronium, morphine) can have a prolonged action in renal failure—use alternatives (e.g. atracurium) if you plan to wake the patient up after surgery.
- Suxamethonium can be used for RSI—avoid if possible if the patient is hyperkalaemic (K^+ >5.5 mmol L^{-1}).
- Maintain renal perfusion with fluids and inotropes/vasopressors to minimize hypoperfusion/ischaemia.
- Aim for a MAP of >70 mmHg to ensure renal perfusion (hypertensive patients may need a higher target).
- Aim to maintain an adequate urine output (if the patient usually passes urine) throughout the case (>0.5 mL kg^{-1} h^{-1}).
- Furosemide and/or mannitol (0.5 g kg^{-1} IV) can be used to induce a diuresis. There is no evidence that this prevents the progression of renal failure.
- If renal replacement is likely to be needed postoperatively insert an appropriate central venous catheter ('vascath') in the operating room (discuss with ICU).
- Analyse blood gases regularly to monitor acid–base status and electrolytes. Pay particular attention to electrolyte imbalance if blood products are being given or in conditions such as rhabdomyolysis.
- Ventilate to avoid hypercapnia and subsequent acidosis as this may exacerbate hyperkalaemia.
- Radiological contrast can worsen renal failure—discuss the risks/benefits with a radiologist.

Postoperative

- Manage on HDU/ICU if possible.
- Use local anaesthetic techniques, paracetamol, or short-acting opioids (e.g. fentanyl PCA, hydromorphone) with care for analgesia.
- Avoid all nephrotoxic drugs (especially NSAIDs and ACEIs).
- Monitor urine output closely. If urine output drops below 0.5 mL kg^{-1} h^{-1} give fluid boluses guided by CVP or non-invasive cardiac output monitoring. Consider inotropes/vasopressors.
- Consider monitoring intra-abdominal pressure if there is a risk of intra-abdominal hypertension. This can be done via the bladder catheter.
- Dosing of antibiotics such as gentamicin and vancomycin should be guided by monitoring antibiotic levels in the blood as their elimination may be significantly delayed.
- Start RRT—anticoagulation requires careful thought, balancing the risks of bleeding and the need for renal replacement.

Management of patients with established renal failure (RIFLE criteria 'F', 'L', and 'E') or kidney transplants

- Discuss management of patients with established renal failure or with kidney transplants with their renal team.
- Patients may be having haemofiltration on ICU, or long-term dialysis via a peritoneal catheter, an indwelling catheter or an arteriovenous fistula.
- In addition to the issues listed for patients with RIFLE 'R' and 'I' criteria, these patients often have multiple comorbidities (e.g. anaemia, hypertension, ischaemic heart disease, diabetes).

- Check usual and current Hb, Na, K, Ur, Cr, Ca, and pH. NB Moderate anaemia, uraemia, hyponatraemia, hyperkalaemia, hypocalcaemia, hyperphosphataemia, and acidosis may all be usual in CRF.
- Arrange appropriate blood products. Avoid transfusing chronic anaemia. This can cause ↑ BP, left ventricular failure, and fistula thrombosis. Transplanted patients may need cytomegalovirus-negative blood products.
- Reverse heparin from haemodialysis for surgery and neuraxial blocks. NB Uraemic platelet dysfunction does not seem to increase risk of neuraxial blocks but may be partly reversed with desmopressin 0.3 micrograms kg^{-1} IV over 20 min.
- Empty any peritoneal dialysis fluid to reduce intra-abdominal pressure. Arrange post-operative RRT if peritoneum compromised by pathology.
- In long-term dialysis patients, plan the need for pre- and postoperative dialysis. This may be on the ICU or in an acute dialysis unit.
- Long-term dialysis patients usually have poor veins and difficult vascular access. They may need a central venous catheter for access. This may also be difficult to insert if they have had previous central venous catheters for dialysis. Senior help (often radiological) is often needed as patients may have stenosed central veins—numerous scars over central veins insertion sites for previous dialysis access is a warning sign.
- Protect any arteriovenous fistulae extremely carefully—the arm must be padded and should not be used for arterial or venous lines or NIBP cuffs. Ensure there is no pressure on the arm during surgery.
- Careful monitoring of haemodynamic status and fluid balance may require invasive arterial and venous monitoring, or a non-invasive haemodynamic monitor.
- Dialysis patients with end-stage renal failure can be given NSAIDs and some other nephrotoxic drugs (e.g. gentamicin) with care when appropriate.
- Check for the correct adjusted dose and frequency for antibiotics, anti-emetics, etc.
- For patients with a renal transplant, some or all immunosuppressants should be continued perioperatively—discuss with a renal specialist.
- The same intraoperative and postoperative concerns apply as for acute renal failure.

Further reading

Hoste EA, Clermont G, Kersten A, et al. RIFLE criteria for acute kidney injury are associated with hospital mortality in critically ill patients: a cohort analysis. Crit Care 2006; **10**:R73.

Joannidis M, Druml W, Forni LG, et al. Prevention of acute kidney injury and protection of renal function in the intensive care unit. Expert opinion of the working group for nephrology, ESICM. Intensive Care Med 2010; **36**:392–411.

Mehta RL, Kellum JA, Shah SV, et al. Acute Kidney Injury Network: report of an initiative to improve outcomes in acute kidney injury. Crit Care 2007; **11**:R31.

Wagener G, Brentjens TE. Anesthetic concerns in patients presenting with renal failure. Anesthesiol Clin 2010; **28**:39–54.

Diabetes mellitus

Key points

- Diabetes mellitus is common and associated with complications that increase perioperative morbidity and mortality.
- Stress and surgery increase gluconeogenesis, insulin resistance, and blood glucose concentration.
- Suboptimal perioperative glucose control is associated with worse outcomes but the optimal control strategy is not known.
- Hospitals should have guidelines for the management of diabetes in the emergency perioperative period. Reasonable targets are $>4\,mmol\,L^{-1}$ and $<10\,mmol\,L^{-1}$.
- Hypoglycaemia ($<4\,mmol\,L^{-1}$) is difficult to detect during GA.
- Severe hypoglycaemia, e.g. $<2.8\,mmol\,L^{-1}$, may cause brain injury and, like hyperglycaemia, may be associated with micro-and macrovascular events.

Background

Perioperative hyper- and hypoglycaemia may be associated with infection, impaired wound healing, anastomotic leak, and exacerbation of any ischaemic injury to the brain, heart, and kidney. Proposed mechanisms include related electrolyte and fluid shifts, abnormal substrate metabolism, protein glycation, and pro-inflammatory effects of glucose. Carefully achieving near normal glucose levels may reduce tissue microvascular damage. Diabetes-associated macrovascular occlusive disease (peripheral, renal or cerebral) also requires careful maintenance of blood flow and pressure for tissue preservation and organ function.

Preoperative

- Obtain a clear history with particular reference to complications associated with diabetes mellitus (coronary, carotid, renal and peripheral vascular disease, neuropathy, retinopathy, obesity-related sleep apnoea).
- Advanced disease is associated with autonomic neuropathy (↓ corrective haemodynamic reflexes to anaesthesia and neuraxial block, ↓ gastric emptying, and ↑ aspiration risk).
- Check glucose, ketones, electrolytes, urea and creatinine for acute disturbance and kidney injury as well as chronic renal impairment.
- Correct hypovolaemia, dehydration, and electrolyte abnormalities (K^+, Mg^{2+}, PO_4^-), which are caused by hyperglycaemic osmotic diuresis. Manage ketoacidosis according to the local hospital guideline.
- If time allows, attempt to bring glucose into target range although surgical disease (e.g. surgical sepsis) can make this difficult.
- A recent glycosylated haemoglobin (HbA1c) level of 6.5–7% suggests good diabetic control over the previous 1–3 months. Higher values correlate with worse control and associated co-morbidities.
- Review drugs: stop biguanides (e.g. metformin) perioperatively. These accumulate if renal function deteriorates (e.g. after IV contrast) and are associated with lactic acidosis in these circumstances.

- Oral hypoglycaemics such as sulphonylureas (e.g. gliclazide, glipizide) or insulin sensitizers such as thiazolidinediones (e.g. pioglitazone) are short acting. Omit these unless emergency surgery is brief and the patient will return to a normal diet rapidly.
- Incretins (e.g. exenatide, liraglutide) slow gastric emptying and increase aspiration risk and postoperative nausea and should be stopped.
- Insulin preparations have various pharmacokinetics. Intermediate, long-acting, and glargine preparations may act for up to 24–36h. Rather than adjusting long-term diabetic regimens it is often easier to temporarily stop all drugs, monitor glucose regularly and start a titrated insulin infusion if blood levels breach a target (e.g. 10mmolL^{-1}).

Intraoperative

- Blood glucose monitoring can be undertaken from capillary, venous, or arterial samples. Normal arterial glucose is greater than venous and capillary values. Capillary glucose values correlate poorly with arterial values in shock and bad peripheral perfusion.
- Low target ranges (4.0–6.0mmolL^{-1}) are no longer recommended. Aim for a blood glucose >4 and <10mmolL^{-1}. This decreases the risk of inadvertent hypoglycaemia associated with targeting lower ranges and avoids significant hyperglycaemia.
- Hypoglycaemia is associated with harm and can be difficult to detect during GA. Tachycardia and sweating may not occur. Treat hypoglycaemia with bolus IV glucose (e.g. 10mL of 20% glucose) and measure the blood glucose again quickly (e.g. 15min).
- Postoperative hyperglycaemia (>11.1mmolL^{-1}) is associated with ↑ mortality in subgroups of surgical patients.
- Short procedures rarely require more intervention apart from monitoring glucose levels. Patients can usually resume a normal diet and take their usual medication rapidly following surgery.
- Longer procedures require insulin infusions if blood glucose values rise.
- Titrate insulin infusion rate hourly to blood glucose. Measure more frequently if hypoglycaemic or severely hyperglycaemic.
- Manage macrovascular disease (atherosclerosis, arteriosclerosis, calcific disease etc.) by maintaining cardiac output with fluids and inotropes and restore usual vascular tone without excessive vasoconstriction.

Postoperative

- Monitor glucose frequently until normal diet and medications are re-established.
- Diabetics are at a relatively ↑ risk of cardiac events (arrhythmias and acute coronary syndromes) that peaks 2 days after major surgery.
- Patients with poor preoperative glucose control should be referred to the local diabetes team for education, drug adjustment, and follow-up.

Further reading

Akhtar S, Brash PG, Inzucchi, SE. Scientific principles and clinical implications of perioperative glucose regulation and control. *Anesth Analg* 2010; **110**:478–97.

NHS Diabetes. *Management of adults with diabetes undergoing surgery and elective procedures: improving standards.* April 2011. Available at: ℛ http://www.diabetes.nhs.uk.

Coagulopathy

Key points

- Preoperative diagnosis of coagulopathy may enable some correction.
- Emergency surgery and rapid volume replacement can delay recognition.
- Coagulopathy may be a laboratory diagnosis or clinically apparent (unusual purpura, petechiae, puncture site bleeding, or surgically uncontrollable oozing).
- Do not allow exsanguination waiting for test results.
- Maintain tissue perfusion and oxygenation whilst managing coagulation.
- Engage cooperation from surgeon, interventional radiologist, haematologist, and lab technician. Organize blood component delivery.
- Stable thrombus needs sufficient thrombin formation, fibrinogen, platelets, and factor XIII but replacement protocols do not reverse all coagulopathies reliably.

Background

See also 📖 Transfusion, p.20.

Acute problems and related coagulopathies (Table 4.3)

- Differentiating DIC from loss or dilution of coagulation components is difficult during trauma and surgery. Both cause progressive ↓ fibrinogen, ↓ platelets, ↑ prothrombin time (PT), ↑ activated partial thromboplastin time (APTT), and ↑ fibrin degradation products (FDP)/D-dimer.
- If no cause is obvious consider undiagnosed von Willebrand's disease (1% prevalence but only 0.1% clinically significant) or acquired coagulation inhibitors (autoimmune, lymphoma, myeloma, peripartum).

Chronic problems and related coagulopathies

- Liver disease (see 📖 Liver failure, p.120) causes reduced factor synthesis and platelet and fibrinogen dysfunction. Terlipressin, vasopressin, and a transjugular intrahepatic portosystemic shunt (TIPSS) can reduce portal hypertension and related bleeding.
- Chronic renal failure causes platelet dysfunction—improve urgently with desmopressin 0.3 micrograms kg^{-1} IV over 20 min and platelet transfusion or less urgently by dialysis. Treatment of severe anaemia aids clotting.
- Reverse warfarin with prothrombin complex concentrate, heparin with protamine, low-molecular-weight heparin with protamine (with difficulty and haematology advice), aspirin with platelets. The effects of clopidogrel are reversed partially with platelets and plasma exchange (takes time). Direct thrombin and factor Xa inhibitors cannot easily be reversed.

Table 4.3 Acute problems and related coagulopathies

Clinical problem	Associated coagulopathy
Hypothermia	↓ coagulation and platelet function
Massive haemorrhage (150 mL min^{-1}; 50% blood volume loss in <3 h or 100% <24 h)	DIC ± fibrinolysis
Massive volume replacement (5 red cell units <1 h or 10 units <6 h)	Dilutional coagulopathy
Trauma (shock; soft tissue injury; crush; fat embolism, burns)	DIC
Obstetric complications (placental abruption, amniotic fluid embolus, retained or infected products of conception)	DIC
Tissue exposure (prostatic, uterine, pulmonary, brain and some malignant tissues)	Local fibrinolysis
Cardiopulmonary bypass	Platelet dysfunction, dilutional coagulopathy, DIC
Transfusion and anaphylactic reactions	DIC
Hypocalcaemia (<0.9 mM Ca^{2+})	Ca^{2+} is a coagulation co-factor
Large volumes of colloid	↓ function of fibrinogen and von Willebrand factor

Preoperative

- The absence of history (or family history) of excessive bleeding with minor trauma, surgery, tooth extraction, or childbirth make congenital problems unlikely.
- Manage pre-existing medical conditions (e.g. von Willebrand's disease; haemophilia) in conjunction with a haematologist.
- Order five essential tests; haemoglobin concentration; PT; APTT; fibrinogen; and platelet count.
- Thromboelastography gives additional useful information on clot stability and fibrinolysis but may take up to 1 h to complete.
- Bleeding time is rarely measured. Clotting around punctures or wounds may give similar information.
- Other tests (platelet function analysis, factor assays, mixing studies) take time and may not be relevant or available.
- If blood products are justifiable, forewarn the haematology department of likely volumes and urgency. FFP and cryoprecipitate take up to 30 min to thaw. Platelets may require urgent transport from another site.
- Consider radiological intervention to stop bleeding from relevant sites.
- Aim for clinically acceptable clotting parameters if time allows. Use early empirical FFP (15 mL kg^{-1}) if bleeding is active and expected to be massive.
- Assemble cell salvage systems if appropriate.

Goals in massive haemorrhage with dilutional coagulopathy
See Table 4.4.

Table 4.4 Goals in massive haemorrhage with dilutional coagulopathy

Goal	Treatment
Fibrinogen >1 g L^{-1} (Fibrinogen ↓ faster than platelet count; <0.5 g L^{-1} is associated with microvascular bleeding)	10 units of cryoprecipitate ↑ fibrinogen >0.5 g L^{-1} in a 70 kg person
Platelet count >100 × 10^9 L^{-1} in multiple trauma or CNS injury; >75 × 10^9 L^{-1} if active bleeding (usually <50 × 10^9 L^{-1} after 2 blood volume replacements)	1 platelet pool should ↑ count by > 20 × 10^9 L^{-1} in a 70 kg person if no ongoing consumption or dilution.
INR and APPT ratio <1.5	15–30 mL kg^{-1} of FFP is recommended in actively bleeding coagulopathic patients
Haemoglobin >8 g dL^{-1} Give red cells if blood volume loss >40%; persistent or recurrent ↓ BP or ↑ heart rate without known Hb; or coronary ischaemia. A reduced haematocrit will reduce platelet margination and thrombus formation	Use un-crossmatched O –ve blood in an emergency. ABO matching is preferable and possible in 20 min; full crossmatching takes 40 min.
Evidence of fibrinolysis (laboratory or clinical or empirical in multitrauma) Monitoring needs thromboelastography or other laboratory tests	Tranexamic acid 1 g IV over 10 min then 1 g IVI over 8 h in trauma.
Factor XIII >60% (requires lab assay)	Contained in cryoprecipitate and FFP

Intraoperative
- Use rapid infusion devices, warmers, radiant heaters, warm operating rooms.
- Get help with fast but safe transfusion product identification.
- In multitrauma (see ▢ The Injured Patient, p.63), minimize fluid to avoid haemodilution and permit hypotension judiciously during vessel repair/ligation, packing and external fixation of fractures.
- If massive transfusion is needed, military and urban experience suggests early plasma, red cell, and platelet transfusion in ratios approaching 1:1:1 and higher fibrinogen values avoid early coagulopathy associated with death. Such strategies are also associated with complications such as transfusion-related acute lung injury (TRALI).

- Recombinant VIIa (90 mg kg^{-1}) may have a place especially in blunt trauma but platelets >30 ×10^9 L^{-1} and fibrinogen >1 g L^{-1} are also needed. Discuss with haematologist.

Postoperative

- If bleeding is persistent, rule out surgically remediable causes quickly.
- Keep warm non-invasively. Consider invasive rewarming if temperature <35°C.
- DIC may slowly resolve if the provoking source has been removed.
- Monitor clinically and check clotting function 4-hourly until acceptable.

Further reading

Association of Anaesthetists of Great Britain and Ireland, Thomas D, Wee M, et al. Blood transfusion and the anaesthetist: management of massive haemorrhage. *Anaesthesia* 2010; **65**:1153–61.

The agitated patient undergoing procedures

Key points
- Agitation is often multifactorial. Agitated patients typically present for investigations and procedures from emergency and critical care areas and are frequently elderly. They present risks to themselves and others.
- Treat reversible causes perioperatively whenever possible.
- Gather skilled and sufficient staff to assist sedation and anaesthesia. Inserting/maintaining IV access and administering all treatment is difficult.
- Perioperative sedation and continuous, close monitoring in an appropriate area may be necessary. Agitation scales/scores may be useful to guide sedation goals.
- When sedating and anaesthetizing agitated patients, their mental capacity and best interests must be taken into account.

Background
Causes of agitation in critical illness (Table 4.5)

Table 4.5 Causes of agitation in critical illness

Drugs	Illicit drugs, opioids (remember patches), benzodiazepines, anticholinergics, antihistamines, corticosteroids
	Withdrawal: alcohol, prescribed or illicit drugs, nicotine or sedatives especially benzodiazepines
	Accidental or deliberate overdose
Physiological disturbance	Hypotension and shock
	Hypoxia (lung injury, pulmonary embolus, exacerbation of or end-stage lung disease)
	Organ failure (renal failure, hepatic encephalopathy)
Intracranial pathology	Head injury, infection, malignancy, intracerebral haemorrhage, cerebral oedema and ↑ ICP, post-ictal states
Acute infection	Septic encephalopathy or CNS infection
Biochemical/ metabolic	Electrolyte disturbances, hypo/hyperglycaemia, hypercalcaemia, hyper/hypothyroidism
Environmental	Pain, positioning, pruritus, immobilization and immobility, wounds, catheters, drains, nasogastric tubes, IV lines, tracheal tubes, patient-ventilator dyssynchrony, full bladder, need to defecate/constipation, sleep deprivation, fear, inability to communicate
Psychiatric/ psychological	Psychosis, autism, dementia, hallucination, ICU psychosis

Legal and ethical issues
- The agitated patient may lack capacity to give informed consent.
- In the absence of capacity, establish that the treatment/procedure is in the patient's best interests. Relatives and carers should be consulted but they cannot give consent on behalf of the patient.
- In emergencies, temporary restraint to provide necessary treatment is not deemed deprivation of liberty.

Agitation scales and scores
The Richmond Agitation Sedation Scale (RASS) is graded from +4 (combative, violent, danger to staff) to −5 (unrousable). The Ramsay Scale is graded from 1 (anxious and agitated) to 6 (non-responsive). These were devised to guide sedation levels in critical care areas.

Preoperative
- Diagnose and treat reversible causes of agitation if possible.
- Establish the need for investigations, treatments, and procedures with medical, surgical, and nursing staff and the patient's relatives and carers.
- Document clearly any discussions.
- Organize sufficient and skilled staff, drugs, and equipment for induction.
- Warn recovery and ward staff to prepare for postoperative agitation.
- Discuss the need for continued postoperative intubation, sedation, monitoring, supervision, and management with critical care staff.
- Consider hospital Level 1 areas for postoperative care if available.

Intraoperative
- Environmental modification (e.g. presence of familiar staff/carers, softer ambient light or noise reduction) may alleviate mild agitation.
- For severely agitated patients a second anaesthetist and the presence of staff trained in safe and legal restraint is advised.
- The choice of induction and maintenance agents should be dictated by the patient's physiological state and presenting condition, and familiarity with the agent.
- If IV access is unavailable and cannulation hazardous consider:
  - Midazolam sedation: intranasal $0.2\,mg\,kg^{-1}$; buccal/rectal $0.5\,mg\,kg^{-1}$; oral $0.5\,mg\,kg^{-1}$ (caution or ↓ dose in liver failure and elderly).
  - Ketamine induction: $5–10\,mg\,kg^{-1}$ PO or $10\,mg\,kg^{-1}$ IM while establishing IV access. Beware emergence phenomena and ↑ ICP.
- Avoid long-acting opioids. These can worsen postoperative confusion.
- RA may be possible with concomitant sedation and may ↓ postoperative opioid use but may mandate ↑ postoperative supervision.

Postoperative
Hand over current problems and future management plans to recovery and ward staff.

Further reading
Mental Capacity Act 2005 http://www.legislation.gov.uk/ukpga/2005/9/contents?view=plain.

General Surgical Emergencies

Rhys Davies and Amit Goswami

Acute appendicitis

Key points
- Appendicitis is common in young, fit patients but it may present at any age.
- Patients range from those that appear clinically well to those that present with profound sepsis and haemodynamic instability.
- Laparoscopic surgical techniques are now commonly used.

Background
- Acute appendicitis is the most common intra-abdominal emergency (44 000 admissions/year in UK). Mortality is low (0.9–2.5/1000 cases at 30 days).
- The peak incidence is between the ages of 10–30 years, although it may present at any age.
- Appendicectomy is the most common non-obstetric surgical procedure performed in pregnancy.
- Key differential diagnoses to consider include bowel obstruction in the older patient and a ruptured ectopic pregnancy in young, female patients.
- Independent determinants for an increase in mortality include: male sex, advanced age, ↑ co-morbidities, open surgery, and perforation.
- Perforation of the appendix increases mortality ~6–10-fold.
- Treatment involves fluid resuscitation followed by appendicectomy. This is usually a relatively short procedure with minimal blood loss.
- Whilst laparoscopic surgery may be associated with improved benefits postoperatively, intraoperatively there may be significant physiological effects caused by the pneumoperitoneum.

Preoperative
- Most patients will be young, with few co-morbidities, and look well despite being significantly ill.
- The combination of anorexia, nausea, vomiting, and fever that occurs in appendicitis often results in dehydration.
- Assess haemodynamic status, including fluid balance, and ensure appropriate fluid resuscitation.
- Review relevant investigations including blood tests (FBC, U&E). Confirm blood sent for group and screen.
- ▶Discuss with the surgeon to clarify the urgency of the procedure and to determine whether the procedure will be open or laparoscopic.
- Rarely regional anaesthesia alone may be considered, if GA is considered too high risk.

Intraoperative
- Ensure large-bore IV access. Reassess haemodynamic and fluid status prior to induction and administer further fluids if necessary.
- In the haemodynamically unstable patient, consider inserting an arterial cannula before induction to enable continuous BP monitoring.
- Patients require a RSI and tracheal intubation.

- Give antibiotics according to local policy.
- Laparoscopy has associated problems (see 📖 Emergency laparoscopic general surgery, p.148).
- Unless contraindicated, consider use of paracetamol (IV or PR), NSAIDS (IV or PR) in addition to titrated doses of opioid.
- At closure, if a regional block has not been performed, ask the surgeon to infiltrate the wound or port sites with LA.

Postoperative

- Reassess fluid balance and prescribe postoperative fluids as appropriate; many will require no further fluids and can eat and drink as soon as they wish.
- Postoperatively, adopt a multimodal strategy to providing analgesia. Unless contraindicated prescribe: regular paracetamol, regular NSAIDs, a weak opioid (e.g. codeine or tramadol) either regularly or PRN depending on if open or laparoscopic, a strong opioid (e.g. morphine, oxycodone) PRN, and at least one antiemetic (e.g. ondansetron) PRN.
- Most patients recover rapidly and are discharged within 24–48 h.

Further reading

Faiz O, Clark J, Brown T, et al. Traditional and laparoscopic appendectomy in adults: outcomes in English NHS hospitals between 1996 and 2006. *Ann Surg* 2008; **248**(5):800–6.

Hospital Episode Statistics. *Primary diagnosis: summary*. Available at: 🔗 http://www.hesonline.nhs. uk/Ease/servlet/ContentServer?siteID=1937&categoryID=202.

Humes D, Simpson J. Acute appendicitis. *BMJ* 2006; **333**:530–4.

Bowel obstruction, perforation, and ischaemia

Key points
- Obstruction of the large and/or small bowel accounts for 20–30% of surgical referrals.
- Bowel ischaemia can present with non-specific abdominal symptoms.
- Emergency laparotomy, especially in the elderly has a high mortality and morbidity.

Background
- In both large- and small-bowel obstruction, fluid and gas is sequestered proximal to the obstruction. Distension of the bowel leads to oedema of the bowel wall, causing fluid to leak into the peritoneum, which can cause peritonitis.
- In more proximal bowel obstruction there is an increase in intra-abdominal pressure, which can impair diaphragmatic movement and cause basal atelectasis. Nausea and vomiting can cause aspiration and pneumonia.
- In more distal bowel obstruction, gas accumulation leads to distension and eventually perforation of the bowel.
- Causes of bowel perforation include: trauma, peptic ulcers, rupture of the appendix, diverticular disease, following bowel obstruction/ischaemia, and following laparoscopy/endoscopy.
- Signs of perforation include haemodynamic instability and peritonism.
- Acute mesenteric ischaemia more commonly affects the small bowel. Causes include: disruption of the arterial blood supply by thrombus or emboli (70% of cases), non-occlusive causes (poor cardiac output) (20%), venous thrombosis (5%), other causes (5%).
- Signs of acute mesenteric ischaemia include: acute severe abdominal pain, the absence of abdominal signs, and haemodynamic instability.
- In all three conditions, fluid sequestration and fluid shifts across compartments, coupled with the poor oral intake and/or vomiting, cause significant dehydration.
- Translocation of gut flora across oedematous bowel wall, pneumonia, perforation leading to peritoneal contamination with bowel contents, and bowel ischaemia cause sepsis (see 📖 Septic shock, p.110). Both the dehydration and inflammatory response make the patient profoundly ill and can cause multiple organ failure.

Advances in perioperative management
Reduced length of stay associated with enhanced recovery programmes is starting to influence the care of emergency cases. Advances include:
- Surgical techniques—the use of smaller and different incisions covering fewer dermatomes as opposed to a large midline laparotomy may be possible, as may laparoscopic assessment and surgery (see 📖 Emergency laparoscopic general surgery, p.148).

- Early postoperative enteral nutrition when possible, whilst accepting this group are at higher risk of ileus.
- Multimodal analgesic techniques aiming to reduce opioid requirements.
- Early mobilization.

Preoperative

- Aim to achieve rapid access to diagnostics, coupled with early fluid resuscitation, timely surgical decision-making, and intervention.
- The spectrum of clinical presentation ranges from the mildly unwell to established multiorgan failure.
- Assess carefully the respiratory, cardiovascular, and renal systems, including an assessment of haemodynamic status and fluid balance.
- Ensure urinary catheterization and hourly urine output monitoring.
- Target fluid resuscitation—this can be achieved using a variety of monitors and clinical endpoints, according to local practices. Fluids used can be crystalloid or colloid; balanced solutions are less likely than 0.9% saline to cause hyperchloraemic acidosis. ABG analysis provides a useful guide to this.
- A nasogastric tube to decompress the bowel may reduce diaphragmatic splinting and improve respiratory function.
- Ensure relevant investigations (FBC, U&Es, liver function tests, clotting screen, ECG, and chest X-ray) have been obtained and reviewed. Confirm the existence of a valid group and save sample and where appropriate ensure compatible blood is available.
- Discuss the case with the operating surgeon to clarify the urgency of intervention, likely intraoperative findings, expected blood loss, and the exact procedure intended.
- Determine the need for invasive monitoring and the likely level of postoperative care required.
- If the patient is seriously unwell, involve the ICU team early to provide assistance with pre- as well as postoperative care. In certain cases preoperative optimization may be appropriate.
- Assess the indications and contraindications for regional techniques (transversus abdominis plane (TAP) block, epidural) to provide intra- and postoperative analgesia.

Intraoperative

- Reassess haemodynamic status before induction and give further fluid boluses as required.
- If haemodynamically unstable insert an arterial cannula before induction for continuous BP monitoring and consider the need for central access to enable infusion of vasopressors and/or inotropes.
- If an epidural is to be placed this can be done before or after induction. There are risks for either: patient discomfort and potential difficulties in positioning while awake versus the asleep patient's inability to describe pain that may indicate neural injury on insertion. If haemodynamically stable, the epidural can be used for intraoperative as well as postoperative analgesia.

- The risk of aspiration is significant and these patients will require a RSI and tracheal intubation. This can be modified, with the use of alternative induction drugs.
- Aspirate the nasogastric tube before fully preoxygenating the patient.
- Avoid using nitrous oxide as it distends the gut.
- If a TAP block is planned, do it before starting the operation to provide intraoperative analgesia.
- Use fluid warmers and forced-air warmers to maintain normothermia (reduced postoperative wound infections).
- Give antibiotics as appropriate before surgical incision. If the patient is septic preoperatively, antibiotics should have been started earlier—ensure doses are not missed and consider top-up doses.
- If a regional technique is not used, provide intraoperative analgesia with boluses of opioid (morphine, fentanyl) or an opioid infusion (remifentanil).
- Following surgical incision, the relief of elevated intra-abdominal pressure may improve respiratory compliance; conversely, at closure, compliance may worsen.
- Abdominal pressures may rise at closure resulting in an abdominal compartment syndrome with hypoperfusion of intra-abdominal organs. It may be necessary to leave the abdominal wall open as a laparostomy as a temporary measure.
- Reassess frequently fluid balance and haemodynamic status intraoperatively. This is achieved by using clinical parameters and ABG analysis.
- Intraoperative blood loss and inflammatory mediator release induced by surgery can cause hypotension. Fluids, vasopressors, and inotropes may all be required to maintain haemodynamic stability.
- If available, oesophageal Doppler or pulse contour analysis devices, may improve outcome in these patients by allowing fluids to be targeted against cardiac output and therefore tissue oxygen delivery.
- Following closure, determine whether the patient is to be extubated or remain intubated and transferred to the ICU. Factors influencing this decision include preoperative co-morbidities, intraoperative findings and the procedure undertaken, intraoperative stability, and current clinical condition.
- Suck secretions from the oropharynx; aspirate the nasogastric tube once more and extubate the patient awake.

Postoperative

- Antibiotics—if perforation has occurred with significant contamination further antibiotics will be needed—discuss with a microbiologist.
- Continue oxygen therapy; consider humidification and postoperative physiotherapy where appropriate.
- Fluids—reassess fluid balance and prescribe postoperative fluids, with additional boluses to be given if observations indicate.
- Ongoing monitoring, hourly urine output, and regular observations, escalated up to repeated ABG's to monitor acidosis and gas exchange. If a central venous catheter is in place, central venous oxygen saturation can be monitored to ensure adequate tissue oxygen delivery targeting a value >75%.

- Nutrition—placement of feeding nasogastric or nasojejunal tubes enables early enteral feeding. If this is not possible, establish whether total parenteral nutrition is required and ensure a dedicated central venous catheter lumen is available.
- Analgesia—adopt a multimodal approach to ensure optimal postoperative analgesia. This should involve regular paracetamol, a regional block (epidural, rectus sheath blocks, TAP blocks, or infusion catheters) and additional opioids if necessary. The level of epidural placement depends on how high the surgical incision will extend. In most cases the epidural is sited at a low/mid-thoracic level. Similarly, abdominal blocks should be appropriate for site of incision. Below the umbilicus TAP blocks provide good analgesia, but for those incisions extending above this additional analgesia can be provided by subcostal TAP blocks or rectus sheath blocks in the upper abdomen. If an epidural is not used post-operatively, prescribe a PCA. Consider carefully the risks and benefits of using NSAIDs; there is likely to be an ↑ risk of postoperative renal dysfunction in these patients and many anaesthetists will avoid them, especially in the elderly.
- If the patient is not transferred to ICU or HDU reassess the patient before discharge from recovery to ensure patient is suitable for ward-level care.

Further reading

Gemmel L, Rincon C. Anaesthetic management of intestinal obstruction. *Br J Anaesth CEPD Rev* 2001; **1**:138–41.

Royal College of Surgeons of England. *Emergency surgery. Standards for unscheduled surgical care. Guidance for providers, commissioners and service planners.* London: Royal College of Surgeons of England, 2011. Available at: ℬ http://www.rcs.ac.uk.

Gastrointestinal haemorrhage

Key points
- Massive acute GI haemorrhage is an emergency associated with a mortality of 5–10%.
- Presentation ranges from compensated hypovolaemia to cardiac arrest.
- Management involves fluid resuscitation and endoscopic and/or interventional radiology and/or surgical intervention.

Background

Upper gastrointestinal haemorrhage
- Acute upper GI haemorrhage has an annual incidence of 40–150 cases per 100 000 people.
- Causes of acute upper GI haemorrhage include: peptic ulceration (44% of all cases), oesophagitis (28%), gastritis/erosions (26%) erosive duodenitis (15%), varices (13%), portal hypertensive gastropathy (7%), malignancy (5%), Mallory–Weiss tear (5%), vascular malformation (3%). Note that some patients have more than one cause and in about 20% of cases no cause is found on endoscopy.
- Independent risk factors for ↑ mortality include: advanced age, co-morbidities, shock on admission, the underlying diagnosis at endoscopy, and rebleeding episodes.
- Endoscopic treatment stops the bleeding in most cases. Treatments include: diathermy, injection of adrenaline, alcohol or sclerosants, and the use of clips, sutures, staples, or bands. When initial endoscopic treatment is unsuccessful in stopping non-variceal upper GI haemorrhage consider repeat endoscopy, selective arterial embolization, or surgery.
- Give terlipressin and antibiotics to patients with suspected variceal bleeding. Balloon tamponade (Sengstaken tube) should be considered as a holding measure if endoscopic control of variceal bleeding fails. TIPSS shunt is recommended for uncontrolled bleeding. When TIPSS fails, surgery is unlikely to be beneficial.

Lower gastrointestinal haemorrhage
- Acute lower GI haemorrhage has an annual incidence of 20–27 cases per 100 000 people.
- Causes include: diverticular disease, colorectal malignancy, acute colitis (infective, ischaemic, and ulcerative), angiodysplasia, radiation enteropathy, and anorectal causes (including anal fissures and haemorrhoids).
- Urgent colonoscopy or angiographic arterial embolization are 1st-line interventions. Consider surgery when these fail or are not feasible.

Preoperative
- Discuss with an endoscopist, radiologist and surgeon to determine the urgency, nature and best location of any procedure. Involve the ICU team.

- Anaesthetic options include sedation or GA. Consider the risk of aspiration (for upper GI endoscopy), and CVS instability and proposed procedure in determining the most appropriate anaesthetic. In the sickest patients GA may be safest.
- Patients presenting with acute GI haemorrhage are commonly elderly with multiple co-morbidities. As excessive alcohol intake is associated with upper GI haemorrhage, a number of patients will have features of alcoholic liver disease (see 📖 Liver failure, p.120).
- Ensure two large-bore cannulae and invasive BP monitoring in unstable patient. Consider inserting a pulmonary artery catheter sheath (8.5 F) in a central vein.
- Review blood tests (FBC, U&Es, LFTs, coagulation screen) and ensure blood is crossmatched. Obtain an ABG sample to provide a rapid measure of haemoglobin as well as acid–base status. Other near-patient testing, such as Hemocue®, may also be useful.
- Haemodynamic status and estimated blood loss will determine the type of fluid required (crystalloid, colloid, blood products). Give fluid through a warming device. Liaise with the blood bank early to discuss the need for blood products (O-negative, type-specific blood, crossmatched blood, FFP, platelets, cryoprecipitate, and recombinant Factor VII). Consider giving tranexamic acid (see 📖 Transfusion, p.20).
- In a patient with major blood loss, aim for the following haematological targets: Hb concentration $>7–8 \, g \, dL^{-1}$, INR <1.5, APTT ratio <1.5, platelets $>75 \times 10^9 \, L^{-1}$, fibrinogen $>1.0 \, g \, L^{-1}$ (see Coagulopathy, p.130).

Intraoperative

Sedation

There are many techniques to achieve this. One such technique involves: patient left lateral, monitored, oxygen via nasal cannulae, IV midazolam 0.5–1 mg as single dose, remifentanil infusion (start at $0.05–0.1 \, micrograms \, kg^{-1} \, min^{-1}$), and topical LA by endoscopist. Once adequately sedated the endoscope is inserted and patient asked to swallow; remind patient to breath. Reduce remifentanil infusion once endoscope passed successfully. Be prepared to convert to GA rapidly if required.

General anaesthesia

- Patients will require a RSI and tracheal intubation. Depending on the degree of haemodynamic instability, the RSI may need to be modified with the use of alternative induction drugs (e.g. etomidate, ketamine) and opioids (e.g. fentanyl, alfentanil). (see 📖 Rapid sequence induction and tracheal intubation, p.6).
- Prepare vasopressors, such as metaraminol, before induction. In more unstable patients, also prepare dilute adrenaline (e.g. 1:100 000).
- Ensure that functioning suction is available. Oropharyngeal soiling may be significant and makes laryngoscopy more difficult.
- Ensure the tube is tied securely, particularly for upper GI endoscopy. Assist the endoscopist to insert the endoscope in the anaesthetized patient (a bite block is also inserted). It may be best to hold the tracheal tube to prevent dislodgement during endoscope movement. Seek help from a 2nd anaesthetist if necessary.

- Be prepared to convert to open surgery if bleeding cannot be stopped.
- If haemostasis is achieved endoscopically, decide whether the patient is to be extubated or to remain ventilated and transferred to the ICU.
- Consider passing a feeding nasojejunal and or nasogastric tube at the time of endoscopy to facilitate nutrition and gastric drainage.
- Ensure the stomach has been emptied and suction the oropharynx before extubation.

Postoperative

- Correct any abnormalities in haemoglobin, platelets, and coagulation.
- Carefully observe the patient for signs of ongoing bleeding. Involve the endoscopist/surgeon early if there are concerns.
- High-risk patients should go to a HDU or ICU for further care.
- Give a proton pump inhibitor (e.g. omeprazole or pantoprazole 80 mg IV bolus followed by 8 mg h^{-1} infusion for 72 h) for major peptic ulcer bleeding.

Further reading

Scottish Intercollegiate Guidelines Network. *Management of acute upper and lower gastrointestinal bleeding. A national clinical guideline.* Guideline number 105. Edinburgh, SIGN, 2008. Available at: http://www.sign.ac.uk.

Emergency laparoscopic general surgery

Key points
- Laparoscopic techniques are used increasingly for emergency surgery.
- Pneumoperitoneum has significant physiological effects on the respiratory and cardiovascular systems.

Background
- Common laparoscopic emergencies include: diagnostic laparoscopy, appendicectomy, cholecystectomy, and bowel resection.
- Laparoscopic procedures require the creation and maintenance of a pneumoperitoneum. This is achieved by inserting a needle or trochar into the peritoneum and insufflating a constant flow of gas, usually carbon dioxide.
- Complications include: organ or vascular damage, gas embolism, severe bradycardia/asystole caused by vagal stimulation, subcutaneous emphysema, pneumothoraces or pneumomediastinum.
- Laparoscopic surgery can take much more time than the equivalent open surgery.
- Physiological effects include:
  - IVC compression and reduction in venous return.
  - Systemic vascular resistance increase, as a result of ↑ intra-abdominal pressure and an increase in circulating catecholamines, causing an ↑ heart rate and BP. This leads to increase in myocardial work and can cause myocardial ischaemia.
  - Pneumoperitoneum causes the diaphragm to move cephalad, thereby reducing the FRC. This may cause atelectasis, V/Q mismatch and hypoxaemia.
  - An increase in airway resistance and a reduction in compliance are also observed. Reduction in minute ventilation leads to hypercarbia.
  - Maintenance of minute ventilation, through ↑ ventilatory pressures, increases the risk of barotrauma.
  - A reduction in renal function and urine output.
  - An increase in ICP.
  - An ↑ intra-abdominal pressure also increases the risk of regurgitation of gastric contents.
- Avoid excessive insufflation pressures (>15 mmHg) to minimize these effects.
- Absorption of the insufflating gas, usually carbon dioxide, also produces physiological effects. Absorption of CO_2 from the peritoneum, coupled with a reduction in minute ventilation leads to a rise in $PaCO_2$. Absorption of gas, particularly over a prolonged period of time, can cause hypothermia.
- There are few absolute contraindications to laparoscopy, relative contraindications that require caution include: severe ischaemic heart disease, significant cardiac valve lesions, conditions resulting in a raised ICP, and hypovolaemia.

Preoperative

Discuss patients with critical illness or significant co-morbidities with the surgeon to balance benefits of minimally invasive surgery and risks of pneumoperitoneum. Discuss the option of conversion to an open procedure if laparoscopic approach tolerated poorly. Involve a senior anaesthetist early if necessary.

Intraoperative

- Avoid nitrous oxide: it increases the size of pneumothoraces or gas emboli—potential complications of laparoscopy.
- Ventilation can be volume or pressure-controlled; both have potential problems when used during laparoscopy. Volume control is easier for $PaCO_2$ control because the minute volume is constant. Pressure control results in lower airway pressures, but tidal volume must be monitored as it can change rapidly with changes in intra-abdominal presssure. Consider PEEP to prevent basal atelectasis.
- Before insufflation, adjust the ventilator to deliver a minute volume that will achieve a low/normal $ETCO_2$. Once the pneumoperitoneum is established, the $ETCO_2$ will rise. Starting with a lower $ETCO_2$ will hopefully prevent a high $ETCO_2$ during surgery. Excessive changes in ventilator settings are often noticed by the surgeon because of changes in intra-abdominal pressure. The surgeon may respond by increasing insufflation pressure and this may worsen ventilation problems.
- During laparoscopy, BP and heart rate often increase. This response can be attenuated by bolus opioids, a remifentanil infusion, or by increasing the depth of anaesthesia.
- During gas insufflation, look for vagally-mediated arrhythmias, including asystole, caused by peritoneal stretching. If severe bradycardia or asystole occur, tell the surgeon to deflate the pneumoperitoneum immediately. Give an anticholinergic (e.g. glycopyrronium or atropine).
- Fluid requirements are reduced for laparoscopic surgery compared with open surgery.
- Laparoscopy is associated with an increased incidence of post-operative nausea and vomiting (PONV). Give one or more anti-emetics.
- Analgesia should include LA, either local port infiltration or a regional block.
- TAP blocks provide analgesia up to T9. To provide analgesia higher up the abdominal wall, subcostal TAP blocks can be used.
- Give IV paracetamol, NSAIDS (if not contraindicated) in addition to titrated doses of opioid.

Postoperative

- Many patients will tolerate oral intake and require limited IV fluids.
- Use a multimodal strategy to providing analgesia. Unless contraindicated prescribe: regular paracetamol, regular NSAIDs, a weak opioid (e.g. codeine or tramadol) either regularly or PRN, a strong opioid (e.g. morphine, oxycodone) PRN, and at least one antiemetic PRN.

Further reading

Perrin M, Fletcher A. Laparoscopic abdominal surgery. Cont Educ Anaesth Crit Care Pain 2004; 4:107–10.

Titu LV, Zafar N, Phillips SM, et al. Emergency laparoscopic surgery for complicated diverticular disease. Colorectal Dis 2009; 11:401–4.

Liver transplantation and resection

Key points
- Hepatic resection is indicated most commonly for isolated colorectal metastases.
- Hepatic transplant is indicated in end-stage liver failure or acute hepatic failure.
- Patients presenting secondary to chronic liver disease often have had extensive preoperative evaluation, and may have significant comorbidities.
- There is potential for major blood loss and physiological disturbance.

Background
- Hepatic resection is used in the management of: primary hepatobiliary tumours, hepatic trauma, donation for hepatic transplantation, and isolated colorectal hepatic metastases. The aim is to resect the diseased part of the liver, leaving enough healthy liver to avoid postoperative liver failure.
- The operative procedure can be divided into three phases: initial phase—when the liver is mobilized; resection phase—when the diseased part of the liver is identified and removed; and closure—following confirmation of haemostasis.
- Hepatic transplant is indicated in end-stage liver failure or acute hepatic failure. Indications for transplantation include: cirrhosis (58% of all transplants in Europe since 1988), carcinoma (14%), acute hepatic failure (8%), and other causes including cholestatic and metabolic diseases (20%).
- Following first liver transplantation, 1-year patient survival is 86%, 10–year survival is 63%.
- Liver transplants can be heterotopic or more commonly orthotopic. In heterotopic liver transplantation, the donor liver is placed in the paravertebral gutter without removal of the diseased liver. In orthotopic liver transplantation the diseased liver is removed and the donor liver transplanted to that site.
- Orthotopic liver transplantation has three distinct operative phases: phase I (pre-anhepatic phase); phase II (anhepatic phase); and phase III (neohepatic, post-anhepatic phase, or reperfusion phase).
- In addition to standard postoperative complications of major abdominal surgery, such as bleeding, sepsis, respiratory failure, and renal dysfunction, postoperative liver failure or dysfunction is a major concern.
- Up to 10% of hepatic transplants have delayed or absent function. In these cases urgent re-transplantation is often indicated. ~3% of hepatic resection patients experience postoperative liver dysfunction or failure.
- In both hepatic resection and transplantation, blood loss is extremely variable with potential for major blood loss.

Preoperative

- Review preoperative investigations. With the exception of trauma patients and those in acute liver failure, patients presenting for hepatic resection or transplantation will usually have had extensive preoperative investigation: echocardiography, cardiac stress test, pulmonary function tests, and cardiopulmonary exercise testing, as well as an ECG and chest X-ray.
- Identify patients with conditions causing raised CVP or right-sided cardiac pressures. A major source of intraoperative bleeding is backflow from valveless hepatic veins; as a result, patients with a higher CVP have greater intraoperative blood loss.
- Patients with hepatic dysfunction often have deranged clotting function as well as thrombocytopaenia, hypoalbuminaemia, and hyponatraemia.
- Confirm that compatible blood products are available. Different centres will have different protocols stating requirements for RBCs, FFP, and platelets preoperatively.
- Ensure cell salvage and rapid infusion devices are available, because blood loss may be massive.

Intraoperative

- Analgesic options include thoracic epidural, paravertebral block, intrapleural catheters, and PCA. An epidural can be sited pre- or post-induction. A mid-thoracic level of insertion is necessary to cover the extent of the incision. Abnormal coagulation is common perioperatively.
- No single anaesthetic technique has been shown to be beneficial but hepatic clearance will be ↓. Current trends are towards shorter-acting agents (e.g. desflurane and remifentanil infusions).
- Avoid PEEP where possible, because it will increase the CVP.
- Insert a nasogastric tube, urinary catheter, and temperature probe.
- For hepatic transplantation, a range of cardiac output monitoring can be used intraoperatively, including PA catheters, pulse contour analysis devices, and transoesophageal echocardiography.
- Use fluid warmers and forced-air warmers to prevent hypothermia.
- Monitor regularly ABGs, FBC, U&E, and coagulation function.
- Aim for a haemoglobin concentration of $7-9\,g\,dL^{-1}$—at this level oxygen delivery is maintained without significantly increasing blood viscosity and the risk of hepatic artery thrombosis.
- Correct hypocalcaemia and hypoglycaemia.
- Use of thromboelastography enables rapid assessment of coagulation.

Hepatic resection

- When performed in specialist centres, blood loss may be minimal. Access to radiofrequency-assisted techniques may further reduce blood loss and parenchymal damage. Those performed for trauma and in non-specialist centres will have a significantly higher blood loss.
- In the initial phase of hepatic resection, where possible, maintain a CVP <5 cmH$_2$O. Observe for signs of end-organ hypoperfusion. In some patients maintaining a low CVP will lead to haemodynamic instability and a higher target CVP may be needed. A high CVP can cause

excessive bleeding; however, a CVP which is too low may result in air embolus. Nitrates and/or diuretics may be needed to reduce the CVP.

- Blood loss can also be reduced by temporarily occluding the blood supply to the liver. Complete occlusion of the portal vein and hepatic artery (the Pringle manoeuvre) can help to minimize blood loss, but has significant haemodynamic effects: causing a reduction in cardiac output of up to 60% and an increase in afterload.
- Vasopressors (e.g. noradrenaline) may be needed to maintain a MAP at 50–75 mmHg during the resection phase.
- Following resection, haemostasis is achieved before closing the abdomen. During this phase, fluid can be replaced because the risk of bleeding is reduced.

Hepatic transplantation
- Hepatic transplant patients are often volume overloaded with a hyperdynamic circulation preoperatively. End-stage liver disease may cause a relative resistance to catecholamines.
- During the pre-anhepatic phase, significant blood loss may occur from abdominal wall varices. Decompression of ascites may cause significant fluid shifts. Manipulation of major vessels can reduce venous return and cause transient arrhythmias.
- The anhepatic phase begins with the clamping of the hepatic artery, hepatic portal vein, and the supra- and infrahepatic IVC. Following cross-clamping, there is a significant reduction in venous return and cardiac output. In certain patients venovenous bypass may be used to improve haemodynamic stability.
- After cross-clamping, the native liver is then removed. Without a functioning liver, hepatic clotting factors are not produced, citrate and lactate are not metabolized, and there is reduced gluconeogenesis and glucose uptake. Monitor closely for coagulopathy, worsening metabolic acidosis, hypocalcaemia, and hypoglycaemia.
- In the final phase, cross-clamps are released from the vascular anastomoses and the new liver is perfused. Following unclamping, cold, hyperkalaemic, acidotic fluid enters the systemic circulation, which can cause profound hypotension and severe arrhythmias.
- Assess suitability for extubation. Transfer postoperatively to a HDU/ICU.

Postoperative
- Persisting metabolic acidosis, failure to produce bile, and coagulopathy are all suggestive of absent or delayed graft function post-transplant.
- After resection, a low serum urea may represent an early sign of liver dysfunction. Jaundice, encephalopathy, and coagulopathy at the 3rd or 4th postoperative day may herald the onset of liver failure.
- Monitor blood glucose levels closely: hypoglycaemia is common postoperatively and may require a glucose infusion.
- Monitor potassium levels closely: hypokalaemia is often seen in the 1st 36 h after liver transplant.
- Aim for a haemoglobin concentration of 7–9 g dL^{-1} in transplant recipients.
- Ensure optimal analgesia, regular chest physiotherapy, and early enteral feeding.

Further reading

European Liver Transplant Registry 1988 – 2009. Available at: ℘ http://www.eltr.org.

Fabbroni D, Bellamy M. Anaesthesia for hepatic transplantation. *Cont Educ Anaesth Crit Care Pain* 2006; **6**:171–5.

Hartog A, Mills G. Anaesthesia for hepatic resection surgery. *Cont Educ Anaesth Crit Care Pain* 2009; **9**:1–5.

Ear, Nose, and Throat Emergencies

Clare Hommers and Tim Cook

Acute airway obstruction

Key points
- Must consider.
  - Speed of onset of symptoms.
  - Urgency of intervention.
  - Level of obstruction.
  - General condition of the patient.
- High-risk cases.
- Communication, plan, back-up plan.

Background
▶ Management of the obstructed airway is one of the greatest challenges in anaesthesia airway management and there may be catastrophic consequences if planning or management is poor.
- Anaesthesia and airway manipulation will often worsen airway obstruction because of loss of airway tone, reflex airway responses, trauma, and bleeding.
- Senior anaesthetic involvement is essential and immediate surgical preparedness is often required.

Assessment
Level of obstruction
- Oropharyngeal—limited mouth opening, tongue protrusion.
- Laryngeal and extrathoracic—(inspiratory) stridor, voice changes.
- Intrathoracic—(expiratory) wheeze.

Severity: consider
- Speed of onset.
- Work of breathing.
- Respiratory distress.
- Stridor.
- Wheeze.
- Drooling.
- Dysphagia.
- Nocturnal or positional panic.
- Effect of posture (sleeping position).
- Hypoxaemia (often related to poor cough—atelectasis, infection).
- Silent chest/exhaustion/obtunded.

Co-morbidity
- Cough.
- COPD.
- Previous radiotherapy and known intubation difficulty.
- Previous tracheostomy.

Head and neck
- Teeth.
- Mouth opening.
- Temporomandibular joint mobility including sliding motion (i.e. jaw protrusion).

- Tongue mobility.
- Neck extension.
- LMA extension.
- Ease of emergency tracheal access.

Investigations

If time allows, further investigations can help delineate the exact nature, site, extent, friability, and severity of the obstructing lesion. It is important to try to establish involvement of related structures.
- Nasoendoscopy (by anaesthetist or jointly with surgeon)—an underused technique.
- CT/MRI.
- Lung function (including flow-volume loops).
- Echocardiogram.

A specific diagnosis may enable shrinking of a lesion with antibiotics, steroids, chemotherapy, or radiotherapy if time allows.

Planning

A large proportion of major harm during airway management by anaesthetists arises during care of the obstructed airway. Poor planning is common. Always discuss with the surgeon the likely extent and friability of the lesion, their surgical plans, and the extent of airway soiling.

Little evidence supports one particular technique and the choices are often determined by the skills and experience of the responsible anaesthetist, as well as individual circumstances. Lack of evidence is partly because all techniques may fail: clearly formulated, back-up plans (plan B, C, etc.) are essential. The skills, equipment, and personnel to carry out both primary and back-up plans must be available in the operating room and the plan communicated clearly to all. If necessary this may require different anaesthetists or transfer of the patient.

Persistence with failing techniques (task fixation, loss of situation awareness) is common in major airway disasters. Whatever technique chosen, all members of team should be aware of the 'break point' at which the primary plan should be abandoned and the patient awoken (default plan) or, if appropriate, Plan B used. Any member of the team should be able to identify the break point. Patient waking may not always be straightforward and may also require a specific plan and a change of technique.

Management

Traditional options include:
- Awake fibre-optic intubation.
- Direct laryngoscopy after deep inhalational anaesthesia.
- Awake tracheostomy under local anaesthesia.

Techniques advocated more recently include:
- Awake intubation using modern videolaryngoscopes.
- Incremental TIVA with spontaneous ventilation as an alternative to gaseous induction.

- IV induction, muscle paralysis and controlled ventilation (perhaps initially via a supraglottic airway) prior to intubation using conventional, video, or fibreoptic laryngoscopy (suitable only in a minority of lesions and requiring definite clear back up plans).

In children many of these options are not available (see 📖 Airway emergencies in children, p.308). In adults the technique selected will predominantly depend upon the level of the obstruction. Whichever technique is chosen it should be performed in the operating room with assistance available, not in isolation in a small anaesthetic room.

▶▶In the acute situation, avoid unnecessary delays and consider buying time with:

- Heliox (21% O_2 in helium—use of a 'Y' connector can increase FiO_2).
- Nebulized adrenaline (5 mg per nebulization).
- Corticosteroids.

Preoxygenation

- Careful and complete preoxygenation is vital before anaesthesia.
- Reverse Trendelenburg (head-up) position for induction in all obese patients.
- CPAP (and note the effect on obstruction).
- Targeted to end-tidal O_2 >90%.

During airway manipulation, attempts to oxygenate remain paramount and should be pursued actively. Continue supplemental oxygen delivery throughout all awake techniques. Consider passive oxygenation with nasal 'specs' during asleep techniques.

Oral/supraglottic/floor of mouth/laryngeal lesions

E.g. trauma, burns, tumour, infections.

- Main concerns are:
  - Precipitating complete obstruction.
  - Anatomical distortion of the airway.
  - Difficulty viewing the larynx and in passing a tracheal tube.
  - Increased risk of failed rescue techniques.
- Nasoendoscopy can be very helpful in assessing whether intubation is likely to be possible.
- Emergency access to the neck is usually unimpeded in these circumstances but previous radiotherapy should raise concerns about this and both mask ventilation and ease of laryngoscopy.
- Consider:
  - Awake fibreoptic or videolaryngoscopy techniques.
  - Induction of anaesthesia maintaining spontaneous ventilation (inhalational or stepwise TIVA induction) and direct or fibreoptic laryngoscopy.
  - Elective awake tracheostomy or cricothyroidotomy.

These choices are not mandatory and other techniques may be appropriate, particularly in skilled hands. New rigid fibreoptic laryngoscopes and optical stylets have a role but only in the hands of those with established skills.

- Awake fibreoptic intubation may be technically very challenging:
  - Anatomically.
  - Vascular/friable lesions can impede vision and cause obstruction.

- Obstruction can occur with the scope ('cork in the bottle') with subsequent inability to pass the tracheal tube.
- Passage of the tube is 'blind' and risks hold-up at the larynx or trauma to the lesion. Careful tube selection (small with non-traumatic tip) lessens this effect.
- Placement of a transtracheal ventilation catheter (e.g. Ravussin®) before induction of anaesthesia is often appropriate and may be used to oxygenate/ventilate in the event of complete obstruction. It is essential to ensure an expiratory path is present during use otherwise barotrauma will occur. If no expiratory route is present, basal oxygen delivery (200–500 mL/min) may provide some oxygenation while a definitive airway is achieved.
- An experienced surgeon should be scrubbed, equipped, assisted, and ready to perform a cricothyroidotomy or very rapid tracheostomy in the event of complete obstruction. This plan should be communicated to all.
- A supraglottic airway device (SAD) (ideally one with a high airway seal: e.g. ProSeal® LMA, possibly Supreme® LMA, i-gel®) may assist ventilation during emergency airway access. In skilled and experienced hands, use of such a device may form part of the primary plan for intubation.
- For laser surgery options include:
  - Supralaryngeal ventilation (via the surgeon's laryngoscope with spontaneous or 'jet' ventilation).
  - Translaryngeal ventilation (e.g. Hunsaker tube).
  - Transtracheal ventilation (cricothyroid cannula).

All jet (i.e. high-pressure source) ventilation requires an expiratory route.
- Inserting a rigid bronchoscope may provide an emergency airway in some laryngeal/upper tracheal cases.
- For a lesion above the larynx, IV induction and attempted laryngoscopy (with or without paralysis) risks a catastrophic 'can't intubate, can't ventilate' situation in a patient unable to breath spontaneously and cannot be recommended without a robust back-up plan.
- Some experts recommend a technique based on IV induction, paralysis, and controlled ventilation for laryngeal lesions but this technique is not recommended outside expert practice.

Upper and mid tracheal lesions

E.g. tumour, bleeding into goitre or thyroid tumour, low pharyngeal abscesses.
- Very different situation to upper airway lesions.
- There are fewer options—the main considerations include:
  - Knowing the site of the lesion is vital.
  - Upper airway usually normal at laryngoscopy (but beware obesity, previous radiotherapy).
  - Difficulty may arise when the tube is inserted into the trachea.
  - Cricothyroidotomy/tracheostomy may be precluded and attempts risk bleeding and complete obstruction.
  - Determine whether the obstruction is fixed or variable: fixed obstructions vary little with respiratory cycle. Variable obstruction (e.g. rapidly growing tumours, infective masses, some haematomas) may be more challenging. Lesions that improve with CPAP may be variable.

- Determine whether the obstruction is extrathoracic or intrathoracic. Extrathoracic obstruction (lesions of upper trachea) tends to worsen during inspiration. Intrathoracic obstruction (mid and lower trachea) tends to worsen with expiration. Anaesthesia likely worsens both. CPAP and positive pressure may be beneficial.
  - May require discussion or involvement of ENT or thoracic surgeons for primary or back-up plans.
- CT scanning is mandatory unless the circumstances are life saving. But note CT images are affected by supine position for scan. Most patients are managed sitting up.
- Pay particular attention to:
  - Exact site.
  - Dimensions.
  - Tracheal lumen size.
  - Tracheal wall invasion.
  - Relation to the carina.

▶Is there space for a tube cuff and bevel to sit below the obstruction and above the carina?

▶Is an emergency tracheostomy an option? (Is it long enough to pass the obstruction?)

▶Standard induction verses awake fibreoptic intubation.
- Inhalational induction may be very slow and difficult if there is severe narrowing of the airway.
- Awake fibreoptic intubation may be indicated if failure to ventilate under anaesthesia is a significant possibility. However:
  - Coughing and distress may cause ↑ obstruction and a cycle of decline.
  - Passage of the fibreoptic scope through the narrowing may hinder spontaneous ventilation and lead to patient panic.
- A smaller tracheal tube or a hollow intubation bougie that enables conventional (e.g. Aintree Intubation Catheter®) or jet ventilation (Cook airway exchange catheter, Hunsaker tube) may pass the narrowing. Jet ventilation always requires an expiratory route.
- IV induction, rapid neuromuscular blockade, and early passage of a rigid bronchoscope may be used for advanced tracheal obstruction requiring thoracic surgery, e.g. resection, laser, or stenting. The rigid bronchoscope establishes a patent airway and can then be used for further assessment, oxygenation, ventilation, and surgery.
- Anaesthesia may need to be maintained with an IV technique.

Lower tracheal/bronchial obstruction
E.g. tumour, trauma, large mediastinal masses.
- Best managed by experienced specialists in a thoracic centre.
- Risks of anaesthesia:
  - Altered respiratory mechanics when switching from spontaneous to positive pressure ventilation.
  - Sudden respiratory obstruction at induction/paralysis.
- IV induction, rapid neuromuscular blockade, and passage of a rigid bronchoscope may be life saving.

- Cardiopulmonary bypass is sometime necessary (e.g. pulmonary artery compression) as primary or even back-up plan. It is time consuming and to be effective requires full preparation prior to instituting airway management.
- For diagnostic purposes in a non-thoracic centre always consider procedures under LA.

Extubation

- Must be planned.
- Re-intubation may be much more difficult due to:
  - Airway bruising and swelling.
  - Airway contamination with clot, pus, or regurgitated material.
- Prepare the same equipment and personnel as for the intubation.
- Communicate with the surgeon.
- Clear the upper airway and ensure good haemostasis.
- Consider adjuncts, empty the stomach if necessary, and ensure reversal of neuromuscular blockade and removal of any surgical packs.
- Optimize patient position, usually sitting up.
- Perform a leak test—deflating the cuff and ventilate to ensure there is a low-pressure leak around the tube.
- Extubate the preoxygenated, awake patient when obeying commands.
- Do not transfer to recovery until stable.
- Monitor closely in recovery for an extended period and ensure suitable supervision and equipment for reintervention during this time.
- Consider:
  - Extended monitoring in a high dependency area.
  - Delaying extubation, ventilating on ICU and reassessing later.
  - Corticosteroid therapy for 24h before extubation to reduce oedema.
  - Elective tracheostomy.
  - Positioning a Cook airway exchange catheter in the trachea before extubation. These devices permit a tracheal tube to be rail-roaded into the trachea and also allow oxygen delivery and jet ventilation if required.

Further reading

Isono S, Kitamura Y, Asai T, et al. Perioperative airway management of a patient with tracheal stenosis: expert opinions and actual clinical management. Anesthesiology 2010; **112**:970–8.

Mason RA, Fielder CP. The obstructed airway in head and neck surgery. Anaesthesia 1999; **54**:625–8.

Nouraei SA, Giussani DA, Howard DJ, et al. Physiological comparison of spontaneous and positive-pressure ventilation in laryngotracheal stenosis. Br J Anaesth 2008; **101**:419–23.

Bleeding tonsil

Key points

- Hypovolaemia—often concealed.
- High risk of aspiration—blood in the stomach.
- Difficult laryngoscopy—bleeding obscuring the view, possible oedema from previous airway instrumentation and surgery.
- Residual anaesthetic.
- Back-up plan.

Background

The incidence of bleeding after tonsillectomy is 0.5–3.5% although only 0.9% need to return to the operating room. Usually caused by venous or capillary bleeding from the tonsillar bed; associated risk factors include older age, male gender, and surgical technique (use of diathermy).

Categorized as primary or secondary haemorrhage:

- Primary—occurs within 24h although most are within 6h.
- Secondary—up to 28 days after surgery; often associated with sloughing of necrotic tissue or infection.

Preoperative

▶Resuscitation is essential to avoid cardiovascular collapse on induction.

- Blood loss is often underestimated because it occurs over several hours and with significant volumes concealed because of swallowing. Spitting blood or excessive swallowing, especially in children, may be a sign of brisk bleeding.
- Look for signs of hypovolaemic shock—↑ heart rate, ↑ respiratory rate, ↑ capillary refill time and ↓ urine output.
- Check haemoglobin, coagulation, and crossmatch.
- Obtain large-bore IV access.
- Give fluids and blood products as required.
- Review the time since previous surgery, last ingestion of food, presence of clots or spitting of blood, and any signs of airway difficulty (respiratory noise and respiratory distress).
- Examine the previous anaesthetic chart—check the tracheal tube size used, grade at laryngoscopy, and analgesia administered. In a significant proportion of cases a flexible LMA may have been used rather than intubation; these patients require careful assessment to detect risks of difficult intubation.
- If thiopental was used in the original anaesthetic within the last 24h, reduce the induction dose to account for residual drug.

Perioperative

These are difficult cases: seek senior anaesthetic help early.

- Prepare standard equipment plus:
  - Selection of tracheal tube sizes.
  - Selection of laryngoscope blades (e.g. videolaryngoscopes if experienced in their use).
  - Two wide-bore suction catheters: checked and turned on.
  - Rescue devices and difficult intubation aids.
- ENT surgeon in the operating room, scrubbed, assisted, and ready with all instruments.
- The safest anaesthetic technique for a bleeding tonsil has been debated for many years. Options include:
  - RSI (generally favoured).
  - Inhalational induction in the left lateral, head-down position.

Rapid sequence induction

Pros

- Supine position.
- Familiar technique.
- Enables rapid airway protection.
- Less stressful for the anxious patient.
- Familiar position for rescue techniques (SAD, front of neck).

Cons

- Adequate preoxygenation may be impossible.
- Laryngoscopy may be difficult if bleeding is profuse.
- Risk of hypoxia if intubation is difficult and spontaneous ventilation has been lost.

Inhalational induction

Pros

- Oxygenation maintained during spontaneous ventilation.
- Blood drains from the airway by gravity.
- May allow more time for laryngoscopy if bleeding is excessive (because they are preoxygenated).
- Suxamethonium may be given prior to intubation (left-lateral or turned supine).

Cons

- Often takes longer.
- Technique unfamiliar to many.
- Technically demanding.
- Risks of laryngospasm during light anaesthesia.
- Risks of aspiration of blood while deepening anaesthesia.

Whichever technique is used, always have a back-up plan—use of a supra-glottic airway that is easy to insert, seals the airway well and protects from regurgitation and aspiration (e.g. ProSeal® LMA, perhaps i-gel®, Supreme® LMA) is a logical part of plan B.

- A smaller tracheal tube than used first time is strongly recommended.
- In children consider using a small cuffed tracheal tube.
- Use controlled ventilation to improve conditions for haemostasis.

- Avoid hypotension as may prevent identification of bleeding points.
- Further fluid and blood should be given guided by clinical signs. Near patient testing of haemoglobin concentration can be useful.
- Consider steroids if oedema present or likely.
- Pass a wide-bore gastric tube under direct vision to empty the stomach.
- Careful suction of the oropharynx and nasopharynx under direct vision at the end of the procedure.
- Ensure full reversal of neuromuscular blockade before extubation.
- Extubate fully awake in the left lateral position.
- If adenoidal bleeding, a nasopharyngeal pack may be left *in situ*.

Postoperative

- Extended recovery with close monitoring for recurrence of bleeding.
- Consider omitting NSAIDs postoperatively. Discuss with surgeon.
- Check the haemoglobin concentration.

Further reading

The Royal College of Surgeons of England. *National Prospective Tonsillectomy Audit 2003*. London: The Royal College of Surgeons of England, 2005. Available at: http://www.rcseng.ac.uk

Severe epistaxis

Key points
- There are local and systemic causes and contributors.
- Consider hypovolaemia.
- High risk of aspiration.
- Laryngoscopy may be difficult.
- Co-morbidities are common in the elderly.

Background
Epistaxis is common, but results in massive bleeding only rarely. Occurring most commonly in men, it has a bimodal distribution of age (<10 and >50 years). It usually follows trauma to the nose but predisposing conditions include:
- Bleeding disorders.
- Hereditary telangiectasia.
- Raised venous pressures.
- Nasal intubation/airway passage especially if no vasoconstrictors used.

Nasal bleeding occurs from:
- Veins of nasal septum (younger patients).
- Anterior nasal cavity—arterial anastomoses of the lower nasal septum, Little's area (older patients, often associated with hypertension).
- Posterior nasal cavity—branches of sphenopalatine artery (rare).

Usually managed conservatively with nasal packing and cautery. May rarely require ligation of the maxillary (via the nose) and/or anterior ethmoidal artery (via the mouth/neck).

Preoperative
- Whilst bleeding from the anterior nasal cavity is obvious, posterior bleeding may be insidious and often concealed because it has been swallowed.
- Assessment of cardiovascular status and fluid resuscitation are vital.
- Actively seek signs of hypovolaemia.
- Assess co-morbidities: pay particular attention to cardiovascular fitness and medications—many elderly patients are on warfarin and have associated hypertension and ischaemic heart disease.
- Identify patients with hereditary telangiectasia: though rare, these patients have ↑ risk of bleeding from airway manipulation and elsewhere.
- Check Hb, coagulation, and crossmatch.
- ECG and biochemistry as indicated by individual patients.
- Large-bore IV access.
- Fluids and blood products as required.
- Consider rapid reversal of coagulopathy with vitamin K, FFP, or prothrombin complex concentrate. Tranexamic acid may have a role.
- Actively assess for signs of airway difficulty.

Intraoperative

- Management reflects the bleeding tonsil (see 📖 Bleeding tonsil, p.162).
- Seek senior anaesthetic help early.
- Prepare standard equipment plus:
  - Selection of small tracheal tubes.
  - Selection of laryngoscope blades (e.g. videolaryngoscopes if experienced).
  - Two wide-bore suction catheters (checked and turned on).
  - Equipment for back-up plan.
- If severe ongoing bleeding the ENT surgeon should be in the operating room, scrubbed, assisted, and ready with all instruments.
- Similar to the bleeding tonsil, the anaesthetic technique depends on individual experience and choice. Options include:
  - RSI.
  - Inhalational induction in the left lateral, head-down position.
- Laryngoscopy may be difficult if bleeding is brisk—always have a back-up plan.
- The nose is usually packed, producing obstruction of the nasal airway.
- Nasal vasoconstrictors often applied (local anaesthetic/adrenaline/ cocaine/Moffett's solution): may have systemic side effects, especially in excessive doses.
- Controlled ventilation to improve conditions for haemostasis.
- Avoid hypotension as it may prevent identification of bleeding points.
- Give further fluid and blood guided by clinical signs. Near patient testing of Hb concentration can be useful.
- Pass a wide-bore gastric tube under direct vision to empty the stomach.
- Carefully suck blood out of the oropharynx and nasopharynx under direct vision at the end of the procedure ('Coroner's clot' behind the soft palate).
- Ensure full reversal of neuromuscular blockade before extubation.
- Extubate fully awake in the left lateral position. Exchange to a SAD at the end of surgery prior to waking the patient may be appropriate for smooth emergence.

Postoperative

- Sit up as soon as awake to reduce bleeding.
- Extended recovery with close monitoring to detect recurrence of bleeding.
- Nasal packs are likely to be left *in situ* and prevent nasal breathing.
- Check Hb concentration and coagulation.
- Avoid NSAIDs postoperatively. Pain is rarely a problem.

Emergency oesophagoscopy

Key points
- The shared airway may challenge the anaesthetist and surgeon.
- There is a risk of regurgitation and pulmonary aspiration.
- Be careful with cricoid pressure or avoid it.
- There is a risk of oesophageal perforation.

Background

Emergency oesophagoscopy is usually performed in the context of an ingested foreign body. Removal often requires general anaesthesia and rigid oesophagoscopy. Flexible fibreoptic oesophagoscopy under light sedation may be an alternative.

Preoperative

- History of indigestion, dysphagia (difficulty swallowing) and odynophagia (pain on swallowing).
- Impaction may occur at any point of physiological or pathological narrowing; most commonly at the level of the cricopharyngeus muscle but also the aortic arch, left main stem bronchus, or diaphragmatic hiatus.
- Commonly found in:
  - Children.
  - High-risk adults, e.g. prisoners, alcoholics, those with learning difficulties or psychiatric illness.
  - Elderly edentulous patients who are unable to chew food fully and who may have underlying pathological oesophageal narrowing or out-pouches (webs, tumours, pouches).
- Rarely may be retained for many years and present with a fistula.
- Obstructive lesions can result in proximal oesophageal dilation.
- Recurrent obstruction and aspiration may precipitate laryngeal oedema, asthma, and chronic chest infection
- Assess carefully for signs of malnutrition, dehydration, and malignancy, as well as risks of regurgitation, aspiration, and low-grade chest infections.

Intraoperative

- Correct dehydration and electrolyte abnormalities.
- Consider antisialagogue if excess secretions.
- IV induction with suxamethonium for rapid control of the airway.
- RSI is generally appropriate but avoid cricoid pressure if foreign body is sharp or in the upper oesophagus.
- Secure the tracheal tube carefully.
- Tape tracheal tube to the left to enable easier access for the endoscopist.
- Ensure adequate depth of anaesthesia and good muscle relaxation:
  - Highly stimulating procedure.

- Aids passage of the oesophagoscope through the cricopharyngeal sphincter (may be impeded by vertebral osteophytes and neck stiffness).
- Proximity of major blood vessels.
- Reduces the risk of perforation.
- Watch for damage to the teeth (consider mouth guard) and compression of the tracheal tube.
- Over-inflated tracheal tube cuff may exacerbate difficulties in passing the endoscope and temporary deflation may be necessary.
- Use of short-acting muscle relaxants and opioids enables rapid return of muscle power and upper airway reflexes.
- Observe endoscopy throughout, particularly at removal, because there is a risk of tracheal tube displacement.
- Ensure pharynx cleared of debris and blood and extubate fully awake in the lateral position or sitting fully upright.

Postoperative
- Routine postoperative care.
- High index of suspicion for oesophageal perforation.
- If suspected:
  - Withhold oral intake and maintain IV fluids.
  - Observe closely for features of mediastinitis—chest pain, pyrexia, and surgical emphysema.
  - IV antibiotics.

Maxillofacial Emergencies

Facial trauma

Key points
- Facial trauma can be associated with airway problems and massive haemorrhage.
- Patients can have other injuries, e.g. head injury.

Background
- The anaesthetist may be involved in the initial resuscitation of the patient with facial trauma and later for repair of facial soft tissue injuries or fractures.
- The incidence of facial fractures has ↓ with use of seat belts and airbags. The main cause now is assault in young males (80% of all cases) and is often associated with alcohol.
- ▶ Unless there is acute airway compromise or uncontrolled haemorrhage, surgery for facial fractures is often delayed until other injuries have been treated, and swelling has subsided. Surgery is as for other fractures including reduction and internal fixation. Lacerations of the face should be cleaned and sutured within 12 h.
- Facial fractures occur along lines of weakness of the facial bones and are classified according to anatomy and displacement: mandibular, midface, orbital.
- Mandibular fractures: vary in incidence and site. 35% occur at the condylar neck. Airway obstruction may occur because of posterior displacement of the anterior insertion of the tongue in bilateral mandibular fractures.
- Midface fractures are classified according to Le Fort fracture lines:
  - *Le Fort I fractures* may be unilateral or bilateral and pass transversely through the maxilla. Posterior displacement of the inferior portion of the maxilla may obstruct the nasopharynx.
  - *Le Fort II fractures* are usually bilateral and extend in a pyramidal fashion to include the maxilla, orbital floor, nasal bridge, and lacrimal bones.
  - *Le Fort III fractures* result in craniofacial dissociation, extending posteriorly from the bridge of the nose, through the orbit and the zygomatic arch.
- Le Fort II and III fractures are associated with cribriform plate fracture resulting in dural tears and CSF leakage. CSF leak often resolves with fracture fixation. Persistent CSF leak needs lumbar CSF drainage or neurosurgical repair.
- Patients may also have significant soft tissue injuries and broken teeth.
- Major haemorrhage can occur if there are tears of the terminal branches of the maxillary artery (will require nasal packing—packs can cause airway obstruction), or tears of the inferior alveolar artery associated with mandibular fracture (will require reduction and fixation of fracture).
- Facial injuries are often associated with underlying head injury and a risk of cervical spine injury. Any CT imaging should include the head and cervical spine. Alcohol intoxication may make neurological assessment difficult.

- Strategies to prevention secondary brain injury must be used in patients with traumatic brain injury (see 📖 Traumatic brain injury, p.98).

Preoperative

Airway assessment

Knowledge of the mechanism of injury should be sought to predict any potential problems with establishing a definitive airway in addition to the likelihood of associated injuries. The presence/absence of the following features should be determined:

- *Airway obstruction*—may be present due to several factors including: disruption of normal facial/upper airway anatomy; presence of teeth, blood, vomit, or other foreign bodies; ↓ conscious level due to head injury, drugs (self-administered or iatrogenic), or alcohol intoxication. Patients who are conscious will tend to self-position for optimum airway patency.
- *Uncooperative patients*—are unlikely to tolerate airway techniques that require cooperation. Lack of cooperation may be due to associated head injury, drug or alcohol effects, pain, or hypoxia.
- *Risk of gastric aspiration*—a full stomach is highly likely in any trauma patient and standard anaesthetic precautions should be undertaken (RSI with cricoid pressure, awake fibreoptic intubation) to prevent this.
- *Disruption of normal facial anatomy*—often leads to problems with obtaining an adequate seal around an anaesthetic facemask. Oropharyngeal and nasopharyngeal airway devices may be ineffective or contraindicated. Mandibular fractures can cause ↓ mouth opening because of pain and trismus. Mouth opening is usually possible after induction of anaesthesia.
- *Cervical spine protection*—must be ensured before, during, and following securing the airway. Manual in-line stabilization should be used. This is likely to increase the difficulty of laryngoscopy.

Discuss with the surgeon airway access and type of tube (oral, nasal, submental, tracheostomy) needed to enable surgery.

Intraoperative

- Adequate preoxygenation followed by RSI with cricoid pressure remains the technique of choice in trauma patients provided laryngoscopy is not predicted to be impossible. Ensure the presence of an experienced anaesthetist who is familiar with the difficult airway adjuncts that are immediately available.
- A back-up plan must be considered if securing the airway proves impossible, together with appropriate equipment and skills for surgical access to the airway and emergency oxygenation (± ventilation).
- If traditional laryngoscopy is predicted to be impossible, use an alternative technique to secure the airway. This may be inhalational induction, awake fibreoptic intubation, and tracheostomy insertion under LA. All these techniques will be difficult in patients with severe facial trauma, particularly if they are uncooperative. The choice of technique is dependant on the experience and skills of the senior anaesthetist present.

- Depending on the type of surgery being performed the original airway device securing the airway may need to be changed to allow surgical access. The options available are fibreoptic nasal intubation, tracheostomy insertion, or submental intubation (the tracheal tube is passed through the floor of the mouth).
- Prevention of secondary brain injury must be considered intraoperatively (normocapnia, avoidance of hypotension and hypoxaemia, head-up tilt).
- Consider prophylactic antibiotics in association with local microbiological protocols and advice.
- Use short-acting anaesthetic and analgesic drugs (e.g. remifentanil), to enable rapid emergence and establishment of airway reflexes after surgery.
- Use a multimodal analgesic technique to avoid large doses of opioids. NSAIDs are particularly useful provided there are no contraindications.
- Consider giving anti-emetic drugs, particularly for patients who have received opioids and/or are likely to have swallowed blood.
- Most patients can be extubated at the end of surgery provided there are no indications for prolonged sedation and ventilation (e.g. severe head injury, acute lung injury, further surgical intervention required in patients with multiple trauma).
- Airway problems occur at extubation with the same frequency as at intubation.
- Ensure appropriate equipment and drugs are immediately available should emergency re-intubation is needed.
- Nasal tubes can be left in until the patient is awake.

Postoperative

- For moderate or severe injuries, patients should receive HDU care unless prolonged ventilation and sedation is required.
- Paracetamol and NSAIDs (if not contraindicated) are usually sufficient for analgesia.
- Sequential GCS assessment is essential in awake patients with an associated head injury.

Further reading

Chesshire NJ, Knight DJ. The anaesthetic management of facial fractures. *Br J Anaesth CEPD Rev* 2001; **1**(4):108–12.
Curran JE. Anaesthesia for facial trauma. *Anaesth Intens Care Med* 2005; **6**(8):258–62.

Dental abscess

Key points
- The patient is usually in severe pain; may be exhausted, dehydrated, and septic—possibly unable to swallow saliva, drinks, or food.
- Careful airway assessment necessary, but may be restricted by pain.
- Trismus (inability to fully open the mouth) is common and may not relax on induction.
- Progression to Ludwig's angina may occur.
- Assume that airway management will be difficult and ensure appropriate equipment and skills are available.
- If circumstances permit, involve an experienced airway anaesthetist.
- Extubation is also potentially hazardous.

Background
- A dental abscess is an acute lesion characterized by localization of pus in the structures that surround the teeth. Pus initially collects around dental roots resulting in severe bony pain. The abscess may rupture into surrounding tissues where it can produce pain, swelling, and erythema of the face, which may extend to the neck. Trismus may develop.
- Ludwig's angina is a rapidly spreading acute cellulitis of the soft tissues and floor of the mouth, which can develop as a result of a dental infection. Although it begins unilaterally, it quickly develops into a bilateral brawny oedema of the suprahyoid region of the neck. The tongue becomes elevated and displaced posteriorly, leading to airway compromise, especially in the supine position.

Differential diagnosis of trismus with facial swelling
Pericoronitis of wisdom teeth—infection in tissue pocket surrounding a partially erupted wisdom tooth, tonsillar abscess or quinsy, granulomas, fractured jaw, or other intraoral trauma, lymphoma, parotiditis (infection, stone or mumps), tuberculosis, tetanus.

Management of dental abscess
The symptoms and signs of dental abscess vary markedly in severity; only the very worst will require hospital surgical intervention. Initial dental management will usually have included antibiotics and mouthwashes. The infection may be associated with recent dental procedures such as root filling. The urgency of surgery will depend on level of airway compromise, and patient's condition.

Preoperative
- Take a history and determine progression of symptoms. Evaluate previous anaesthetic records, especially if previous maxillofacial surgery.
- Airway assessment, especially mouth opening—Mallampati and gape may be obscured. Assess severity of facial/neck swelling—neck movement may be reduced.
- Look at any scans that are available.
- Stridor or voice change may indicate tongue or laryngeal swelling.

- Check for signs of dehydration/systemic infection—IV access and rehydrate as required.
- Make operating room staff and surgeon aware of potential for airway difficulty. Involve senior anaesthetist experienced and familiar with planned airway management techniques. Discuss airway plans and back-up plans with anaesthetic assistant and surgeon. Ensure difficult airway trolley available (see also 📖 Acute airway obstruction, p.156 and 📖 Failed tracheal intubation, p.356).
- Surgical airway may be difficult in patients with anterior neck swelling.

Intraoperative

- Induce anaesthesia in head-up position.
- Pre-oxygenate for at least 3 min.
- The technique for securing the airway used in any individual case will depend upon the clinical presentation of the patient, together with the skill and experience of the anaesthetists. Back-up plans are essential in case of failure of first-choice technique. Options available:
  - IV induction—can be used if no evidence of airway compromise. If history of trismus is present for <72 h, jaw will usually relax on induction. This can never be guaranteed, especially with longer histories.
  - Gas induction.
  - Awake fibreoptic intubation—the patient is likely to be distressed, in pain, and unable to swallow. LA may be difficult to establish in the presence of infection. Reserve for patients with evidence of airway compromise. Ensure anaesthetist confident with technique.
- Confirm correct airway placement: capnography, auscultate bilaterally to ensure good air entry with patient in surgical position. Secure airway and connections firmly—ensure position of tracheal tube to enable surgical access to mouth and neck. Protect patient's eyes.
- Maintain anaesthesia with vapour or IV propofol.
- Give IV antibiotics—seek microbiology advice especially for those patients who have already been on antibiotics.
- If surgeon unable to drain pus, ensure biopsies taken to look for lymphoma, infection, or granulomas.
- Record details of intubation clearly on anaesthetic chart in case of need to return to the operating room.
- Consider nasogastric tube placement for feeding if postoperative swallowing problems anticipated.
- Extubation can be more hazardous than intubation. The potential for airway compromise remains. Ensure equipment and personnel available for reintubation should the need arise. Consider placing catheter before extubation to enable reintubation if problems occur. Extubate awake. Ensure neuromuscular blockade fully reversed (may be short procedure). Head-up position. Ensure leak around tube before removal. Consider dexamethasone (4–8 mg IV) to help decrease airway oedema.
- If concerns about airway oedema, consider delayed extubation and transfer to ICU sedated. Return to operating room for extubation with surgical team present if necessary.

Postoperative
- Assess need for ICU/HDU/close monitoring on specialist head and neck ward depending on airway difficulty and potential for worsening of condition.
- Nurse head-up.
- Continue regular antibiotics based on microbiology advice.

Cardiovascular Emergencies

Emergency abdominal aortic aneurysm repair

Key points

- A ruptured abdominal aortic aneurysm (AAA) requires immediate surgery to control bleeding and has a high mortality.
- At least two anaesthetists are needed.
- Emergency endovascular repair is becoming increasingly common.
- Postoperative ICU is needed to treat complications of bleeding, and ischaemia-reperfusion injury.

Background

AAAs are common, with 7–8% prevalence in men aged >65 years. Ideally, patients with AAA should be identified and considered for treatment before rupture. In the UK, ~5000 patients die of ruptured AAA per year.

Presentation

The classic triad of a ruptured AAA is abdominal or back pain, hypotension, and a pulsatile abdominal mass. There may be minimal cardiovascular instability or complete cardiovascular collapse depending on the type of leak and extent of blood loss. The mortality of patients with a ruptured AAA surviving to hospital admission is as high as 50%. Patients should be treated by vascular specialists, even if this requires transfer to another hospital.

Preoperative

- There is limited time to optimize or investigate the patient and expedient assessment of the patient is required. Co-morbidities and prior functional capacity, as well as current cardiovascular state are relevant to the decision to proceed for operative repair.
- Several scoring systems (e.g. Hardman index) are available to help clinicians identify those patients who are unlikely to benefit from intervention.

Hardman index

Score 1 point for each of the following:

- Age >76 years.
- Loss of consciousness after presentation.
- Creatinine >190 µmol L^{-1}.
- Haemoglobin <9 g dL^{-1}.
- Acute myocardial ischaemia. (Depressed ST segments > 1 mm and/or T wave changes.)

Score of 3 or more is associated with a 100% mortality in most series.

Data from Hardman DTA, Fisher CM, Patel MI, et al. Ruptured abdominal aortic aneurysms: Who should be offered surgery? J Vasc Surg 1996; **23**:123–9.

- Significant co-morbidities associated with ruptured AAA include: coronary artery disease, impaired ventricular function, hypertension, renal impairment, diabetes mellitus, and smoking-related chest disease.
- If significant cardiovascular collapse, immediate transfer to the operating room is required. In most patients there is time to perform CT angiography to confirm the diagnosis and assess the morphology of the AAA. This requires patient monitoring and accompanying personnel as collapse may occur. Minimize rolling and moving of the patient.

Initial resuscitation of collapsed patient

- Permissive hypotension—allow limited fluid resuscitation with crystalloid or colloid to maintain organ perfusion (MAP 60 mmHg) but avoid aggressive fluid resuscitation to achieve a higher BP as this may exacerbate blood loss by raising BP, disrupting clot and causing dilutional coagulopathy.
- A blood sample should be sent to the blood bank so that at least 6 units of group confirmed RBCs and FFP 15 mL kg^{-1} can be sent to the operating room.
- Get help—senior input is needed and two anaesthetists.

Intraoperative

Procedure

- Ruptured AAA is generally treated by open repair via midline laparotomy requiring aortic cross-clamping and insertion of a graft to bypass the aneurysmal segment of aorta.
▶ The immediate goal is control of haemorrhage by the surgeon cross-clamping the aorta.
- It is possible to perform endovascular repair of a ruptured AAA (EVAR) in centres equipped with the necessary expertise and infrastructure. 80% of ruptured AAA may be anatomically suitable for EVAR. There appears to be a survival benefit with EVAR; however, this has not been proven in a randomized trial.

Induction of anaesthesia

- Induction of anaesthesia results in loss of abdominal tone, which can exacerbate intra-abdominal bleeding. The patient should therefore be induced once the surgeon is scrubbed and the abdomen is prepared and draped.
- Ideally use a 5-lead ECG with CM5 positioning to enable best assessment of myocardial ischaemia.
- Poor peripheral perfusion may make pulse oximetry unreliable.
- Invasive BP monitoring is ideal. Do not delay induction for arterial access if the patient is unstable. Put arms out on boards for access.
- Have warmed fluids pressurized and ready to run through a large-bore IV cannulae.
- RSI with a high dose of opioid and small dose of induction drug is an appropriate technique. Ketamine will provide greater cardiovascular stability. Have vasopressors, inotropes, and vasodilators drawn up— you will need them!
- Patient instability, time constraints, and active bleeding almost always prevent the use of RA.

Maintenance of anaesthesia

- Volatile anaesthetics provide cardioprotection against ischaemia. Isoflurane has the most evidence for cardioprotection. Desflurane may be associated with less diastolic dysfunction during ischaemia compared with sevoflurane, but should be avoided in concentrations >1.5 MAC because of ↑ sympathetic activity.
- Establish invasive arterial and central venous monitoring if not already in place.

Cardiovascular

- Once the cross-clamp is in place initiate aggressive fluid resuscitation using warmed, pressurized fluid (e.g. Level 1 system). Crystalloid or colloid fluid replacement is suitable initially, but blood products are required early to replace Hb and clotting factors.
- Aim for normotension and adequate fluid resuscitation with cross-clamp in place. CVP is commonly used as a marker of cardiac filling but may be unreliable. Consider non-invasive cardiac output monitoring.
- Noradrenaline may be the initial vasopressor of choice to increase the systemic vascular resistance (SVR) because, despite the cross-clamp, these patients often have significant collateral blood flow. Adrenaline may increase myocardial oxygen demand significantly.
- Risk of intraoperative myocardial ischaemia is high because of coronary artery disease, hypotension, anaemia, and cross-clamping. Consider IV nitrate infusion if signs of ischaemia present on ECG.
- ABG analysis is helpful to monitor adequacy of resuscitation (improving lactate and metabolic acidosis).

Haematological

- Early use of blood products and plasma can restore circulating volume and correct anaemia and coagulopathy. Use O-negative or group specific blood if fully cross-matched not immediately available.
- Intraoperative red cell salvage reduces use of bank blood. The cell saver collecting system needs to be set up and ready to use when surgery starts.
- Use near patient testing of haemoglobin (HemoCue® or ABG analysis). Aim for a target Hb ≥10 g L^{-1}.
- Near-patient testing of coagulation (thromboelastography) is ideal but rarely available in the UK. Laboratory testing of clotting, including INR, fibrinogen, and platelets is therefore used but will give delayed results. Give plasma, cryoprecipitate, and platelets guided by the clinical situation and results when available (see ▢ Transfusion, p.20 and ▢ Coagulopathy, p.130).

Other intraoperative issues

- Hypothermia caused by fluid resuscitation and patient exposure can exacerbate coagulopathy. Use upper body forced-air warming and warmed fluid. Do not warm the lower limbs this can exacerbate peripheral ischaemia.
- A urinary catheter with hourly monitoring is essential. A suprarenal clamp will cause kidney injury from acute ischaemia but even an infrarenal clamp will reduce renal blood flow via the renin–angiotensin–aldosterone system.

Removal of aortic cross-clamp
- This can result in marked hypotension because of a reduction in the SVR, sequestration of blood in reperfused organs, and release of vasoactive cytokines and metabolites from ischaemic tissues which directly depress the myocardium.
- Ensure the patient is intravascularly filled and cardiovascularly stable before cross-clamp release.
- ▶ Good communication with surgeon is essential—the cross-clamp may be released slowly or even replaced temporarily if needed.
- Increase minute ventilation to remove additional CO_2 generated by acidotic blood returning from the legs. Give vasopressors. Additional fluid filling may be required.

Anaesthesia for EVAR
- Patients are resuscitated and prepared as previously described and anaesthesia is performed with an equivalent technique and monitoring in case of conversion to open repair.
- RA is not used because of haemodynamic compromise, coagulopathy, and time constraints; however, it may be possible to perform some cases under LA alone.
- Access is achieved via the femoral artery.
- An aortic occlusion balloon may be required if the patient is cardiovascularly unstable.

Postoperative
- If the blood loss has been limited and the patient is warm, with minimal acidosis and inotrope requirement, extubation may be appropriate. However most patients are likely to be hypothermic, acidotic, and require significant cardiovascular support—these patients should remain ventilated.
- All patients require transfer to ICU for further care. Patients are at high risk of respiratory and kidney failure and may have a prolonged ICU stay.
- Monitor lower limbs for signs of ischaemia.

Further reading
Howard-Alpe G, Stoneham M. Anaesthesia for vascular emergencies. *Anaesth Intens Care Med* 2010; **11**:187–90.

Metha M. Endovascular aneurysm repair for ruptured abdominal aortic aneurysm: How I do it. *J Vasc Surg* 2010; **52**:1706–12.

Moll FL, Powell JT, Fraedrich G, et al. Management of abdominal aortic aneurysms clinical practice guidelines of the European society for vascular surgery. *Eur J Vasc Endovasc Surg* 2011; **41**(Suppl. 1):S1–S58.

Telford RJ. Anaesthesia for abdominal vascular surgery. *Anaesth Intens Care Med* 2010; **11**:174–8.

Carotid endarterectomy

Key points
- GA or LA can be used.
- Perioperative control of BP is important to minimize risk of further stroke.

Background
- In the UK, the National Stroke Strategy recommends carotid endarterectomy (CEA) is performed within 48 h of a transient ischaemic attack (TIA) or minor stroke if the patient is neurologically stable. As such, CEA is becoming a vascular emergency.
- CEA reduces the incidence of fatal and disabling stroke in patients with carotid stenosis. Symptomatic patients present with TIA, or stroke, or transient mono-ocular blindness. It is now recognized that further neurological events occur generally within days or weeks of initial symptoms. In some high-risk groups the risk of further stroke may be as high as 12% at 1 week; therefore, the sooner a patient undergoes CEA after symptoms, the greater the benefit.
- The benefits of CEA can be realized only if the mortality and morbidity of the procedure are low. The combined risk of stroke, death, or myocardial infarction (MI) following CEA is around 5% (GALA trial).

Procedure
Exposure of the internal, external, and common carotid is achieved by an incision along the anterior border of sternocleidomastoid. Following systemic heparinization and arterial control, endarterectomy is performed. Adjunctive shunting may be required.

Indications
- Symptomatic patients with a >50% internal carotid stenosis (North American Symptomatic Carotid Endarterectomy Trial (NASCET) criteria) benefit from CEA.
- There is more benefit for greater degrees of stenosis, but there is no benefit for occlusion or subocclusion: 50–69% stenosis—7.8% absolute risk reduction (ARR) at 5 years; 70–99% stenosis—15.6% ARR at 5 years.

Preoperative
- Patients are in general, elderly arteriopaths. 2/3 are hypertensive and many will have diabetes, ischaemic heart disease, and cardiac failure. 50% of deaths following CEA are related to the cardiovascular system.
- Quantify cardiovascular and respiratory disease—this should include an assessment of exercise tolerance.
- Uncontrolled hypertension may be problematic but acute BP control may not be beneficial.
- Document any neurological deficits.
- Assess the patient's ability to lie flat and still if 'awake' CEA is planned.
- Measure the BP in both arms—use the higher of the two for intraoperative comparison.
- Blood loss is often minimal, but a group and screen sample should be taken.

Intraoperative

- The GALA trial showed little difference in outcome whether CEA is performed under GA or LA. The decision will take into account surgical, anaesthetic and patient factors/preferences.
- Arterial line—ideally in the ipsilateral arm—to allow function testing in the contralateral arm.
- Cerebral monitoring techniques are sometimes used with GA.
- Ensure vasoactive drugs available (vasopressors and beta-blockers).
- Maintain systolic BP (SBP) within 20% of baseline.
- Cross-clamping may result in marked hypertension and this should not be reduced aggressively.
- Use of LA blocks if using a GA may improve intraoperative fluctuations.

General anaesthesia

- Careful induction—haemodynamic instability compromises cerebral blood flow.
- Most anaesthetists use a tracheal tube because of inaccessibility of the airway and the possibility of the cuff from a laryngeal mask reducing carotid blood flow.
- Maintain normocarbia.
- A remifentanil/propofol technique gives rapid waking without coughing and has beneficial effects for cerebral blood flow.

Local anaesthesia

Blockade of the C2–C4 dermatomes is required for adequate anaesthesia. Even with a 'perfect' block, ~50% of patients will require supplementary LA. Previously, both superficial and deep cervical plexus blocks have been used. Meta-analyses show that the rate of conversion to GA and complications with a superficial cervical plexus block are less than with deep block.

Superficial cervical plexus block

- Prior full explanation to the patient is essential.
- Patient should empty bladder just prior to surgery. Give only enough fluid to replace losses.
- Remifentanil/propofol sedation can be used during block placement.
- The patient's head should be turned to the contralateral side.
- Draw a line from the mastoid process to the tuberosity of the transverse process of C6. At the midpoint between these two landmarks, insert a 22-G needle and inject 10–15 mL 0.5% bupivacaine in a fan across the posterior border of sternocleidomastoid (SCM).
- Infiltration along the jaw line will help with pain from the retractor.
- Supplementary LA is usually required for dissection around the carotid sheath.
- Give supplementary oxygen, ensure patient is comfortably positioned and surgical drapes/screen do not make patient claustrophobic. Have someone hold the patient's hand.

Monitoring cerebral function

Monitor the patient's cerebration, speech and contralateral limb function.

A change in cerebral function is an indication for shunt placement. Neurological recovery should take place rapidly after shunt placement. GA is indicated only for airway compromise and not for neuroprotection which has been advocated in the past. Maintaining BP above baseline may also improve cerebral blood flow via collateral vessels.

Postoperative

- Observe the patient closely with invasive BP monitoring for 2–4 h in the postanaesthesia care unit.
- Complications include airway oedema (5–10%) and neck haematoma.
- If re-exploration is indicated, GA is often required.
- If the patient develops new neurological symptoms, obtain an urgent surgical review in case a return to the operating room is required.
- Haemodynamic instability can occur. Hypotension predisposes to cerebral ischaemia. Maintain SBP >90 mmHg. Fluids and vasoconstrictors are useful. Hypertension may cause hyperperfusion syndrome; an area of brain previously not exposed to high arterial pressures (due to a carotid stenosis) is now subjected to these. Symptoms are of headaches and ultimately neurological deficit. Ideally maintain SBP <140 mmHg. Beta-blockers and calcium channel blockers reduce systolic pressure without affecting cerebral blood flow.

Further reading

Department of Health. National Stroke Strategy. London: DH, 2007. Available at: ℜ http://www.dh.gov.uk/en/Publicationsandstatistics/Publications/PublicationsPolicyAndGuidance/DH_081062.

GALA Trial Collaborative Group. General anaesthesia vs local anaesthesia for carotid surgery (GALA): a multicentre, randomized controlled trial. *Lancet* 2008; **372**:2132–42.

Howell SJ. Carotid endarterectomy. *Br J Anaesth* 2007; **99**:119–31.

Stoneham M. Anaesthetic techniques for carotid surgery. *Anaesth Intens Care Med* 2010; **11**:184–6.

Stoneham MD, Thompson JP. Blood pressure management and carotid endarterectomy. *Br J Anaesth* 2009; **102**:442–52.

Emergency limb revascularization

Key points
- Patients have a high risk of cardiovascular disease and postoperative cardiac complication.
- There is limited time for investigation and optimization when the patient has an acutely ischaemic limb.
- Patients often require perioperative anticoagulation.

Background
- Acute limb-threatening ischaemia may be caused by thrombosis (atherosclerotic plaque, peripheral aneurysm, previous bypass graft, hypercoagulable states), embolism, or intimal dissection.
- The aetiology of the ischaemia influences the *type* of intervention; however, the *urgency* of intervention is dependent on the severity of the lower limb ischaemia.

Procedure
An embolism can usually be managed by thromboembolectomy, whilst most other causes require some form of bypass. If there is time to obtain vascular imaging before revascularization there is likely to be a clear operative plan; if not, both surgeon and anaesthetist must be flexible as a procedure could start with simple embolectomy and may finish with a bypass. Communication between the anaesthetist and vascular specialist is key. The following should be discussed:

Urgency
A patient presenting with a potentially salvageable acutely ischaemic limb, in whom there is both sensory and motor loss should undergo revascularization at the earliest opportunity, without delaying for preoperative arterial imaging.

Heparin
Most patients will usually be systemically anticoagulated with unfractionated IV heparin, *contraindicating neuroaxial blockade*. Determine whether this should be continued postoperatively.

Operative plan
- Thromboembolectomy—what is the site of incision? The usual sites are groin (femoral), medial calf (popliteal), or antecubital fossa (brachial). What is the next step if thromboembolectomy fails? This may include on-table angiography, bypass distal to the initial incision, or bypass to allow adequate inflow from above the initial incision.
- Bypass operations—bypass from where to where? What type of conduit is going to be used (prosthetic or autologous vein)? A bypass using prosthetic material requires only two incisions to expose the inflow and target vessels. Alternatively, a bypass using autologous material may require incisions in the ipsilateral leg, the contralateral leg, and/or the arm to obtain adequate vein.
- Fasciotomies—what is the likelihood that a fasciotomy will be required?

- Once these issues have been clarified it should be clear which patients can have a procedure performed using LA infiltration, which patients may subsequently need GA and which patients will definitely require GA.

Preoperative

The mortality rate following peripheral limb revascularization may be as high as 25%. The risks are highest in the elderly, those with proximal (aortic) disease or a history of angina, congestive cardiac failure, or a recent MI. Assessment and optimization are limited by the need to proceed quickly to salvage a limb.

- Do not delay for starvation—use a RSI if GA indicated.
- Take a detailed cardiorespiratory history—only 8% of these patients will have normal coronary arteries, 60% will have significant coronary artery stenosis
- Atrial fibrillation—aim for rate control or consider cardioversion if acute onset.
- In emergency cases do not delay surgery for prolonged cardiovascular investigation.
- Assess for risk of size of reperfusion injury—size of ischaemic area and ischaemic time period.
- Embolectomy requires a 'group and screen' sample and bypass cross matching of 2 units of blood.

Intraoperative

- Have a low threshold for arterial line insertion.
- Acidosis, hyperkalaemia, renal impairment, arrhythmias, and myocardial depression can occur on limb reperfusion.
- Insert lines in the contralateral arm for axillobifemoral grafts.
- Heparin bolus (3000–5000 units) may be required on clamping.
- Cardiac output monitoring could be considered in high-risk patients for bypass surgery.

Postoperative

- Oral analgesics are usually sufficient for pain relief after embolectomy. Opioids may be required for bypass procedures.
- Monitor renal function, serum potassium, acid–base, and myoglobin.
- Fasciotomies are associated with ↑ blood and fluid loss—prescribe fluids accordingly.
- Continued anticoagulation is often required.
- Patients will benefit from postoperative HDU care.

Further reading

Tovey G, Thompson JP. Anaesthesia for lower limb revascularisation. *BJA CEACCP* 2005; **5**:89–92.

Lower limb amputation

Key points
- Amputation has a 30-day mortality of 16.8%.

Background
Minor or major lower limb amputations are often performed on non-elective lists and 25% are performed out-of-hours (National Vascular Database). Major lower limb amputation in the UK is associated with a 30-day mortality of 16.8%.

Procedure
- Minor amputation—digital, metatarsal/ray, forefoot. Often performed urgently for sepsis—particularly in the diabetic. Can be life and limb saving.
- Major amputation—below-knee, through-knee, above-knee, or more complex proximal level. May be associated with significant blood loss, especially with chronic venous insufficiency.

Preoperative
- Some independent risk factors for poor outcome after amputation are useful for assessment of preoperative risk: level of amputation (above-knee worse than below-knee), age, female sex, diabetes, hypertension, coronary heart disease, cardiac failure, prior cerebrovascular event, chronic airways disease, renal failure, and malignancy.
- Surgical urgency may limit time available for preoperative optimization. Preoperative investigation of cardiovascular or respiratory disease will need to be guided by the urgency and the patient's condition.
- Some independent predictors of poor outcome after amputation may be modified and should therefore be investigated and treated prior to surgery: haematocrit (>45%), electrolyte disturbances (hypokalaemia), and sepsis.
- Crossmatch blood if major amputation.

Intraoperative
General, neuraxial, or regional anaesthesia may be appropriate for amputation. The significant perioperative mortality and patient co-morbidity associated with amputation requires that these patients receive anaesthetic input similar to that for peripheral revascularization.

Peripheral nerve blocks
Amputations in patients with peripheral arterial disease are most often performed without a tourniquet and this makes minor amputations amenable to RA blocks (digital, ankle, or popliteal block), provided there is no clotting disturbance or sepsis at the site of blockade.

Neuraxial anaesthesia
Spinal or epidural anaesthesia is often used in combination with sedation or GA and this may be beneficial due to:
- Reduction in tachycardia and hypertension associated with the stress response.

- Improved postoperative analgesia.
- Evidence of reduction in postoperative respiratory complications is seen in lower limb revascularization but no evidence is available for amputation.

General anaesthesia

May provide improved cardiovascular stability compared with RA and enables controlled ventilation. A balanced technique with high-dose opioid is ideal. Consider remifentanil infusion.

Postoperative

- High-risk patients benefit from postoperative HDU care.
- Pain after amputation can be severe. Effective postoperative analgesia is imperative in patients undergoing amputation to enable early movement and reduce risk of stump contracture.
- Epidurals—provide excellent analgesia and avoid opioid side effects. There is limited evidence indicating that preoperative placement may reduce phantom limb pain.
- Perineural catheters—continuous infusion of LA via a catheter placed alongside transected nerves (sciatic or tibial) at surgery is a safe and effective method of reducing post operative pain.

Further reading

Feinglass J, Pearce WH, Martin GJ, et al. Postoperative and late survival outcomes after major amputation: findings from the Department of Veterans Affairs National Surgical Quality Improvement Program. Surgery 2001; **130**:21–9.

Emergency coronary artery bypass grafting

Key points
- The perioperative mortality associated with emergency coronary artery bypass grafting (CABG) is eight times more than for elective CABG.
- Patients with decompensated heart failure may require a period of medical optimization before surgery.
- Assess risk factors and optimize those that can be treated without delaying surgery.
- A high-dose opioid technique minimizes perioperative ischaemia and improves perioperative cardiovascular stability.

Background

Perioperative mortality for emergency CABG is increased from <1.0% for patients with stable angina to 8.3% for emergency surgery (defined as operative care provided immediately) and it may be advisable to delay surgical intervention whenever possible. However, in the presence of refractory symptoms, haemodynamic instability, or in patients with ST-elevation myocardial infarction (STEMI), immediate surgical revascularization may be indicated.

Patients aged >70 years (odds ratio (OR) 3.2), with left main stenosis (OR 4.4), or with cardiogenic shock (OR 17.8) are at highest risk of death. Patients transferred directly to the operating room from the cardiac catheter laboratory following failed percutaneous coronary intervention (PCI) have a mortality of 29% (50% of these patients are in shock and 36% have left main stenosis).

Indications for emergency coronary artery bypass grafting
- Unstable acute coronary syndrome, refractory to medical therapy (unsuitable for PCI).
- Failed PCI with evolving disease (e.g. coronary artery dissection).
- In conjunction with acute myocardial disease:
  - Acute mitral regurgitation (secondary to chordae rupture).
  - Infarct ventricular septal defect.
  - Free wall rupture with tamponade.
  - Aortic dissection.

Determining the best window for intervention is challenging. Patients with decompensated heart failure may require a period of medical optimization before surgery.

Preoperative
- Patients presenting for emergency surgery may have significant, non-optimized co-morbidities and be taking a range of medication with significant haemodynamic and coagulopathic effects; there is little opportunity to optimize the patient and stop medications before surgery.
- Assess risk factors and optimize those that can be treated without delaying surgery:
  - Age >60 years.
  - Arterial and/or pulmonary hypertension.

- BMI <20 or >35 kg m^{-2}.
- Congestive cardiac failure.
- Peripheral vascular disease.
- Aortic atheroma.
- Diabetes mellitus.
- Renal insufficiency.
- Chronic pulmonary disease.
- Neurological disease.
- Previous cardiac surgery.
- Preoperative viewing of the echocardiogram (transthoracic or transoesophageal) and angiogram gives a useful indication of ventricular and valve function.
- Assess for drugs that interfere with coagulation (aspirin, NSAIDs, clopidogrel, glycoprotein IIb/IIIa antagonists, thrombolytics, heparin, warfarin).
- Consider preoperative thromboelastogram (TEG)/Multiplate® analysis. Liaise with blood bank about need for platelets and other clotting factors as appropriate.
- If time permits, reverse warfarin with 1–2 mg vitamin K IV. If more urgent, give human prothrombin complex (e.g. Beriplex®), titrated against INR (see Table 8.1):

Table 8.1 Beriplex dose for urgent warfarin reversal

Initial INR:	2.0–3.9	4.0–6.0	>6.0
Beriplex dose units kg^{-1}:	25	35	50

- Assess for drugs affecting the cardiovascular system:
  - Beta-blockers—may require postoperative pacing.
  - ACEIs—increase the need for vasoconstrictors during, and on separation from, cardiopulmonary bypass (CPB).
- Consider intra-aortic balloon pump (IABP) insertion in severe left ventricular (LV) dysfunction, congestive heart failure, cardiomyopathy, or anticipated prolonged bypass. The IABP decreases afterload and increases cardiac output, which increases coronary and systemic perfusion pressures and facilitates weaning from CPB.

Premedication
Although a heavy opioid-based premed reduces sympathetic-induced tachycardia and hypertension to minimize the risk of anxiety-induced ischaemia, critically ischaemic patients depend on endogenous catecholamine release to maintain their cardiovascular status. A heavy premed may therefore accelerate cardiovascular collapse in some patients. The urgency of the surgery may also preclude premed administration.

Operative
- Ensure the patient is consented, ICU staff are aware of the impending admission, and the operating room team are briefed and present in the operating room (including the surgeons!).

- Use standard cardiac monitoring:
  - ECG—lead V5 and II.
  - Radial arterial line (check that radial arterial grafts are not required).
  - Central venous line (consider PA catheter sheath for postoperative monitoring).
  - Urinary catheter.
  - Core temperature.
  - Transoesophageal echo is useful to detect wall motion abnormalities and is a more sensitive indicator of myocardial ischaemia than ECG or invasive pressure monitoring.

Induction

- A high-dose opioid technique (50–100 micrograms kg^{-1} fentanyl) minimizes perioperative ischaemia and improves perioperative cardiovascular stability.
- Propofol and thiopental may cause more hypotension on induction than midazolam, especially in the presence of poor LV function.
- Vecuronium avoids CVS side effects associated with other neuromuscular blockers, but mild tachycardia induced by pancuronium may be useful to offset the bradycardia caused by high-dose opioids.
- Use small boluses of vasoconstrictor (e.g. phenylephrine 50–100 micrograms mL^{-1}) to minimize inevitable hypotension.

Maintenance

- Minimize use of drugs causing myocardial depression, i.e. use high-dose opioids to reduce the dose of volatile anaesthetic.
- Maintain coronary perfusion pressure using fluids, vasoconstrictors, and inotropes as appropriate.
- For internal defibrillation use 10–20-J shocks.

Anticoagulation

- Use 3 mg kg^{-1} heparin (= 300 units kg^{-1}) for activated clotting time (ACT) >400.
- Anti-fibrinolytics (e.g. tranexamic acid 2 g IV on induction, 2 g in CPB prime, 1 g IV post-bypass) reduce postoperative bleeding.
- Reverse heparin with protamine at 1 mg for every 100 units heparin. Protamine may cause hypotension and may also increase pulmonary vascular resistance (PVR) causing right ventricular failure.
- Order clotting products in good time. Remember that a normal platelet count does not mean normal function. Assess platelet function using a Multiplate® assay/TEG if available.

Weaning from bypass

- Ensure adequate core (36.5–37.5°C) and peripheral (>34.5°C) rewarming.
- May require inotrope infusion to wean from bypass, which is continued in the immediate postoperative period.
- Common causes of failure to wean are:
  - Ischaemia (graft failure—clot, air bubble, kink, inadequate coronary blood flow, coronary spasm, inadequate coronary perfusion pressure).
  - Valve failure.

- Inadequate gas exchange (low FiO_2, bronchospasm, pulmonary oedema).
- Hypovolaemia.
- Reperfusion injury.
- Electrolyte or acid–base imbalance.
- Pre-existing LV failure.

Postoperative

- A period of haemodynamic stability is often of benefit in these patients—achieve this before attempting to awaken and extubate.
- Consider postoperative echocardiogram, PA catheter, and correctable causes in haemodynamically unstable patients.
- Monitor for pneumonia, pulmonary embolism, renal failure, and neurological events, which are more common following emergency surgery.

Further reading

Barnard M, Martin B. (eds) *Cardiac Anaesthesia*. Oxford: Oxford University Press, 2010.

Anaesthesia for urgent valve replacement

Key points
- Comorbidities are common.
- If valve disease is caused by infective endocarditis there may be associated septic shock.

Background
Although progressive valve disease usually manifests as clinical symptoms over several months/years, allowing planned surgery, urgent valve replacement is indicated in patients with sudden decompensated valve failure or infective endocarditis. It is unusual for the pulmonary or tricuspid valves to require urgent repair or replacement.

Preoperative
- Comorbidities are common, particularly diabetes, previous stroke/TIA, and chronic renal failure. Optimize as best as possible preoperatively.
- In patients with infective endocarditis, assess for signs of sepsis because active infections are associated with vasodilation and hypotension, and established or impending multiorgan failure.
- These patients are likely to need appropriate antibiotic cover and perioperative vasoconstrictors (noradrenaline, vasopressin). Septic shock causes impairment of myocardial contractility and inotropic support is also likely to be needed.

Indications for urgent valve replacement
Aortic valve
- Aortic stenosis causing decompensated LV failure.
- Aortic regurgitation causing decompensated LV failure.
- Infective endocarditis causing acute aortic regurgitation and/or embolic phenomenon (cerebrovascular accident (CVA)/TIA/septic emboli, etc.)
- Aortic dissection involving the valve structure, causing acute aortic regurgitation.

Mitral valve
- Mitral stenosis causing decompensated LV ± RV failure.
- Mitral regurgitation causing decompensated LV ± RV failure secondary to:
  - Acute ischaemic chordae rupture.
  - Dilated valve ring (fluid overload, valve failure, dilated cardiomyopathy, etc.).
  - Valve degeneration.
  - Infective endocarditis (and/or embolic phenomenon).

Perioperative management
Aortic stenosis
- May present acutely as syncope and acute LV failure, usually when valve area <2 cm^2; gradient >70 mmHg is severe (~0.6 cm^2).

- Results in a low cardiac output state, with cardiac output determined by heart rate; therefore, bradycardia causes hypotension. Tachycardia is also tolerated poorly as it reduces LV filling time, and the diastolic time during which coronary perfusion occurs.
- Aortic diastolic pressure must be maintained to preserve coronary blood flow. Ischaemia occurs even with normal coronaries.
- Atrial contraction is important to fill a poorly compliant LV.
- Decrease in SVR is tolerated poorly. Therefore, maintain both pre- and afterload and avoid regional techniques.

Aortic regurgitation

- Presents as an overloaded and failing LV, progressing to acute pulmonary oedema.
- Optimize with diuretics and inotropic support (e.g. dopamine) if time permits.
- Avoid low aortic diastolic pressure, which impairs coronary perfusion pressure.
- Aim for a slight tachycardia, which reduces regurgitant time and reduces LV cavity size (Laplace's law), improving LV efficiency.
- A slight reduction in afterload (SVR) also reduces regurgitation, but may reduce coronary perfusion pressure further.

Mitral stenosis

- Becomes severe when value area <1 cm^2. Results in poor LV filling with a cardiac output dependent on heart rate.
- A low cardiac output is made worse by tachydysrhythmias, e.g. atrial fibrillation/flutter.
- Bradycardia is of benefit by increasing the diastolic time for ventricular filling.
- A high pulmonary venous pressure risks pulmonary oedema, particular with excessive volume overload, but it is important to maintain adequate filling nevertheless.
- A decrease in afterload (SVR) is tolerated poorly so use vasoconstrictors as required and particularly on induction of anaesthesia.
- Consider inotropes and pulmonary vasodilators (milrinone, nitric oxide).

Mitral regurgitation

- Often well tolerated, unless it has occurred acutely as a result of chordae rupture or valve incompetence secondary to infective endocarditis.
- Optimize patients with acute pulmonary oedema preoperatively if time permits (diuretics, inotropes, etc.).
- Aim for a slight tachycardia and reduced afterload to minimize regurgitation.
- GA is usually well tolerated unless pulmonary hypertension has developed, when inotropic support and pulmonary vasodilators (milrinone, nitric oxide) may also be indicated.

Postoperative

- Postoperative management aims to optimize haemodynamic parameters (filling, contractility, heart rate), ensure adequate haemostasis, rewarming the patient and support renal function.
- When performed as an emergency, these patients may arrive on the ICU with ongoing morbidity from their original presentation, e.g. unresolved pulmonary oedema, ongoing sepsis (worsened by the inflammatory response induced by cardiopulmonary bypass) and worsening acute renal failure.
- Early wakening and extubation that is aimed for with elective patients may be delayed in emergency cases until these comorbidities have been addressed. A period of haemodynamic stability may also benefit the patient by minimizing shear stress on suture lines, minimizing the sympathetic response, and assisting with clot formation in coagulopathic patients.

Further reading

Frogel J, Galusca D. Anesthetic considerations for patients with advanced valvular heart disease undergoing noncardiac surgery. *Anesthesiology Clin* 2010; **28**:67–85.

Blunt aortic injury and aortic dissection

Key points
- These are challenging cases for the anaesthetist.
- Endovascular stenting may be available for some patients, avoiding surgical intervention, but is relatively limited in its availability and suitability of patients.
- Systemic heparinization is used—stop the bleeding from any other sites before proceeding to aortic surgery.

Background
Most patients with significant blunt aortic injury or acute aortic dissection die before reaching the operating room. Those that get to the operating room present significant challenges for the anaesthetist:
- Cardiac tamponade.
- Haemothorax.
- Aortic regurgitation with acute LV failure.
- Compression of large airways.
- Occlusion of aortic vessels:
  - Right/left coronary artery ostia, causing myocardial ischaemia.
  - Head and neck vessels.
  - Subclavian arteries.
  - Gut and renal vessels causing gut infarction and acute renal failure respectively.
- Hypotension (25%).
- Hypertension (36%).
- Chest pain.
- Co-morbidities (medical patients).
- Multiple trauma (trauma patients).

Aortic dissection results from a tear in the aortic intima, through which blood penetrates into the deeper media layer (smooth muscle and elastic fibres). The media is torn apart by the high pressure, splitting the inner 2/3 and the outer 1/3 of the media apart. The dissection may progress retrograde back to the aortic root and antegradely as far as the aortic bifurcation.

Classification
- Type A—involves the ascending aorta and/or aortic arch/descending aorta. The tear originates in the ascending aorta, the aortic arch, or less commonly, in the descending aorta. These may dissect retrogradely to occlude coronary artery ostia or disrupt the aortic valve structure, causing acute aortic regurgitation. Rupture through the aortic wall may result in a contained haemopericardium (tamponade).
- Type B—involves the descending aorta beyond the left subclavian artery origin, and does not involve the ascending aorta or aortic arch.

Traumatic dissection
Caused by sudden deceleration, causing the heart and anterior arch to move forward and tear away from the tethered posterior arch at the junction of the ligamentum arteriosum.

Preoperative

- Trauma patients—ensure a thorough primary and secondary survey (significant head, chest, and abdominal injuries are common in these patients).
- Liaise with neurosurgeons if indicated (systemic heparinization of patients for CPB is disastrous in the presence of CNS trauma). Consider heparin-bonded CPB circuit to avoid systemic heparinization in these patients.
- Cross match 8 units of blood. Warn blood bank that significant amounts of FFP, cryoprecipitate, platelets, etc. may be required.
- Measure baseline electrolytes, clotting (TEG and Multiplate® if possible) and ABGs.
- Assess and optimize comorbidities where time permits (hypertension, diabetes, ischaemic heart disease, chronic renal failure, etc.).
- View CT/MRI scans with the surgeon to understand what procedures are planned.
- Pseudohypotension (falsely low BP measurement) may occur due to involvement of the brachiocephalic artery (supplying the right arm) or the left subclavian artery (supplying the left arm). Compare left and right arm BPs. Liaise with surgeons about location of arterial monitoring (usually right radial artery and left femoral).
- Control hypertension using glyceryl trinitrate or sodium nitroprusside infusion.

Perioperative

- Obtain good vascular access (14-G cannulae; PA catheter sheath provides good large-bore access).
- Set up blood warmers/fluid infusion devices and position a warming blanket around the patient.
- If total circulatory arrest is planned (usually while anastomosing head/neck vessels), once CPB is established, give dexamethasone 0.5 mg kg^{-1} IV, ± thiopental 10 mg kg^{-1} IV, and pack head in bags of ice (take care to avoid orbit compression).

Postoperative

Most trauma patients are relatively young with little co-morbidity. Most postoperative problems relate to:

- **Haemostasis**—patients have often had long periods on bypass, significant manipulation of core temperature, and massive transfusion resulting in a coagulopathic state. Early, aggressive control of haemostasis is important to avoid return to the operating room and prevent comorbidity.
- **BP control**—following aortic surgery, hypertension is not uncommon, which risks disruption of suture lines and catastrophic haemorrhage. Alpha/beta blockers, nitrates, and nitroprusside are all appropriate for control of BP.

Further reading

Neschis DG, Scalea TM, Flinn WR, Griffith BP. Blunt aortic injury. *N Engl J Med*. 2008; **359**:1708–16.

Nagy K, Fabian T, Rodman G, *et al.* Guidelines for the diagnosis and management of blunt aortic injury: an EAST Practice Management Guidelines Work Group. *J Trauma*. 2000; **48**(6):1128–43.

Cardiac tamponade

Key points
- As little as 100 mL of pericardial fluid may cause cardiac tamponade.
- It presents as progressive hypotension with a CVP.
- Anaesthetic induction may cause cardiac arrest.
- Surgeons usually drain the tamponade by forming a pericardial window.

Background

Acute accumulation of fluid in the pericardial sac is tolerated poorly because the pericardium is unable to stretch and the atria and ventricles are subsequently compressed, impairing cardiac filling, stroke volume, and cardiac output. Acutely, as little as 100 mL fluid may cause tamponade.

Usually presents as an emergency due to:
- Physical trauma (penetrating trauma involving the pericardium or blunt chest trauma).
- Pericarditis.
- Bleeding following cardiothoracic surgery.
- Myocardial rupture (usually in association with myocardial infarct).
- Type A aortic dissection.

Presents as:
- Progressive hypotension.
- Rising CVP.

The absence of blood drainage from chest drains does not exclude tamponade because blood clots may block drains. Most effectively diagnosed using transthoracic echocardiogram.

Preoperative

- If caused by trauma, perform a careful primary and secondary survey. Cardiac tamponade is likely to be associated with significant cardiothoracic injuries that may also need surgical repair. Tamponade caused by blunt myocardial rupture is associated with significant myocardial contusion and impaired function.
- If the tamponade has a medical cause (e.g. acute MI), assess and optimize other co-morbidities where time permits (hypertension, diabetes, ischaemic heart disease, chronic renal failure, etc.)
- By definition, patients are in a state of haemodynamic collapse. Optimize by ensuring optimal filling (preferably assessing using echocardiography as right-sided pressures are misleading). Inotropic support (e.g. dopamine 2.5–10 micrograms kg^{-1} min^{-1}) may assist a tired myocardium.
- In patients who are bleeding after cardiac surgery, it is necessary to distinguish between surgical and coagulopathic bleeding. Assess coagulation (INR, APTT, TEG, Multiplate®, etc). Optimize the haemoglobin concentration (anaemia reduces platelet margination), platelets, and fibrinogen levels. Ensure core temperature >36.0°C because hypothermia impairs the clotting cascade. In patients who are bleeding at more than 200 mL h^{-1}, surgical re-exploration is necessary.

- Pericardiocentesis is of little benefit in acute tamponade secondary to bleeding, and risks myocardial injury.

Perioperative

- Anaesthetic induction is high risk, because further haemodynamic collapse may cause cardiac arrest. Ensure surgeons are scrubbed in the operating room before induction. Ensure cardiac arrest drugs/ defibrillator is available and the anaesthetic team is fully briefed.
- Use anaesthetic induction drugs that minimize cardiovascular instability (e.g. ketamine or etomidate), together with boluses of vasoconstrictor (e.g. phenylephrine 50–100 micrograms IV).
- Use a ventilation strategy that minimizes the mean intrathoracic pressure, which will further impair myocardial filling.
- Maintain filling pressure to overcome diastolic filling restriction. CVP >20 mmHg may be needed. Avoid bradycardia as cardiac output is rate dependent.
- Surgeons usually drain the tamponade by forming a pericardial window. Ensure good communication with surgeons because release of tamponade at this stage is associated with sudden rebound hypertension (usually transient) as impaired ventricular filling is relieved.

Postoperative

- Relief of tamponade may result in hypertension as cardiac output returns to normal in a vasoconstricted patient. Be prepared to control postoperative BP.
- Consider pre-existing myocardial dysfunction if patient remains hypotensive, e.g. mitral valve disease, myocardial ischaemia.

Further reading

O'Connor CJ, Tuman KJ. The intraoperative management of patients with pericardial tamponade. *Anesthesiol Clinics* 2010; **28**:87–96.

Pulmonary embolism and surgical embolectomy

Key points
- Early diagnosis and severity assessment of pulmonary embolism (PE) determines treatment.
- Most cases of PE are treated by anticoagulation with low-molecular-weight heparin (LMWH) or unfractionated heparin.
- PE associated with severe haemodynamic compromise may require immediate thrombolysis or rarely, in selected patients, percutaneous or surgical embolectomy.

Background
- Occlusion of the pulmonary circulation by a thromboembolus leads to acute life-threatening RV failure.
- Although an acute PE can be caused by air, fat, or amniotic fluid, the commonest cause is embolism from a deep vein thrombosis (DVT) of the pelvis or proximal leg.

Risk factors
- Immobility—secondary to neurological disease, cardiac and respiratory conditions.
- Surgery—particularly major abdominal and pelvic surgery, limb fractures, joint replacement, postoperative intensive care.
- Obstetrics—late pregnancy, Caesarean section, puerperium.
- Also—malignancy, hypercoagulable states, previous DVT/PE, thrombotic disease, air travel, obesity, hormone therapy (oral contraceptive pill (OCP)/hormonal replacement therapy (HRT)), elderly, heart failure.

Presentation
- Dyspnoea (80%), chest pain (pleuritic 52%, substernal 12%), cough (12%) haemoptysis (11%), syncope (19%).
- Sudden onset—can lead to rapid deterioration and cardiac arrest (usually PEA).
- On examination there may be tachypnoea ($>20\,min^{-1}$), cyanosis, tachycardia ($>100\,min^{-1}$), hypotension, raised jugular venous pressure/CVP, dysrhythmias, pleural rub, RV gallop, loud pulmonary component of 2nd heart sound, reduced $ETCO_2$, ↑ A–a gradient, fever ($>38.5°C$), engorged neck veins, signs of DVT.

Investigations
- ECG—RV strain, deep S wave lead I, Q wave lead III, T wave inversion lead III (S1, Q3, T3), right bundle branch block (RBBB).
- Chest X-ray—useful to exclude other causes of symptoms e.g. pneumonia.
- ABGs—hypoxaemia, hypercapnia, metabolic acidosis, ↑ A–a PO_2 gradient.
- A normal D-dimer level generally excludes a thrombotic PE.

- A transthoracic echocardiogram may show a full, tired RV with a relatively empty LV. Akinesia of the mid-free wall of the RV but normal motion of the apex has 77% sensitivity and 94% specificity for the diagnosis of acute PE (McConnell's sign).
- The definitive test is a computed tomography pulmonary angiography (CTPA) using IV contrast.
- Compression venous ultrasonography may identify DVT.
- Ventilation–perfusion scintigraphy (V/Q scan)—not useful in acute situation.
- Pulmonary angiogram: reliable but invasive.
- Differential diagnoses to exclude include acute MI, pneumothorax, cardiac tamponade, acute valvular dysfunction, hypovolaemia, pneumonia, sepsis.

Determine PE severity to guide investigations and treatment

- Massive PE—severe haemodynamic compromise, ventilatory impairment, marked RV dysfunction, cardiopulmonary arrest. Echocardiography if feasible; resuscitate; thrombolysis or surgical embolectomy.
- Submassive PE—haemodynamically stable but RV strain/dysfunction, chest pain, dyspnoea. Investigate with CTPA, and echocardiography. Treat with anticoagulation. Consider thrombolysis.
- Non-massive PE—stable circulation and right heart. Investigate with CTPA and start anticoagulation.

Non-surgical treatments

Anticoagulation

- Heparin 80 units kg^{-1} loading; 18 units kg^{-1} infusion (aim for APTT twice normal).
- LMWHs inhibit Factor Xa, require less monitoring, e.g. enoxaparin 1.5 mg kg^{-1} SC once a day (needs dose adjustment in renal failure).
- Fondaparinux has similar effects and cautions as LMWH (i.e. high bleeding risk or severe renal dysfunction). It has less risk of heparin-induced thrombocytopaenia.
- Patients also need to start warfarin for long-term anticoagulation.

Thrombolysis:

- Streptokinase: 250 000 units loading over 30 min; 100 000 IU h^{-1} for 12–24 h or rapid regime 1.5 million units over 2 h.
- Urokinase: 4400 units loading over 10 min; 4400 units kg^{-1}h^{-1} for 12–24 h.
- Alteplase (rTPA) 100 mg over 2 h or 0.6 mg kg^{-1} over 15 min (max. 50 mg dose) followed by remainder of 100-mg infusion at 50 mg h^{-1}.

Percutaneous embolectomy and caval filters

- Percutaneous catheter embolectomy or fragmentation of clots in the proximal pulmonary artery can be considered if surgery is not available or where there is an absolute contraindication to thrombolysis or if it has failed. These patients usually require intensive care support including sedation, tracheal intubation, and ventilation.
- Placement of an IVC filter can be considered at this point, but not routinely recommended. They may be considered if absolute contraindication to anticoagulation or high risk of recurrence.

Surgical embolectomy

Preoperative

- This is very rare and dependent on local service provision. Optimize the patient as best you can.
- Patients requiring emergency thromboembolectomy usually require intubation and ICU admission in order to optimize the failing cardiovascular and respiratory status.

Intraoperative

- Anaesthetic induction is high risk and may cause cardiac arrest. Ensure surgeons are scrubbed before induction. Ensure cardiac arrest drugs/defibrillator is available and the anaesthetic team is fully briefed.
- Optimize patient while the operating room is prepared. Ensure adequate filling but avoid worsening any RV strain. Low-dose inotropes (e.g. adrenaline) will help a failing RV.
- Use anaesthetic induction drugs that minimize cardiovascular instability (e.g. ketamine, etomidate), together with boluses of vasoconstrictor (e.g. phenylephrine 50–100 micrograms IV). Small boluses of adrenaline (20–50 micrograms) may be required on induction to maintain cardiac output.
- Thrombectomy is usually performed on bypass. In these patients, separation from bypass is likely to require inotropic support as the right ventricle is exhausted.
- Pulmonary haemorrhage can occur.

Postoperative

- Postoperative complications associated with a preoperative prolonged low cardiac output state (or cardiac arrest) are common and patients may remain haemodynamically unstable.
- Consider cooling if patient has had a cardiac arrest at any stage (32–34°C for 12–24h).
- Optimize blood sugar and metabolic status. Renal dialysis may be necessary if acid–base status is deranged in the presence of acute renal failure.
- Consider systemic heparinization if there is a risk of further pulmonary emboli.

Further reading

British Thoracic Society Standards of Care Committee Pulmonary Embolism Guideline Development Group. British Thoracic Society guidelines for the management of suspected acute pulmonary embolism. *Thorax* 2003; **58**:470–84.
ESC Task Force for the Diagnosis and Management of Acute Pulmonary Embolism. Guidelines on the diagnosis and management of acute pulmonary embolism. *Eur Heart J* 2008; **29**:2276–315.

Anaesthesia for electrical cardioversion

Key points
- The patient requiring urgent cardioversion may have very low BP and cardiac output, and a full stomach.
- The challenge is to induce anaesthesia and secure the airway without causing cardiovascular collapse and then to achieve rapid recovery.

Background
- Urgent electrical cardioversion is likely to be required if a tachycardia is causing cardiovascular instability (see 🕮 Fig. 16.5, p.372), defined by:
  - Reduced conscious level.
  - Chest pain.
  - SBP <90 mmHg.
  - Heart failure.
- Depending on the rhythm and the type of defibrillator, electrical cardioversion will require the delivery of a shock/s of 100–360 J, which would be very painful in the conscious patient. A tachycardia causing profound hypotension may render the patient unconscious, negating the need for sedation or anaesthesia—this would be typical of the peri-arrest setting.

Preoperative
- The commonest arrhythmias requiring urgent cardioversion are:
  - Fast atrial fibrillation.
  - Regular broad complex tachycardia (ventricular tachycardia, supraventricular tachycardia with aberrant conduction).
  - Regular narrow complex tachycardia (supraventricular tachycardia).
- The urgency of the cardioversion will depend on the extent of haemodynamic compromise and this will be determined by the precise rhythm, rate, myocardial function, intravascular filling, and SVR. In many cases patients will not be fasted. Those who are hypotensive because of the arrhythmia and yet remain conscious enough to require full GA are potentially the most challenging.
- The most common locations for urgent electrical cardioversion requiring GA are: the emergency department, coronary care unit, ICU; rarely, this procedure may have to be undertaken on a ward. Most of these locations should be properly equipped to enable GA to be given safely and the staff will be familiar with the support that is required. This will not be true of a standard hospital ward.
- Try to obtain any relevant history: previous anaesthetics, current drug treatment, co-morbidities (particularly other cardiovascular or respiratory disease), allergies, last oral intake. The patient may have been cardioverted previously.
- Ensure any electrolyte abnormalities are being corrected (e.g. K^+, Mg^{2+}).
- Record a 12-lead ECG.
- Confirm who is going to be undertaking the cardioversion and ensure that they are familiar with the equipment and the procedure.

Intraoperative

- Confirm or obtain IV access. Make a rapid assessment of the patient's intravascular volume and give fluid if this is likely to improve the haemodynamic state.
- Apply ECG electrodes, pulse oximeter, and NIBP cuff. In the haemodynamically unstable patient, if the facility is available, consider inserting an arterial cannula to enable continuous BP monitoring. This is in anticipation of a significant reduction in BP when anaesthesia is induced.
- The most common practice is to use self-adhesive defibrillation patches instead of manual paddles for cardioversion. Chest hair can be shaved and the self-adhesive patches applied before induction of anaesthesia.
- The ideal drug for inducing anaesthesia for electrical cardioversion would be cardiovascular stable and enable rapid loss and then recovery of consciousness. No drug is ideal but options include:
  - *Propofol* is particularly popular for elective cardioversion because it enables rapid recovery of consciousness but it invariably causes hypotension particularly in the cardiovascularly unstable patient.
  - *Midazolam* is a popular choice among clinicians who are not experience with anaesthetic induction drugs (e.g. emergency physicians). Emergence is prolonged in comparison with propofol.
  - *Etomidate* provides cardiovascular stability but is associated with myoclonus and a high incidence of nausea and vomiting; it also causes adrenal cortical suppression for at least 24 h, which may be harmful in critical patients.
  - *Thiopental* causes less hypotension than propofol but the recovery is more prolonged.
  - *Ketamine* is less likely to cause hypotension than other induction drugs. Its emergence phenomena have probably been overstated but its sympathomimetic properties may exacerbate tachyarrhythmias.
- Patients who are not fasted will require a RSI and tracheal intubation. In haemodynamically unstable patients, the RSI can be modified (described later in this list). Although suxamethonium has many disadvantages it remains the 1st choice neuromuscular blocker when the airway needs to be secured rapidly. Emergency cardioversion should be a very short procedure and as soon as a satisfactory rhythm has been restored the relatively rapid recovery from suxamethonium is an advantage. Rocuronium 1 mg kg^{-1} enables intubation just as quickly as suxamethonium but, after this dose, recovery from neuromuscular blockade would normally take >1 h. Sugammadex, which has recently become available, enables full reversal of rocuronium with recovery of muscle power in even less than time then it takes to recover spontaneously from suxamethonium. Unfortunately, sugammadex is very expensive and few clinicians use it in this scenario.
- A small dose of an opioid, such as fentanyl 1 micrograms kg^{-1} or alfentani 10–20 micrograms kg^{-1}, will reduce the dose of induction drugs required, which will reduce the extent of any hypotension. The opioid will also reduce the tendency for laryngoscopy and intubation to worsen any tachyarrhythmia. The shorter time to onset of action

(1 vs. 3 min) and shorter duration (10 vs. 40 min) gives alfentanil advantages over fentanyl for this short procedure.
- Prepare a vasopressor, such as metaraminol, before induction: this can be used to offset any hypotension caused by the induction drug.
- Ensure that suction is immediately available and functions well.
- Fully preoxygenate—given the likely environment, this will typically be undertaken with a bag–mask device with oxygen reservoir. Inject the opioid. After 1 min, inject the induction drug slowly, titrating to achieve loss of consciousness. These patients will have a considerably reduced cardiac output and prolonged circulation time. If RSI and tracheal intubation is required, inject a relatively small, predetermined dose of induction drug; on loss of consciousness, apply cricoid pressure and inject the muscle relaxant to enable intubation. If the patient has profound cardiovascular instability because of the arrhythmia, experienced practitioners may elect to undertake 'modified RSI'—the induction is injected slowly and, once cricoid pressure is applied, the lungs are inflated gently until the onset of full muscle paralysis enables intubation to be achieved. The experienced practitioner must weigh the risks of aspiration associated with this 'modified RSI' against the risks of profound cardiovascular collapse caused by rapid injection of an excessive dose of induction drug.
- Once the airway is secure, quickly check the BP—give a dose of vasopressor if the patient is hypotensive.
- Select the synchronization button and the appropriate initial energy level on the defibrillator (broad complex tachycardia and atrial fibrillation 120–150 J biphasic; atrial flutter and regular narrow complex tachycardia 70–120 J biphasic). Ensure that there is no high-flow oxygen within 1 m of the patient's chest—the oxygen delivery system can be left attached to a supraglottic airway or tracheal tube. Once the defibrillator is charged, ensure no one is touching the patient before delivering the shock. Increase the energy level if the first shock is unsuccessful. Give small additional doses of IV anaesthetic, as required, to maintain anaesthesia. Consider an anti-arrhythmic drug, such as amiodarone, if sinus rhythm is not restored after a 3rd shock.

Postoperative
- Once sinus rhythm and haemodynamic stability has been restored, allow the patient to regain consciousness and, if intubated, extubate in the left lateral position.
- Repeat the 12-lead ECG. Continue oxygen by facemask and full monitoring until the patient is well enough to be transferred to a ward.

Further reading
Benger J, Nolan J, Clancy M. (eds). *Emergency Airway Management*. Cambridge: Cambridge University Press, 2008.

Anaesthesia in the catheter laboratory

Key points

- The remote location of the cardiac catheter lab necessitates adequate assistance, drugs, and equipment before starting anaesthesia.
- Careful assessment of the patient and understanding of the procedure planned enables anticipation of possible complications.
- Arterial and central venous monitoring is appropriate for patients with established or anticipated myocardial dysfunction.
- Pacing lead extraction risks ventricular rupture causing significant haemorrhage or cardiac tamponade, which requires emergency CPB.

Background

Patients requiring emergency anaesthesia in the catheter lab may present with a wide range of cardiac disorders and associated co-morbidity:

- PCI, particularly following cardiac arrest.
- Arrhythmia mapping and ablation (including induction and cardioversion of malignant arrhythmias).
- Implant/explant of pacemaker or implantable cardioverter-defibrillator (ICD) ± associated endocardial leads.
- Percutaneous closure of atrial septal defect.

There are several issues that may impact on emergency GA.

- Poor ventricular function (left/right/biventricular).
- Ischaemic heart disease.
- Congenital heart disease (cyanotic circulations, left-to-right and right-to-left shunts).
- High incidence of dysrhythmias (dysrhythmias worsen cardiac function and vice versa; a vicious cycle of clinical deterioration may ensue).
- Associated co-morbidities (previous CVA/TIA, diabetes, COPD, renal failure, etc.).

Preoperative

Establish the following:

- Is the cardiac anatomy normal? If not, understand the effects of brady/tachycardia, changes in SVR and filling on cardiorespiratory function.
- Is the haemodynamic state affected by rhythm disturbance or impaired ventricular performance?
- What drugs is the patient taking that may affect haemodynamic status (e.g. ACEIs, beta-blockers, nitrates, calcium channel blockers, anti-arrhythmics, etc.).
- Are the potassium and magnesium values within a normal range?
- What is the coagulation status?
- Is the patient fitted with an implanted pacemaker and/or defibrillator? What is it programmed to do and is it turned on/off?
- Understand how to use any mechanical cardiopulmonary resuscitation devices that may be available (e.g. Autopulse®/LUCAS® device).

Perioperative

- Usually a remote location, away from the main operating suite, often with reduced available equipment and assistance. Ensure adequate assistance and equipment is present before starting any procedure.

- Insidious hypothermia is common. Monitor core temperature in prolonged procedures and establish forced air warming early.
- Limited access to the patient's airway and vascular lines means particular care must be taken with lines and monitoring.
- ECG lead/defibrillation pads must be positioned to avoid interfering with imaging or surgical access.
- Moving patient and equipment to and from the imaging table has the potential to dislodge the tracheal tube and vascular access.
- If X-ray screening is being used, ensure a correctly fitting lead apron is available before the procedure commences.
- Tracheal intubation is generally more appropriate in these patients who may deteriorate rapidly. Positive pressure ventilation enables better control of cardiovascular and metabolic status.
- In addition to standard monitoring (NIBP, SaO_2, ECG, partial pressure of $ETCO_2$), establish invasive (radial artery) monitoring if ventricular arrhythmia induction or ventricular lead extraction is planned. At least one large-bore cannula is vital. Consider central venous access for CVP monitoring and inotropes if haemodynamic instability is likely.

Specific procedures
- PCI following cardiac arrest—cool as soon as possible ($30\,mL\,kg^{-1}$ IV cold (4°C) saline lowers core temperature 1.5°C). Optimize metabolic status, avoid hyper/hypoglycaemia. Consider intra-aortic balloon pump/inotropes/pulmonary artery catheter monitoring in unstable patients.
- Arrhythmia mapping/ablation—induction of atrial tachyarrhythmias does not generally cause significant haemodynamic instability unless the patient has left/right ventricular failure. Induction of ventricular tachyarrhythmias is usually associated with significant haemodynamic instability. Resultant myocardial ischaemia may require inotropic support.
- Pacemaker/ICD lead extraction—lead tips are embedded in endocardium and often require laser extraction to remove. There is a significant risk of ventricular wall rupture resulting in rapid tamponade and cardiac arrest. Patient requires immediate surgical intervention (usually CPB) to achieve surgical haemostasis. Ensure all CPB drugs are available preoperatively (e.g. heparin), adequate IV access, and arterial monitoring.
- ICD insertion—usually requires two inductions of ventricular fibrillation to test the device. Ensure an external defibrillator is available for rescue shocks, and amiodarone to treat refractory ventricular fibrillation.

Postoperative
Patients should be haemodynamically stable at the end of a procedure. On occasion, the repeated induction of malignant arrhythmias may result in a temporary worsening of myocardial function, necessitating inotropic support and high care/intensive care postoperatively.

Adequate analgesia is required for patients having had tunnelled procedures or implanted devices as subcutaneous tissues are inflamed and very sore.

Further reading
Braithwaite S. Anaesthesia in the cardiac catheterisation laboratory. *Curr Opin Anaesthesiol* 2010; **23**:507–12.

Neurological Emergencies

Carl Gwinnutt, Craig Carroll, and Joe Sebastian

Status epilepticus

- Defined as seizure activity lasting >30 min, or frequent seizure activity over 30 min without a return to consciousness.
- It is associated with a high morbidity and mortality (up to 20%) if untreated.
- ▶Terminate seizures as quickly as possible.

Background
Prolonged fitting is associated with multiple complications. The metabolic stress of repeated muscular convulsions can lead to rhabdomyolysis and lactic acidosis. The continuously fitting patient is at risk from aspiration pneumonitis, neurogenic pulmonary oedema, and cardiac injury due to a massive catecholamine release. Neuronal death can occur after as little as 30 min of uninterrupted fitting.

The diagnosis of tonic–clonic status is usually straightforward, but non-convulsive status and pseudo-status epilepticus may be challenging and may require EEG monitoring.

Causes
- Occurs most commonly in known epileptics having low plasma concentrations of antiepileptic drugs.
- Febrile convulsions are a common precipitator in children.
- Withdrawal syndromes associated with cessation of alcohol, barbiturates, or benzodiazepines.
- Acute structural brain injury such as stroke, brain tumour, subarachnoid haemorrhage (SAH), head trauma, anoxic or hypoxic damage.
- Previous structural brain injury such as prior head injury, neurosurgery, or arteriovenous malformations.
- CNS infection—encephalitis, meningitis, abscess.
- Metabolic abnormalities: hypoglycaemia, hyponatraemia, hypocalcaemia, hypomagnesaemia, and uraemia.
- Proconvulsant drugs such as beta-lactam and quinolone antibiotics, antidepressants (theophylline, lithium), LAs, some immunosuppressants.
- Eclampsia.

Investigations
- Blood investigations—bedside and laboratory glucose, U&Es, calcium, magnesium, FBC, therapeutic drug levels, toxicology screen, ABGs.
- Septic screen (blood and urine cultures), lumbar puncture if infection suspected.
- EEG.
- CT scan—the possibility of intracranial pathology is high if this is the first presentation of epilepsy.

Emergency management

- ABC, 100% high-flow oxygen (note—pulse oximetry often does not work during seizure).
- Establish IV access and take blood for immediate glucose analysis; correct hypotension and fluid resuscitate.

1st-line therapy

IV lorazepam up to $0.1 \, mg \, kg^{-1}$ at a rate not exceeding $2 \, mg \, min^{-1}$.

2nd-line therapy

If seizures continue for a further 10 min give IV phenytoin $15 \, mg \, kg^{-1}$ at a rate of $\leq 50 \, mg \, min^{-1}$ *or* fosphenytoin $22.5 \, mg \, kg^{-1}$ at a rate of up to $225 \, mg \, min^{-1}$. Monitor the ECG.

Refractory status epilepticus

- Intubate and ventilate if seizures continue.
- Continuous EEG recordings are desirable.
- Maintain GA with propofol (bolus of $1 \, mg \, kg^{-1}$ followed by maintenance infusion $2–12 \, mg \, kg^{-1} \, h^{-1}$) *or* thiopental (IV bolus of $2–4 \, mg \, kg^{-1}$ followed by maintenance infusion $2–5 \, mg \, kg^{-1} \, h^{-1}$) *or* consider midazolam if haemodynamically unstable: $0.2 \, mg \, kg^{-1}$ IV bolus followed by $0.05–0.5 \, mg \, kg^{-1} \, h^{-1}$.
- 3rd-line therapy: phenobarbital $20 \, mg \, kg^{-1}$ at a rate of $<100 \, mg \, min^{-1}$ followed by an infusion of $1–4 \, mg \, kg^{-1} \, h^{-1}$.

Specific management points

- When treating hypoglycaemia with 50% glucose IV 50 mL, consider also giving thiamine 250 mg IV if alcoholism or poor nutrition suspected (risk of Wernicke's encephalopathy).
- If there is a suspicion of intracerebral tumour causing oedema, give dexamethasone 8 mg IV.
- Fosphenytoin is a water soluble prodrug of phenytoin, which can be given at a faster rate. Fosphenytoin 1.5 mg is equivalent to phenytoin 1 mg and its dosage is expressed in phenytoin equivalents.
- If the patient is anaesthetized, EEG monitoring is desirable to enable titration of anticonvulsant drugs. Avoid use of long-acting muscle relaxants especially if not using EEG monitoring. This may stop the visible seizure activity but not the electrical seizure activity in the brain.
- Inotropes may be required to support the BP when using general anaesthesia.

Subsequent management

It is important to establish and treat the underlying cause. As soon as seizures are controlled, start oral drugs and this may require expert guidance by a neurologist.

Further reading

National Institute for Health and Clinical Excellence. *The epilepsies: the diagnosis and management of the epilepsies in adults and children in primary and secondary care.* London: NICE, 2004. Available at: ℘ http://guidance.nice.org.uk/CG20.

Evacuation of traumatic intracranial haematoma

Key points
- Intracranial haematomas can be extradural (EDH), subdural (SDH), or intracerebral (ICH).
- EDHs and SDHs have an effect due primarily to the volume of the haematoma; small volume intracerebral haematomas can be catastrophic if they occur in vital areas of the brain.
▶Patients with life-threatening signs require immediate emergency measures (including neurosurgery) to lower intracranial pressure.

Background
Extradural haematomas
- Result from arterial bleeding, usually from the middle meningeal artery.
- ~20% present with the classical signs of loss of consciousness following trauma, followed by a lucid interval and eventually deterioration secondary to the increasing volume of the haematoma.
- In the temporal region they can be associated with rapid deterioration as the medial aspect of the temporal lobe herniates across the free edge of the tentorium compressing the IIIrd cranial nerve, motor tracts, and brainstem.
- Mortality increases as conscious level decreases, reaching 20% in patients in coma.

Subdural haematomas
- Originate either from tears of bridging veins between dura and cortex or direct cortical injury.
- Divided into:
  - Acute SDH—usually a result of high-energy trauma with a high mortality (60%).
  - Chronic SDH—associated with trivial injury in the presence of other risk factors, ↑ age (>50% in over 60 years of age), chronic alcohol excess, brain atrophy, coagulopathy (pharmacological and pathological). Mortality is ~5%.

Intracerebral (intraparenchymal) haematomas
- Result from either high-energy transfer, typically vehicle deceleration, falls, or as a result of spontaneous haemorrhage secondary to hypertension, or a bleed from an aneurysm, or arteriovenous malformation or into a tumour.
- Traumatic lesions (cerebral contusions) may mature over days with ↑ volume caused by the associated peri-trauma oedema.
- Haematoma in the posterior cranial fossa can cause life-threatening intracranial hypertension secondary to hydrocephalus (see 📖 Management of acute hydrocephalus, p.228). As with temporal clots, mass effect may cause rapid deterioration.

Preoperative

Surgery for evacuation of intracranial haematoma is the most effective way of reducing raised ICP. The decision to operate will depend upon the size and location of the clot, the clinical and radiological signs and the potential for acute life-threatening deterioration. Avoid unnecessary delays.

Assessment of the patient

In the presence of a traumatic haematoma, in addition to the standard anaesthetic assessment, particular attention should be paid to:

- Time and mechanism of injury.
- Additional injuries identified, treatment given, and response.
- GCS at scene.
- The presence of hypoxia, hypotension, or seizures.
- Use of illicit drugs.
- If the cervical spine has not been cleared, treat as unstable.

In the case of spontaneous haematomas, consider premorbid status and pre-existing medical problems.

On examination, document the vital signs, current neurological status: GCS score, pupillary size and reactivity to light, lateralizing signs. Life-threatening signs include:

- Unilateral or bilateral pupillary dilatation.
- Extreme hypertension with bradycardia.
- Coma.
- Extensor posturing.

Identify all other injuries; complete a secondary survey.

Investigations

- CT head ± CT cervical spine.
- FBC, coagulation screen, U&Es; crossmatch 2 units packed cells.
- Patients with chronic SDH may have a coagulopathy, and are prone to hyponatraemia.

Do not delay surgery by performing or requesting investigations that will not alter outcome. Where surgery is potentially life saving, ensure operating room staff are aware and suitably prepared, in order to prevent delaying surgery.

Control of blood pressure, intracranial pressure, and seizures

In addition to routine checks of equipment and drugs:

- Do not attempt to normalize hypertension; this is an indication of ↑ ICP.
- In the presence of life-threatening signs, lower ICP with:
  - Mannitol 20%—IV bolus of 0.5 g kg⁻¹.
  - Moderate hyperventilation—aim for $PaCO_2$ 4.5–5.0 kPa.
  - Hypertonic saline—IV bolus (250 mL 7.5% saline)—avoid in hyponatraemic patients (risk of central pontine myelinolysis).
  - Furosemide—IV bolus, 10–15 mg.
- Seizure activity is best managed by inducing anaesthesia.

Confirm planned procedure, position, and anticipated complications with surgeon. In patients with intracerebral and subdural haematomas, ascertain risk of underlying vascular lesion causing the haematoma.

Intraoperative

Anaesthesia

- Consider risk:benefit of any actions that will delay surgical evacuation of clot.
- Monitoring in accordance with AAGBI guidelines.
- Intra-arterial BP monitoring preferable, but not essential. Enables:
  - Real-time BP measurement.
  - Measurement of $PaCO_2$ (potential for significant A–a gradient).
- Central venous access is *rarely* necessary.
- If diuretics used, insert a urinary catheter after surgery has commenced.
- Avoid head-down position.

If not already intubated, trauma patients should have RSI. The choice of drugs used is less important than therapeutic principles:

- Rapid induction, avoiding hypo- and hypertension; use drugs that do not increase ICP:
  - Thiopental, propofol—reduce dose if comatosed.
  - Fentanyl, alfentanil.
  - Avoid ketamine if BP very high.
- Optimal intubation conditions: suxamethonium 1–2 mg kg^{-1} or rocuronium 1 mg kg^{-1}.
- Maintenance: propofol infusion; volatile anaesthetics; remifentanil infusion; neuromuscular block.
- Maintain $ETCO_2$ at 4.5–5.0 kPa unless life-threatening signs preoperatively. Once dura opened, aim for normocapnia unless there is gross brain swelling.
- Adjust ventilation to keep mean intrathoracic pressure as low as possible.
- Keep MAP >90 mmHg (or cerebral perfusion pressure (CPP) 60–70 mmHg if ICP monitored).
- Maintain euvolaemia; keep haemoglobin above 8.0 g dL^{-1} unless known cardiac disease.
- Avoid hyperglycaemia—measure blood sugar regularly in diabetics.
- There is no evidence to support the use of hypothermia in these patients intraoperatively but hyperthermia must be avoided.
- At more than 1.5 MAC, volatile anaesthetics cause cerebral vasodilation, which increases ICP. In the presence of hypocapnia and hypotension, propofol can cause cerebral hypoperfusion.
- Remifentanil reduces the concentration of volatile anaesthetic required thereby reducing the degree of cerebral vasodilatation.
- There is no place for nitrous oxide in intracranial neuroanaesthetic practice.

Intraoperative problems

- Tight dura—if does not improve with surgical manoeuvres (clot removal, CSF drainage):
  - Optimize position (reverse Trendelenburg).
  - Optimize ventilation: pressures, CO_2.
  - Optimize BP.
  - Check degree of neuromuscular block.
  - Consider bolus of mannitol, thiopental, hypertonic saline, furosemide.

- Brain herniation through craniotomy may be an unsalvageable complication or may require decompressive craniectomy.
- Be alert to the risk of coagulopathy; seek clinical signs to confirm clot formation at wound edges.
- Intraoperative seizure: thiopental bolus, neuromuscular blocker to prevent movement at operative site and patient trauma, anti-convulsant therapy (phenytoin infusion 15 mg kg^{-1} IV over 30 min).
- Extreme cardiovascular instability:
  - Exclude hypovolaemia, seizure, depth of anaesthesia issues.
  - May be indicator of brainstem compression and coning.
  - Utilize emergency ICP controlling measures and alert surgeon.

Postoperative

Where possible, plan to extubate. This enables evaluation of neurological function, but limits therapeutic control of ICP, cerebral metabolic rate and cerebral perfusion; the post-head injury patient may be agitated and confused.

If extubated, the patient must be observed closely and equipment readily available to re-intubate and sedate.

Continued ventilation in a critical care environment will be influenced by:
- Low GCS score on admission (<9), extent of primary brain injury.
- Hypotension or hypoxia following trauma.
- Prolonged seizures.
- Requirement for ICP rescue therapies.
- Brain herniation.
- Preoperative intoxication (alcohol, illicit drugs).
- Presence of other injuries.
- Degree of residual sedation (opioids, benzodiazepines, anticonvulsants).

Patients with non-survivable head injuries may be candidates for organ donation (see 📖 Anaesthesia for organ retrieval, p.244).

Analgesia following craniotomy
- Avoid NSAIDs for the first 24 h.
- Opioids may be necessary.
- Give IV paracetamol; it has an opioid sparing effect.
- If there is increasing pain, consider haemorrhage, hydrocephalus, or CNS infection.

Further reading

Brain Trauma Foundation Guidelines for the management of severe traumatic brain injury 2007. *J Neurotrauma* 2007; **24**(Suppl. 1):S1–S106.
Matta BF, Menon DK, Turner JM (eds). *Textbook of Neuroanaesthesia and Critical Care*. London: Greenwich Medical Media, 2000.
The Brain Trauma Foundation Guidelines. Available at: 🖰 http://www.braintrauma.org.

Subarachnoid haemorrhage

Key points

- Spontaneous (non-traumatic) SAH has a spectrum of severity, from mild headache with no neurological deficit to coma and sudden death.
- Re-bleeding from an aneurysmal SAH carries a high mortality.
- ↓level of consciousness at presentation may be caused by primary brain injury but can be confounded by hydrocephalus and seizures.
- Delayed neurological deficit (vasospasm) can occur from 3–21 days post bleed and can cause focal and global hypoperfusion injury.
- In 25% of cases, SAH is associated with myocardial dysfunction.
- Following a SAH, patients are prone to respiratory dysfunction and lower respiratory tract infection.
- Admission may be delayed after a SAH and patients are at risk of dehydration and electrolyte abnormality.

Background

Causes of subarachnoid haemorrhage

The most common cause of non-traumatic SAH is rupture of a cerebral artery aneurysm. Most subarachnoid aneurysms are associated with atheromatous disease, which is associated with hypertension and smoking. There may be strong family history. Other risk factors for SAH include:

- Connective tissue diseases:
  - Marfan's syndrome, Ehlers–Danlos, fibromuscular dysplasia.
  - Familiar polycystic kidney disease.
  - Coarctation of the aorta.
- Arteriovenous malformations (and flow-related aneurysms).

Other causes of SAH include:

- Non-aneurysmal SAH (usually hypertensive para-mesencephalic bleeds).
- Mycotic (infective emboli—usually located in the middle cerebral artery).
- Cerebral vasculitis.
- Acute head injury.
- Cocaine abuse.

Severity of subarachnoid haemorrhage

Primary brain injury is caused by hypoperfusion injury, possibly accompanied by parenchymal clot; injury can be worsened by acute hydrocephalus, seizures and hypoxia.

The severity of a SAH is most commonly classified clinically using the World Federation of Neurological Surgeons (WFNS) scoring system:

- Grade 1:   GCS 15 with no motor deficit.
- Grade 2:   GCS 13–14 with no motor deficit.
- Grade 3:   GCS 13–14 with motor deficit present.
- Grade 4:   GCS 7–12 (motor deficit absent or present).
- Grade 5:   GCS 3–6 (motor deficit absent or present).

Cardiac dysfunction

Cardiac dysfunction is probably caused by the direct toxic effects of the release of large quantities of catecholamines at the time of the initial bleed. Pulmonary oedema and cardiogenic shock may occur; however, marked hypertension (>190 mmHg systolic) is not uncommon following SAH.

Delayed neurological deficit

Delayed neurological deficit (DND) can occur from 3–21 days post bleed:
- It is most common in the first 2 weeks post bleed.
- There is reduced blood flow through affected vessels resulting in focal/global perfusion deficit and neurological dysfunction.
- DND can occur in the absence of angiographic evidence of vessel spasm.

DND risk is correlated with the subarachnoid blood load; this can be quantified from the head CT using the Fisher Grading system:
- Group 1: no blood detected.
- Group 2: diffuse deposition of subarachnoid blood, no clots, and no layers of blood >1 mm.
- Group 3: localized clots and/or vertical layers of blood 1 mm or greater in thickness.
- Group 4: diffuse or no subarachnoid blood, but intracerebral or intraventricular clots are present.

Treatment of delayed neurological deficit

- Dehydration and hypovolaemia increases the risk of DND; patients are routinely treated with IV crystalloid 3 L day^{-1} and normovolaemia maintained. Minimally-invasive cardiac output monitoring may be useful.
- Optimize haematocrit (30–40%) and correct electrolyte abnormalities.
- Nimodipine 60 mg 4-hourly is given orally for 21 days following the primary SAH. It may cause hypotension; if so, optimize fluid status and consider splitting the dose to 30 mg 2-hourly.
- Novel agents such as magnesium have shown promise but level 1 data are awaited.

Preoperative

Identify the reason for surgery and the urgency:
- Prevention of rebleeding—open surgical or endovascular procedure.
- Treatment of raised ICP:
  - Insertion of external ventricular drain (EVD).
  - Clot evacuation.
  - Decompressive craniectomy.
- Treatment of vasospasm—endovascular angioplasty/intra-arterial vasodilator.

Principles of anaesthetic management

- Minimize risk of further bleeding.
- Prevent secondary brain injury by avoiding:
  - Hypoxia and hypotension.
  - ↑ICP.
  - ↑CMRO$_2$.
  - Preoperative delay.

- Anaesthetic management will be governed by whether the aneurysm is secured and the presence or absence of intracranial hypertension.
- For endovascular procedures, raised ICP may require surgery (EVD/clot removal) before attempting coil embolization.
- Suspect raised ICP in the awake patient if there is worsening headache and/or a decrease in GCS.
- Perform trial of supination to assess ICP in ventilated ICU patients before transfer to angiography suite (if ICP being measured).

Assessment of the patient

Obtain a routine anaesthetic history with additional specific information:
- Time since ictus.
- Initial WFNS score.
- Complications at ictus (seizure, aspiration, cardiac instability).
- GCS and rate of decline.
- Check for CT evidence of hydrocephalus.
- Known cardiorespiratory conditions.

Examination of the patient

- Vital signs, GCS score, and pupillary response.
- Evidence of hypoxia and/or pulmonary oedema.
- Evidence of sepsis.

Investigations

- FBC, U&Es, Mg, coagulation screen, group and screen.
- ECG (if signs of focal ischaemia or global ischaemia (non-vascular territory T-wave abnormalities), measure troponin—if raised consider echocardiography and exclude LV/RV dysfunction.
- CT (if clot evacuation is planned a CT angiogram may be performed).
- For aneurysm surgery: crossmatch of 4 units of red blood cells and consider intraoperative cell salvage.

Intraoperative

General principles

- Apply standard principles for the use of RSI.
- Maintain normocapnia unless danger signs (see 📖 Evacuation of traumatic intracranial haematoma, p.218).
- Aim for pre-induction BP, especially if signs of focal/global neurological deficit.
- Avoid hypovolaemia, anaemia, hypo/hyperglycaemia, hyperthermia (no evidence to support hypothermia except in uncontrolled raised ICP).
- Treat life-threatening ICP.
- Avoid hypotension or attempt reduce SBP rapidly to normal; this may cause cerebral hypoperfusion injury because the ICP may be high and the patient may normally be hypertensive and with right-shifted autoregulation of CBF.
- An increase in CPP may encourage collateral flow, reduce watershed hypoperfusion, and increase flow through spastic arteries.

Anaesthesia for evacuation of intracerebral clot and emergency clipping
Follows similar principles to that for intracerebral haemorrhage; however, underlying vascular abnormality increases risk of brisk haemorrhage. Ensure:
- IV access—two large-bore cannulae (easily accessible perioperatively).
- Rapid fluid infusion and warming device is available in the operating room.
- Arterial BP monitoring pre-induction.

Consider enlisting the assistance of a second anaesthetist.

Induction of anaesthesia
- Avoid surges in BP.
- Induction and maintenance follows the principles outlined in
  📖 Evacuation of traumatic intracranial haematoma, p.218.
- In the absence of *raised* ICP, the cerebrovasodilation caused by volatile agents may be an advantage.
- A remifentanil infusion reduces the dose of hypnotic and reduces unwanted effects on cerebral perfusion.
- There is no definitive evidence on maintenance agents and outcome in SAH; however, volatile preconditioning may *reduce* ischaemic neuronal injury.
- Propofol may have a free radical scavenging role in prevention of reperfusion injury.

Lines
Central venous access enables infusion of vasoactive drugs. Assessment of circulating volume is achieved best with some form of arterial waveform analysis. Urinary catheterization is required.

Positioning
- Mayfield pins and the head position secured (ensure adequate depth of anaesthesia/analgesia when clamp applied).
- Head may be turned; place sandbag under shoulder on occipital side to prevent brachial plexus injury. Position head-up.

Intraoperative problems
- Guidance on BP specific to clipping is given in 📖 Evacuation of traumatic intracranial haematoma, p.218.
- Bleeding can occur on opening the dura, during dissection, and at the time of clipping.
- Techniques for reducing bleeding include:
  - Temporary clip before definitive clipping—this may render an area of the brain ischaemic; bolus thiopental ($2\,mg\,kg^{-1}$) is given to cause burst suppression just before clip application.
  - Surgical preference during temporary clipping may be for:
    (a) circulatory arrest (32 mg adenosine); (b) extreme hypotension, (sodium nitroprusside 10 mg in 50 mL glucose at $10–30\,mL\,h^{-1}$); (c) hypertension—to encourage collateral flow.
  - Exposure of carotid in neck.

Anaesthesia for endovascular neuroradiological procedures (embolization)

- Take precautions to limit radiation exposure.
- Endovascular treatment may not be technically possible and there is a risk of rupture.
- Induction and maintenance is as for operative procedures.
- A central line is not indicated except in the following cases when hypertensive therapy may be necessary: vasospasm and DND evident; WFNS grade 3 or above; large blood load on CT.

Positioning

- Flat on radiology table with head neutral. Arms at the side with groins exposed for endovascular access.
- Beware of the following:
  - The table will be moved during the procedure; ensure lines, tubes, and monitoring do not come under tension.
  - The X-ray C-arms will rotate and can snag IV lines, EVD, ventilator tubing.

Procedure

- Anticoagulation will be necessary (heparin).
- Deployment of coils requires passage of electrical current, causing transient ischaemic appearance on ECG.
- Significant fluid load and contrast media will be injected.

Procedural complications

- Vessel rupture can cause extreme cardiac instability and arrest.
- Vessel dissection (usually treated conservatively).
- Aberrant coil deployment.
- Thrombus formation/embolus- (consider aspirin 500 mg IV, heparinization, IIb/IIIa antagonist—abciximab 10 mg).
- Puncture site haematoma.
- Contrast-induced nephropathy.

Postoperative

Where possible, plan to extubate—this enables evaluation of neurological function, but limits therapeutic control of ICP, cerebral metabolic rate, and cerebral perfusion. Try to avoid coughing during extubation. Agitation and confusion is common on emergence. Once extubated, observe the patient closely and ensure equipment is available to re-intubate and sedate.

The decision to continue ventilation in a critical care environment will be influenced by:
- A low GCS score on admission (<9).
- Extent of primary brain injury.
- Prolonged seizure.
- Requirement of ICP rescue therapies;
- Brain herniation;
- Unsurvivable brain injury where organ donation is being considered (see 📖 Anaesthesia for organ retrieval, p.244).

Analgesia

- Avoid NSAIDs for the first 24 h.
- Give IV paracetamol; it has an opioid-sparing effect, although opioids may still be required.
- Patients undergoing endovascular treatment will have mild groin discomfort.
- Headache will be similar to preoperatively; worsening headache suggests hydrocephalus or rebleed.

Further reading

Bederson JB, Connolly ES, Batjer HH, *et al.* Guidelines for the management of aneurismal subarachnoid haemorrhage. A statement for healthcare professionals from a special writing group of the Stroke Council, American Heart Association. *Stroke* 2009; **40**:994–1025.

Matta BF, Menon DK, Turner JM (eds). *Textbook of Neuroanaesthesia and Critical Care*. London: Greenwich Medical Media, 2000.

van Gijn J, Kerr RS, Rinkel GJ. Subarachnoid haemorrhage. *Lancet* 2007; **369**:306–18.

Management of acute hydrocephalus

Key points
- Patients with acute hydrocephalus will require a drainage procedure, either an EVD or ventriculoperitoneal (VP) shunt.
- These patients are often hypertensive, bradycardic, and have a reduced level of consciousness.
- The anaesthetic challenge is to induce and maintain anaesthesia without compromising CBF by causing either hypotension of further increases in ICP.

Background
Hydrocephalus is a condition in which there is accumulation of CSF within the ventricles and CSF spaces of the brain. It is usually described as either (a) communicating, where flow through CSF pathways is normal but reabsorption is impaired, or (b) non-communicating where there is obstruction to flow.

Causes
- Communicating—SAH, ICH, meningitis, head injury.
- Non-communicating—tumours (ependymoma, choroid plexus papilloma, posterior fossa lesions, pituitary tumours, metastases); congenital; malfunction of an existing VP shunt (infection, disconnection).

~30% cases are idiopathic. Insertion of a CSF shunt is the commonest paediatric neurosurgical operation.

Preoperative
- The increase in ICP initially causes headache, nausea and vomiting, and then progressive drowsiness and confusion. This in turn leads to a fluid deficit and dehydration.
- Untreated, further increases will cause unconsciousness with evidence of brainstem compression; dilated and unreactive pupils, hypertension and bradycardia (Cushing's response), and irregular respiration.
- These patients are at high risk of aspiration, which can be severe as the raised ICP can increase gastric acid secretion. This may also cause gastric ulceration (Cushing's ulcer) and haemorrhage.
- As with any unconscious patient, assessment, especially of the airway, will be difficult.
- In addition to the standard anaesthetic assessment, pay particular attention to the cause of the hydrocephalus as this may indicate other problems, for example; following SAH there may be an unprotected aneurysm, in a head-injured patient there may be injury to the cervical spine and with posterior fossa lesions bulbar problems (impaired swallowing, aspiration, chest infection).
- The surgical plan may also be to insert an EVD followed by definitive treatment of the cause, e.g. clipping or endovascular coiling of an aneurysm, excision of a posterior fossa tumour.
- Patients with an altered level of consciousness will require urgent treatment aimed at reduction of ICP in order to maintain cerebral perfusion (CPP = MAP–ICP). This should start preoperatively with an

IV bolus of 20% mannitol, $0.5 \, g \, kg^{-1}$. This may be given in conjunction with $0.5 \, mg \, kg^{-1}$ of furosemide. The diuresis induced mandates the insertion of a urinary catheter.
- Do not treat hypertension; this is an indication of the severity of raised ICP.

Intraoperative

The principles of anaesthesia are: a RSI to secure the airway and reduce the risk of aspiration, maintenance of stable cerebral and cardiovascular haemodynamics, and rapid recovery.
- Monitoring—in accordance with AAGBI guidelines, IV access.
- Emergency drugs available—atropine, vasopressors.
- All invasive procedures with strict asepsis because of the high risk of infection; give prophylactic antibiotics.
- Preoxygenate and induce with thiopental or propofol in a reduced dose. Give an opioid to reduce pressor response to laryngoscopy and intubation.
- Neuromuscular block: suxamethonium or rocuronium. Faster onset but transient ↑ ICP, versus slower onset with no change in ICP. May be slightly ↑ risk of failed intubation because of lack of ability to assess airway preoperatively. Have sugammadex available to enable rapid reversal of rocuronium.
- Ensure oxygenation, mild hyperventilation to help reduce CBF and ICP.
- Maintain anaesthesia with either IV infusion or inhalational drugs.
  - IV—obtunds response to surgery, particularly when inserting shunt-passer, reduces $CMRO_2$ and CBF, reducing ICP. May cause hypotension. Rapid recovery from remifentanil. Risk of pain postoperatively if pre-emptive opioids not given. May be short procedure (EVD).
  - Inhalational—all are vasodilators so may increase CBF and ICP. Sevoflurane has least effect (max. 1 MAC). Cerebral reactivity to hypocapnia retained. Good recovery.
  - Nitrous oxide has no place in neuroanaesthesia.
- Positioning—avoid extremes of neck rotation—risk of venous occlusion and ↑ ICP. Head-up.
- Ventilation—minimize intrathoracic pressure.
- Beware of potential fall in BP when CSF drained and rapid reduction in ICP.
- May progress to definitive surgery, consider need for additional monitoring—arterial line, CVP, temperature.
- At end—reverse residual block.
- Extubation or ICU for ventilation. Tracheostomy if bulbar dysfunction.

Postoperative

- Oxygen and analgesia (see 📖 Evacuation of traumatic intracranial haematoma, p.218).
- Neurological assessment, to identify complications: ICH (misplaced shunt), subdural due to rapid decompression.
- Care with height of EVD, check with surgeon before leaving the operating room.

Further reading

Fàbregas N, Craen RA. Anaesthesia for endoscopic neurosurgical procedures. *Curr Opin Anaesthesiol* 2010; **23**(5):568–75.

Craniotomy for urgent decompression of tumours

Key points

- Management of the patient with a CNS tumour presenting for emergency craniotomy, requires the early recognition of the signs and symptoms of raised ICP.
- The anaesthetic technique used must maintain haemodynamic stability whilst not further increasing ICP.

Background

Brain tumours are either primary (neoplasms arising from different cells within the CNS), or secondary, arising mostly from the lung and breast. In adults the commonest tumours are gliomas, metastases, and meningiomas; most (80%) lie in the supratentorial compartment. They cause symptoms by invasion of functional brain tissue, adjacent structures and ↑ ICP.

Brain tumours cause a raised ICP as a result of the surrounding oedema occurring from a disruption of the blood–brain barrier, allowing protein-rich fluid to accumulate in the extracellular space. Occasionally tumours may present acutely because of haemorrhage or the development of hydrocephalus.

Most symptoms of raised ICP associated with oedema around the tumour may be managed initially with steroids. A patient presenting with a low GCS score either from peritumoral oedema or associated haemorrhage requires an urgent craniotomy to decompress the tumour.

Preoperative

Assessment

In addition to the standard anaesthetic assessment, pay particular attention to:

- General symptoms of raised ICP—headaches, seizures, nausea and vomiting, syncope, cognitive dysfunction, and drowsiness.
- Focal symptoms of raised ICP—weakness, aphasia, visual dysfunction.
- Speed of deterioration of conscious level.
- Drug history—is patient on steroids/antiepileptics/antiplatelet drugs/ anticoagulants?
- Premorbid status.
- Pre-existing medical problems—such as chronic lung disease in the case of brain metastases?

Examination

- Document vital signs and assess accurately neurological status—GCS score, pupillary size and reactivity to light, papilloedema, lateralizing signs.
- Life-threatening signs—unilateral or bilateral pupillary dilatation; extreme hypertension with bradycardia; coma; extensor posturing.

Investigations

- CT head ± MRI—gives information about size of lesion, presence of focal or diffuse oedema, hydrocephalus or haemorrhage, likely position of patient in the operating room and ease of surgical access.
- U&Es; FBC and coagulation screen; crossmatch 2 units packed cells (meningiomas may be vascular).
- ECG (there may be acute changes associated with raised ICP).

These investigations should not delay surgery if the patient is deteriorating rapidly. Confirm with the surgeon the planned procedure, position and anticipated complications.

Control of intracranial hypertension and seizures

- Nurse the patient in a 15–30° head-up position with neck in the neutral position.
- If the patient is not already on steroids, load with dexamethasone 8 mg orally (IV if patient obtunded) followed by a regular dose of 4 mg four times daily.
- If the patient exhibits life-threatening signs of raised ICP, surgery must not be delayed. Reduce ICP with mannitol 20% ($0.5\,g\,kg^{-1}$). Furosemide $0.5–1.0\,mg\,kg^{-1}$ intravenously may be given to potentiate the effect of mannitol.
- If the patient is fitting, treat promptly (see 🕮 Status epilepticus, p.216), but this is best managed by inducing anaesthesia.

Intraoperative

- Apply standard monitoring in accordance with AAGBI guidelines.
- An arterial line may be useful before induction for beat-to-beat measurement of BP and ABG analysis.
- Anaesthetic induction should be smooth with the aim of avoiding a rise in ICP secondary to laryngoscopy:
  - Undertake a RSI using suxamethonium ($1\,mg\,kg^{-1}$) if the patient is not starved. Suxamethonium may cause a transient increase in ICP but this is not clinically significant because it is offset by the effect of the induction drug. Alternatively, give rocuronium $1\,mg\,kg^{-1}$.
  - The usual choice of induction drugs includes propofol, thiopental, with fentanyl or alfentanil. Reduce the dose if the patient is comatose.
  - Lidocaine $1\,mg\,kg^{-1}$ IV can also used to obtund the ICP response to intubation.
- After induction the following may be inserted—a central venous line is useful if there is anticipated blood loss and as a route for inotropes; a urinary catheter is useful if diuretics have been given; a nasopharyngeal temperature probe.
- Anaesthesia may be maintained using:
  - Propofol infusion.
  - Volatile anaesthetics—above 1.5 MAC these cause cerebral vasodilatation, which increases ICP (halothane >isoflurane >sevoflurane), so they are often used with MAC-sparing drugs such as remifentanil.
  - Do not use nitrous oxide.

- Deepen anaesthesia while the Mayfield head clamp is applied; the aim is to avoid the associated hypertensive and raised ICP response.
- Aim for the following targets:
  - Ventilation—PaO_2 >13.5 kPa and $PaCO_2$ 4.5–5.0 kPa.
  - Keep MAP >90 mmHg (or cerebral perfusion pressure >60 mmHg if ICP measured).
  - Maintain normovolaemia with fluids (choice not important but avoid glucose containing and hypotonic fluids).
  - Normoglycaemia.
- If the patient is hypotensive despite adequate fluid resuscitation inotropes may be required.
- The optimal intraoperative temperature is debatable. Some anaesthetists let the temperature drift down to 34–36°C. This has not been shown to improve outcome.
- Possible intraoperative problems (see anaesthesia for intracranial haemorrhage in ☐ Evacuation of traumatic intracranial haematoma, p.218)

Postoperative

- Extubate where possible—an awake patient enables neurological status to be monitored.
- Aim for a smooth emergence with minimal straining and coughing.
- Postoperatively, nurse the extubated patient on a level 2 ward where frequent neurological assessment can be performed.
- Obtunded consciousness on presentation and intraoperative problems such as brain swelling, difficult haemostasis, and postoperative homeostatic disturbances may require the patient to be ventilated postoperatively, which will also enable therapeutic control of ICP.
- Postcraniotomy analgesia (see ☐ Evacuation of traumatic intracranial haematoma, p.218).

Acute spinal cord compression

Key points

- Patients with acute spinal cord compression will require anaesthesia for surgery to decompress the cord or stabilize the spine. This may take place as an emergency, or several days after presentation.
- Spinal cord compression may present with a spectrum of signs and symptoms, in particular, varying degrees of neurological deficit and often severe pain.
- ▶ Ensure that injuries to the spinal cord are neither caused nor exacerbated by mechanical or physiological mismanagement during anaesthesia and surgery.

Background

Acute spinal cord compression can be caused by trauma, infection, degenerative disease of the intervertebral discs, or malignancy. This topic concentrates on the latter, although the same principles apply when managing patients with infection or disc problems. Acute compression of the cervical cord is managed as described in 🕮 Cervical spine fractures, p.238.

- Direct pressure, vertebral collapse, or instability from metastatic spread or direct extension of a malignancy causing neurological disability is estimated to occur with an incidence of up to 80 cases per million population per year in England and Wales.
- There is a move towards early surgery because this is more effective than radiotherapy in maintaining mobility in those who can still walk.
- Oncologists may request debulking of the tumour before starting radiotherapy treatment.
- Surgery is often carried out as an emergency, can be extensive, and cause massive haemorrhage.
- Many of these patients will be systemically unwell because of the widespread effects of the disease and drug therapy, particularly immunosuppressants.
- Patients should not be denied surgery where it may help pain control, even if life expectancy is limited.

Preoperative

In addition to the standard anaesthetic assessment, pay attention to the following:

- Extent of the disease:
  - Locally—what neurological deficit is present, is the spine stable?
  - Systemically—bony involvement with risk of or presence of pathological fractures, anaemia and thrombocytopaenia, liver metastases affecting function, especially coagulation, cerebral metastases.
  - Pain—severity, effect on movement, ventilation, coughing.
- Medication:
  - Analgesics—type, dose, and route of administration.
  - Anticoagulation—patient are high risk for DVT/PE; reverse any warfarin with prothrombin complex.
  - Immunosuppressants—steroids, risk of intercurrent infections.

- Gut function—risk of ileus.
- Surgical plan:
  - Approach—anterior, posterior, or both; transthoracic.
  - Extent—number of levels, decompression with instrumentation.
  - Positioning—need to turn the patient during the procedure.
- Blood products: crossmatched blood, platelets, FFP.
- Postoperative planning:
  - Airway management—extubation, leave intubated, or perform a tracheostomy. This will depend on several factors including extent and duration of surgery and respiratory and bulbar function.
  - Location—patients will require level 2 or 3 care postoperatively.
  - Analgesia and venous thromboembolism prophylaxis.

Intraoperative

- Monitoring in accordance with AAGBI guidelines:
  - ECG electrodes dependent on position of patient (avoid lying on them).
  - Arterial and CVP lines if significant blood loss anticipated or thoracotomy planned—arterial line enables rapid identification and treatment of hypotension as this may jeopardize cord perfusion.
  - Regular ABG analyses to assess ventilation and tissue perfusion.
- IV access: size and number of cannulae dependent on anticipated blood loss.
- All invasive procedures require strict asepsis because of the high risk of infection; give prophylactic antibiotics.
- Ensure emergency drugs are available: atropine, vasopressors.
- Check blood is crossmatched, blood warmer primed, rapid infusion device available.

Anaesthesia

- Preoxygenation and induction with thiopental or propofol, in a reduced dose. Give an opioid to reduce pressor response to laryngoscopy and intubation.
- Neuromuscular block—if high risk of regurgitation, use RSI with suxamethonium. If presentation delayed >5–7 days, suxamethonium may cause hyperkalaemia because of denervation injury. Alternatively, use rocuronium $1\,mg\,kg^{-1}$; its prolonged duration could cause difficulties in the event of a 'can't intubate, can't ventilate' scenario; therefore, ensure an adequate dose of sugammadex ($16\,mg\,kg^{-1}$) is immediately available.
- Intubate with a double lumen tube or bronchial blocker if thoracotomy and lung deflation required.
- Maintenance—aim to maintain oxygenation and perfusion of the spinal. Avoid hypotension caused by induction. The choice is between a volatile anaesthetic and TIVA.
- Ventilation: pressure control with a low level of PEEP.

Spinal cord monitoring

See 📖 p.243.

Positioning of the patient

Many patients with spinal compression will need to be turned prone for surgery, either at the start of the procedure or after the completion of anterior surgery. This is a critical and high-risk manoeuvre:

- Ensure that the airway is secure. Consider disconnecting from the ventilator tubing during the turn to reduce the risk of accidental extubation.
- Ensure all cannulae are secure; consider short extensions to enable disconnecting while turning.
- All equipment must be in place e.g. chest, pelvic supports, and Montreal mattress.
- Ensure sufficient people—a minimum of six.
- The most experienced person takes the head.

Once prone, check:

- Airway patent and secure, tube in trachea (not dislodged or endobronchial).
- Ventilation re-established, adequate ($ETCO_2$), oxygenation.
- Haemodynamic status, BP, pulse. Venous return is easily compromised reducing cardiac output.
- Anaesthesia adequate, end-tidal volatile, cannulae reconnected, infusions running.
- Patient safe—a 'top-to-toe' check:
  - Eyes protected to prevent corneal injury (ingress of skin prep, drying); avoid pressure as this can cause retinal artery thrombosis.
  - Abdomen free from pressure to maintain venous return and not impede ventilation.
  - Peripheral nerves in arms and legs not under pressure or stretch.
  - Male genitalia not squashed.

Spinal cord monitoring

See 📖 p.243

Management of bleeding

- Monitor blood loss using point-of-care device (e.g. HemoCue®).
- Controlled hypotension may be required to help reduce blood loss.
- Avoid hypothermia.
- Regular check of acid–base status if surgery prolonged or massive transfusion required.

At end of surgery

- Reverse residual neuromuscular block and ensure the patient is normothermic.
- Ensure lung fully inflated, chest drains swinging.
- Return safely to supine position.
- Check neurological function.

Postoperative

- Adequate analgesia—paravertebral catheter, opioid infusion, or PCA with regular paracetamol.
- Avoid NSAIDs for at least 24 h because of the risk of postoperative haematoma around the cord.
- Safe transfer to recovery area or direct to level 2/3 care.

Cervical spine fractures

Key points
- Patients with cervical spine fractures will require anaesthesia for surgery either to the spine or to other injuries. This may take place as an emergency, or several days after injury.
- They may present with a spectrum of injuries ranging from simple fractures with no neurological deficit, to those with high spinal cord damage rendering them quadriplegic and ventilator dependent.
- ▶ Ensure that injuries to the spinal cord are neither caused nor exacerbated by mechanical or physiological mismanagement during anaesthesia and surgery.

Background
- The incidence of cervical spine injury (CSI) in blunt trauma is 2–6%; around 40% of fractures occur at C6/7.
- Most patients with CSI have other injuries; only 20% have an isolated CSI. 25–50% of patients with CSI will have traumatic brain injury (TBI) and around 5% of patients presenting with TBI have associated CSI.
- ~10% of CSI patients will have a ligamentous injury, in association with joint subluxation and 4% have a cord injury without subluxation or a fracture. This is often referred to as spinal cord injury without radiological abnormality (SCIWORA). A proportion of these are unstable.
- Many of these patients are at risk of hypoxaemia and hypotension and will require airway intervention, both of which predispose to secondary injury.

▶ All patients with the potential for CSI must be treated with spinal immobilization until injury has been excluded or definitive management initiated—this is discussed in more detail in 🕮 Spinal injury, p.104.

Preoperative
Use an ABC approach:
- **Airway**—examine the type of spinal immobilization and its effect on the patient's airway, particularly mouth opening. A semi-rigid collar, blocks, and tape restricts movement to 5% of normal, reduces mouth opening, and impedes airway management. A halo jacket and frame restricts movement and access, but with less effect on mouth opening. Assess the patient's dentition and view obtained of the pharynx. Aim to predict problems with laryngoscopy and intubation. If fibreoptic bronchoscopy (FOB) for intubation is planned, check the patency of the patient's nostrils. Obtain informed consent for the procedure if planning to do this awake.
- **Breathing**—the level of cord injury may compromise ventilation. Injury between C4–C7 will result in loss of intercostal function. The patient will be dependent on their diaphragm. If the injury is above C4, they will have no intrinsic respiratory muscle activity and be intubated and ventilated. A tracheostomy may have been performed.

- *Circulation*—hypotension and bradycardia suggest neurogenic shock. The loss of sympathetic tone following cord injury above C7 causes vasodilatation and loss of cardio-accelerator fibres. A relative hypovolaemia exists that may require intravascular volume replacement, inotropes, and vasopressors. Other causes of hypotension, e.g. occult blood loss, must be excluded.
- Current neurological status—check the level of injury and whether the cord injury is complete or incomplete.
- Identify all other injuries, particularly to the brain. If not done, perform a secondary survey.
- Identify other co-morbidities, previous anaesthetics, allergies, drugs, family history.
- Check the results of investigations and availability of crossmatched blood.
- CSI patients have a high risk of delayed gastric emptying increasing the risk of regurgitation. This is due to the development of an ileus, compounded by the stress of trauma and use of opioids.

Assess radiology
Check the level of lesion(s) and the degree of spinal cord injury. Determine if the injury is stable or unstable. Look at the pharyngeal soft tissues to check for the presence of a prevertebral haematoma.

Discuss with surgeon
- The stability of spine.
- The type of operation planned. This may be either an anterior or posterior approach to decompress the spinal cord with fixation of the fracture, or a combination of both.
- The approach will determine the position of the patient and whether they will need to be turned prone for surgery.

Postoperative planning
- Airway management—extubation, leave intubated, or perform a tracheostomy. This will depend on several factors including extent and duration of surgery and respiratory and bulbar function.
- Patients will require level 2 or 3 care postoperatively.
- Analgesia and venous thromboembolism prophylaxis.

Transfer
- Patients with a high cord injury will be on the ICU, intubated and ventilated, and will be monitored invasively.
- Transfer patients to the operating room with close attention to their haemodynamic status. Loss of sympathetic tone can cause marked swings in BP, particularly hypotension.

Intraoperative
- In the anaesthetic room, confirm or obtain wide-bore IV access.
- Secure all cannulae and catheters so they are not pulled out if turned prone.
- Prepare drugs, including those required in an emergency.
- Monitoring:
  - ECG (electrodes dependent on positioning), SpO_2, temperature.

- Intra-arterial BP; allows rapid identification and treatment of hypotension as this may jeopardize cord perfusion.
- If anterior surgery is planned, use the opposite side for an internal jugular central line.
- Urinary catheter if surgery likely to be prolonged.
- Equipment for intubation must be checked and immediately available, including:
  - Laryngoscopes and blades of different sizes and types, McCoy®, Airtraq®, Glidescope®, etc.
  - Tracheal tubes, usually reinforced; range of sizes.
  - Bougie, exchange catheter.
  - Supraglottic airway of choice, intubating laryngeal mask (ILM).
  - Fibreoptic laryngoscope or bronchoscope.
  - Cricothyroidotomy kit, including a high-pressure gas source.

Anaesthesia

The aim is to maintain perfusion of the spinal cord:
- Avoid hypotension during induction.
- Prevent the hypertensive response to laryngoscopy and intubation.
- The choice is IV induction and volatile anaesthetic for maintenance; TIVA; or inhalation induction and maintenance with volatile anaesthetic.

Whichever technique is used, thorough preoxygenation is essential.

The choice of neuromuscular blocking drug for direct laryngoscopy and intubation is between:
- Suxamethonium—rapid onset, but there is the theoretical (unlikely) potential for the fasciculations to cause movement and cord injury. After 5–7 days it may cause hyperkalaemia due to denervation injury. Most commonly used in the emergency situation where high risk of regurgitation.
- Rocuronium 1 mg kg^{-1}—slightly slower onset but avoids the problems of suxamethonium. Its prolonged duration may cause difficulties in the event of a 'can't intubate, can't ventilate' scenario, but the availability of an adequate dose of sugammadex (16 mg kg^{-1}) negates this problem.

Airway management

Secondary cord injury in CSI patients may be precipitated when management is suboptimal. Despite optimal management, deterioration occurs in 2–10% of patients; this is probably an inevitable consequence of the pathophysiology of CSI.
- There is no evidence that one technique is superior to another with respect to neurological outcome.
- The most skilled operator available should perform intubation, using the technique with which they are most competent and confident.
- It is inappropriate to be practising FOB intubation on these patients.

Direct laryngoscopy and tracheal intubation

Replace with manual in-line stabilization (MILS) any lateral blocks, collar and tape. The purpose of MILS is to apply sufficient downward force to the head to oppose the upward movement generated by the laryngoscope during intubation. Reinforced (armoured) tubes are often used for prone patients to prevent kinking. These tubes cannot be shortened and are easily inserted too far.

- MILS is applied by an experienced operator, maintaining the head and neck in a neutral position. Once MILS is applied, remove the anterior portion of the collar or fold it to one side.
- Preoxygenate the patient, induce anaesthesia, inject a neuromuscular blocker, and apply cricoid pressure if indicated.
- Undertake direct laryngoscopy with a McCoy® levering laryngoscope (or suitable videolaryngoscope if experienced in its use).
- Using the least possible force, aim for a view that enables introduction of bougie into larynx.
- While leaving the laryngoscope in position, railroad a size 7 tracheal tube over the bougie, rotating 90° anticlockwise to ease through larynx.
- Inflate cuff, check position, and secure.

In comparison with leaving the blocks, collar, and tape *in situ* during laryngoscopy, MILS reduces the incidence of grade 3 view from 64% to 22%. Cricoid pressure does not cause excessive movement of the spine. There is little evidence that the type of blade used for direct laryngoscopy has a significant effect on spinal movement; however, it may affect the view at laryngoscopy. If the patient is in a halo jacket and frame, this is left in place and MILS is not required. The advantages of this technique are:

- It is generally quicker.
- It does not require specialized equipment.
- The skill is widespread amongst anaesthetists.
- It eliminates the risk of coughing and retching.

The disadvantages are the theoretical potential for greater movement if MILS is applied poorly or excessive force is used and the risk of creating a 'can't intubate, can't ventilate' scenario.

Failure to intubate
- Reoxygenate patient; consider an alternative blade.
- Release cricoid pressure and apply backward, upward, and rightward pressure (BURP) manoeuvre to the larynx.
- Consider different technique, e.g. insert LMA or intubating LMA, FOB.

Intubation using a fibreoptic bronchoscope
- Usually performed with the patient awake, but in combination with LA (spray as you go, nebulized LA or nerve blocks) with or without sedation.
- The nasal route is the most popular and avoids the need to remove the collar.
- If the oral route is used, replace spinal immobilization with MILS.
- Ask the patient to protrude their tongue, or get an assistant to pull the tongue forward to enable a better view of the larynx.
- There is no evidence that tracheal intubation with a FOB is any safer than direct laryngoscopy.
- Most of the evidence for the efficacy of FOB comes from its use in elective cases, usually in patients with degenerative disease of the spine.
- FOB is used widely in planned cases particularly when the patient has had a halo jacket fitted and access is limited.

Advantages:
- Head and neck left in a neutral position, assuming the patient does not cough or retch.
- Little spinal movement to achieve a view of the larynx.
- Protective reflexes are intact, providing excessive sedation is not required.
- Neurological assessment may be possible after intubation.

Disadvantages:
- Hypoxia, hypercapnia.
- Failure.
- Coughing and retching.
- Bleeding.
- Equipment required.
- Skill/training.
- ↑ICP may not be prevented by sedatives or the use of LAs.
- Excessive sedation.
- Intolerance.

Positioning of the patient

▶ A significant proportion of patients with CSI will need to be turned prone for surgery, either at the start of the procedure or after the completion of anterior surgery. This is a high-risk manoeuvre. The surgeon may wish to apply a Mayfield clamp either before or after turning to fix the head and neck in position. During positioning ensure that:
- The airway is secure—consider disconnecting from the ventilator tubing during the turn to reduce the risk of accidental extubation.
- All cannulae are secure—consider disconnecting while turning.
- All equipment is in place, e.g. chest and pelvic supports, Montreal mattress.
- There are sufficient people—a minimum of six.
- The most experienced person takes the head.

Once prone, check:
- Airway patent and secure, the tube is in trachea (not dislodged or endobronchial).
- Ventilation and oxygenation is adequate (ETCO$_2$ and SpO$_2$).
- Haemodynamic status, BP, pulse. Venous return is easily compromised, which decreases the cardiac output.
- Anaesthesia adequate, end-tidal volatile agent, cannulae reconnected, infusions running.
- Check that the patient is safe:
  - Eyes protected to prevent corneal injury (ingress of skin prep, drying)—avoid pressure as this can cause retinal artery thrombosis.
  - Abdomen free from pressure to maintain venous return and not impede ventilation.
  - Peripheral nerves in arms and legs not under pressure or stretch.
  - Male genitalia not squashed!

Spinal cord monitoring

This may be used to provide warning of iatrogenic cord injury during surgery, particularly if the spine is instrumented.

- Somatosensory evoked potentials (SSEPs) work on the principle of applying a peripheral electrical stimulus and monitoring the response in the cerebral cortex via scalp electrodes (amplitude and latency). This enables the integrity of the afferent pathways in the posterior columns to be monitored. A 50% increase in amplitude or 10% increase in latency is usually taken as indication of deteriorating cord function.
- Volatile anaesthetics cause a dose-dependent decrease in both amplitude and latency while SSEPs are well preserved using TIVA. Motor evoked potentials (MEPs) monitor efferent pathways usually by stimulating the cord above the level of the lesion and monitoring electromyographic (EMG) potentials in the leg muscles. They are much more sensitive to volatile anaesthetics and therefore TIVA is required for adequate signal quality.

Problems at extubation

Airway obstruction occurs in ~1% of patients as a result of pharyngeal oedema. It does not appear to be related to technique used for intubation. Re-intubation is usually required, and can be more difficult as a result of surgery (fusion) and airway oedema. It occurs more frequently when surgery is prolonged and involving multiple levels via an anterior approach.

Postoperative

- Posterior cervical spine surgery is very painful and the patient will require opioids.
- If hand function and mental state allows, a PCA with regular paracetamol is usually adequate.
- Avoid NSAIDs for at least 24h because of the risk of postoperative haematoma around the cord.

Further reading

Bonhomme V, Hans P. Management of the unstable cervical spine: elective versus emergent cases. *Curr Opin Anaesthesiol* 2009; **22**:579–85.

Crosby ET. Considerations for airway management for cervical spine surgery in adults. *Anesthesiol Clin* 2007; **25**:511–33.

Gercek E, Wahlen BM, Rommens PM. In vivo ultrasound real-time motion of the cervical spine during intubation under manual in-line stabilization: a comparison of intubation methods. *Eur J Anaesthesiol* 2008; **25**:29–36.

Houde BJ, Williams SR, Cadrin-Chênevert A, et al. A comparison of cervical spine motion during orotracheal intubation with the trachlight or the flexible fiberoptic bronchoscope. *Anesth Analg* 2009; **108**:1638–43.

Manninen PH, Jose GB, Lukitto K, et al. Management of the airway in patients undergoing cervical spine surgery. *J Neurosurg Anesthesiol* 2007; **19**:190–4.

Stephens CT, Kahntroff S, Dutton RP. The success of emergency endotracheal intubation in trauma patients: a 10-year experience at a major adult trauma referral center. *Anesth Analg* 2009; **109**:866–72.

Anaesthesia for organ retrieval

Key points
- Although there has been a gradual increase in the proportion of organ donations from living relatives and donation after circulatory death (DCD) donors, the majority come from patients whose families consent to donation after a patient has been declared brainstem dead (donation after brain death (DBD)).
- After brainstem death there is a gradual decline in cardiovascular stability that results in loss of homeostasis, reduced oxygen delivery, and organ failure.
- In order to maximize donor organ function, the anaesthetist caring for the DBD donor must maintain the physiological support provided in the ICU. Failure to provide this support while waiting for organ retrieval accounts for the loss of up to 25% of transplantable organs.

Background
- Following brainstem death, a wide range of physiological changes occur, which if left untreated will result in organ damage and reduce the chance of a successful transplantation. These changes take place within the cardiovascular, endocrine, respiratory, and renal systems leading to metabolic disturbances and failure of homeostatic mechanisms e.g. coagulation, temperature control, and water and electrolyte balance.
- The longer the period between brainstem death and organ retrieval, the more severe the organ dysfunction. Specific treatment to reduce organ damage and dysfunction must start on ICU and continue en route to, and within, the operating room until the point where the circulation ceases and the organs are removed. During this period, these patients will need continuous cardiovascular and respiratory support, invasive monitoring, metabolic management, strict infection control, and treatment with dignity.
- Brainstem death occurs as a result of ischaemia secondary to ↑ ICP. Initially, BP increases in an attempt to maintain cerebral perfusion. Midbrain ischaemia results in a bradycardia and when the pons becomes ischaemic there is sympathetic activation causing hypertension (Cushing's reflex). As the medulla becomes involved, there is a further massive increase in sympathetic activity and a loss of baroreceptor reflexes, often referred to as an autonomic storm. This results in intense vasoconstriction causing global end-organ ischaemia. Finally the sympathetic outflow abates and the loss of vasomotor control causes hypotension.

Cardiovascular system
There is marked cardiovascular instability, often with hypotension that is exacerbated by hypovolaemia because of:
- Prior treatment of cerebral oedema with diuretics to control ICP.
- Myocardial dysfunction due to ischaemia.
- Pituitary dysfunction and failure of secretion of vasopressin (see following section).
- An osmotic diuresis (see later section).

Cardiac arrhythmias are common, occurring in ~25% donors.

Endocrine system

Failure of the posterior pituitary results in very low plasma concentrations of vasopressin (in up to 90% donors). This causes:

- Vasodilatation (V1 receptors).
- Diabetes insipidus, with loss of water and hypernatraemia (V2 receptors).
- Reduced secretion of adrenocorticotrophic hormone (ACTH) (V3 receptors).

Deficiencies of the anterior pituitary are less consistent but many donors have reduced levels of T_3, T_4, ACTH, thyroid stimulating hormone (TSH), and human growth hormone (HGH). Hyperglycaemia is common, secondary to insulin resistance. Donors with severe TBI may exhibit a stress response and adrenal insufficiency.

Renal system

The kidneys are susceptible to both immunological and non-immunological injury after brainstem death. The latter is exacerbated by hypotension (SBP <80mmHg) and the use of high doses of dopamine (>10 micrograms kg^{-1} min^{-1}) to treat this, which increases the risk of acute tubular necrosis and graft failure.

Respiratory system

Impaired oxygenation may be caused by ARDS compounded by pulmonary infection.

Hepatic system

Donor hypernatraemia (plasma Na^+ >155mmol L^{-1}) must be corrected because otherwise sodium accumulates in the donor liver and after transplantation intracellular water accumulation and cell death may occur.

Hypothermia

- Loss of hypothalamic function and the reduced metabolic rate will tend to cause hypothermia in the donor.
- Hypothermia further compromises the oxygenation of organs by increasing the risk of arrhythmias, inducing a left-shift of the oxygen dissociation curve and predisposing to a coagulopathy.
- Donors often need a lot of fluid (including FFP and blood), an arginine vasopressin infusion or bolus doses of desmopressin, along with vasopressors to maintain SVR and inotropes to maintain cardiac output and urine output.
- Most donors will be given infusions of T_3 and insulin, along with methylprednisolone, as 'hormonal resuscitation'.
- Invasive monitoring is essential and a lung protective strategy is used for ventilation: limiting FiO_2 and inspiratory pressures, use of PEEP.

Preoperative

- Confirm certification of death:
  - Cause of death.
  - Correct procedure and documentation for determination of brainstem death.
- Confirm documentation of consent from the family for organ donation.

- Review donor physiological status:
  - Cardiovascular—observations, fluids, drugs.
  - Respiratory—observations, ventilatory strategy, oxygenation.
  - Metabolic—FBC, U&Es, ABGs, blood sugar, drugs.
- Check equipment for transfer to operating room:
  - Ventilator, oxygen supply.
  - IV pumps—battery life, syringe contents.
  - Monitors—ECG, SpO_2, $ETCO_2$, CVP, BP, temperature, ventilator.
  - IV lines, fluids.
- Preparation of anaesthetic equipment and drugs in the operating room:
  - Anaesthesia machine.
  - Monitors.
  - Drugs—anaesthesia, vasopressors, inotropes, heparin, those requested by transplant team.
  - Defibrillator.
  - Warming devices.
  - Blood available if heart, liver, and kidneys being harvested.

Transfer

Ensure a safe transfer to the operating room and try to maintain haemodynamic stability: pulse 60–120 min^{-1}; MAP 80–90 mmHg; CVP 8–12 mmHg; urine output 100 mL h^{-1}; cardiac output 4–8 L min^{-1}; ScvO$_2$ >75%; and temperature 36.5–37.5°C.

Intraoperative

- Aim to maintain optimal organ perfusion and tissue oxygenation while blunting the effects of the spinal, cardiovascular, and adrenal medullary reflexes.
- Give neuromuscular blockers to prevent reflex activity and facilitate surgery.
- Give opioids to control haemodynamic response to surgery.
- Anaesthetic drugs, e.g. volatile drugs, whilst not essential, are often given to help control the haemodynamic reflexes, at the same time providing psychological assurance that the donor is not suffering any stress.
- Anticipate fluid shifts and blood loss, maintain drug infusions and prevent hypothermia.
- Measure regularly ABGs, clotting, U&Es, and blood glucose.
- Ventilation: aim for a PaO_2 of 12–20 kPa; maintain normocapnia—brain death reduces CO_2 production; normal minute volume may cause severe hypocapnia and vasoconstriction.

Arrhythmias

- Ventricular arrhythmias may need amiodarone.
- Bradycardia is usually resistant to treatment with atropine and may need an adrenaline or isoprenaline infusion.
- Ensure a defibrillator is immediately available (with internal paddles).

Lung donors

- Control FiO_2 to reduce oxygen toxicity—0.4 is usually adequate.
- Aim for PEEP <7.5 cmH_2O.
- Mediastinal and tracheal dissection may cause problems with ventilation.
- Pulmonary perfusate may cause hypotension—once it is given, reduce ventilation. Suction the trachea before extubating.

Heart donors

- Heparinization is required.
- Anaesthesia ends with aortic cross-clamping and infusion of cooling/cardioplegia solution.
- Note aortic cross-clamp time.
- Stop anaesthesia and withdraw any CVP/PA catheters.

Records

Document the anaesthetic; any drugs given at request of transplant team and the timings of all events.

Postoperative

Debrief the staff; they may not want an immediate debrief, but the opportunity must be made later if required. It is essential to enable all of those involved in the procedure the opportunity to express their thoughts about what has happened. Many donors are young and this can be distressing, particularly for those with children.

Further reading

Academy of Medical Royal Colleges. A code of practice for the diagnosis and confirmation of death. London: Academy of Medical Royal Colleges, 2008. Available at: ℬ http://www.aomrc.org.uk/reports-guidance.html.

McKeown DW, Bonser RS, Kellum JA. Management of the heartbeating brain-dead organ donor. *Br J Anaesth* 2012; **108**(S1): i96–i107.

UK Donation Ethics Committee guidance. Available at: ℬ www.aomrc.org.uk/committees/uk-donation-ethics-committee/work-programme.html.

Plastic Surgery

Rhys Davies and David Windsor

Major burns

Key points

- Anaesthetists will be involved in resuscitation, transfer, intensive care, and multiple operating room episodes.
- Assess airway and gain vascular access early.
- Burns can be associated with other injuries—road traffic crashes, blasts.
- Pay attention to temperature regulation, fluid and electrolyte balance, and blood loss.
- Involve burn specialists early.
- There are associations with psychiatric illness, poverty and extremes of age.

Background

- Burns account for 175 000 ED attendances each year in the UK. Of these, 13 000 require admission and 1000 require fluid resuscitation. Half of all burns admissions are children.
- Burns can be thermal (hot or cold), chemical (acid or alkali), or electrical. Skin conditions can also give burn-like injury (e.g. Stevens–Johnson syndrome, staphylococcal scalded skin, epidermolysis bullosa). Most adult burns are flame burns. Scalds account for 70% of paediatric burns (70% between 1 and 3 years old).

Burn assessment

- Classified as type, depth of injury and percentage of total body surface area (TBSA).
- Using 'rule of nines' for % burn estimate in adults (head 9%, front of chest 9%, front of abdomen 9%, upper/mid/lower back and buttocks 18%, each arm 9%, groin 1%, each leg 18%). The patient's palm is ~1%. Erythema should not be included as part of the estimate. Formal calculation should be done using Lund and Browder charts (Fig. 10.1).
- Burn depth (Table 10.1)
- A burn may consist of different depths within its area.
- Specialist burns input needed if: TBSA (adult >10%, child >5%), age (<5 or >60 years), site (face, hands, feet, perineum, circumferential), inhalational injury, mechanism (chemical with >5% TBSA, ionizing radiation), co-morbidities, associated injuries (e.g. open fractures, tissue loss), or suspected non-accidental injury.

% Total Body Surface Area Burn
Be clear and accurate, and do not include erythema
(Lund and Browder)

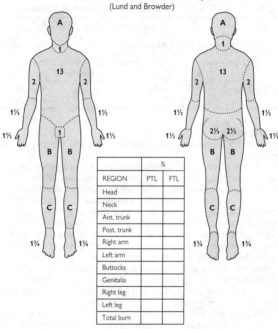

	%	
REGION	PTL	FTL
Head		
Neck		
Ant. trunk		
Post. trunk		
Right arm		
Left arm		
Buttocks		
Genitalia		
Right leg		
Left leg		
Total burn		

AREA	Age 0	1	5	10	15	Adult
A = ½ OF HEAD	9½	8½	6½	5½	4½	3½
B = ½ OF ONE THIGH	2¾	3¼	4	4½	4½	4¾
C = ½ OF ONE LOWER LEG	2½	2½	2¾	3	3¼	3½

Fig. 10.1 Lund and Browder chart. Reproduced from *British Medical Journal*, 'ABC of burns: Initial management of a major burn: II—assessment and resuscitation', Shehan Hettiaratchy and Remo Papini, **529**, p.101, 2004, with permission from BMJ Publishing Group Ltd.

Table 10.1 Characteristics of burns according to depth

Depth	Appearance	Sensation	Scarring
Superficial	Red, erythema	Yes	No
Partial thickness—superficial	Red, blistering	Yes	Less
Partial thickness—deep	Pink, mottled	May be reduced	More
Full thickness	White, leathery	Absent	Yes, with contracture

Pathophysiology
Major thermal injury causes tissue damage and a SIRS affecting all organ systems:
- *Respiratory* effects include upper airway injury and progressive airway oedema and obstruction. Swelling can last several days. Lower airway thermal injury from smoke inhalation causes mucosal damage, inflammation, oedema and ARDS. Consider carbon monoxide and cyanide poisoning from inhalation of toxic gases.
- *Circulation* effects include tissue destruction and thrombosis of blood vessels. SIRS causes ↑ capillary permeability (maximal in the first 8 h but can last days) resulting in oedema proportional to the size of the burn. Hypovolaemia is common. Cardiac output is initially low with vasoconstriction; later it is high because of vasodilation from SIRS.
- *Gastrointestinal* capillary leak causes gut oedema. Delayed gastric emptying is common early, as is ileus later. Hypercatabolism generates high calorific requirements—start enteral feeding early.
- *Dermal* loss leads to massive heat and fluid loss and ↑ risk of local and systemic infection. Ensure meticulous infection control from all team members to prevent hospital-acquired infections.
- *Musculoskeletal* damage occurs initially from burn and trauma, and later due to infection and surgical debridement. Muscle destruction will cause myoglobin release. Contractures can occur either early or late, and may require escharotomy or fasciotomy if causing respiratory or vascular compromise.
- *Renal* impairment can be prerenal (hypovolaemia) or renal (rhabdomyolysis—check creatine kinase and dip urine for myoglobin).

Preoperative resuscitation
Use an ABCDE approach.

Airway/breathing
- Assess immediately and repeat frequently.
- Give oxygen to maintain normal saturation.
- Carbonaceous deposits to nose, mouth, and sputum, singeing of eyebrows/nasal hair, voice changes/hoarseness, facial/airway swelling, a history of contained explosion or prolonged entrapment should raise suspicion of airway and lung injury.

- Analyse ABGs with co-oximetry to diagnose carbon monoxide poisoning.
- Early tracheal intubation is indicated if there is airway injury, respiratory failure, or reduced level of consciousness. Leave the tracheal tube uncut to accommodate ongoing facial/airway swelling. The risk of difficult intubation is high. Access to airway adjuncts, rescue devices and senior help is recommended.

Circulation

- Large-bore IV access should be obtained and bloods taken (including group and save, U&Es, FBC, carboxyhaemoglobin, creatine kinase, and consider cyanide levels).
- Infuse warmed resuscitation fluids if >20 %TBSA (see 📖 Fluid therapy, p.26).
- Central venous (multilumen and antimicrobial if available) and arterial lines must be placed with strict asepsis, ideally through unburned skin.
- Insert a urinary catheter and monitor urine output (dip urine for myoglobin/haemoglobin).
- High fluid and protein losses mean hypovolaemia and subsequent cardiovascular instability is common.
- Aggressive fluid resuscitation guided by the Parkland formula (IV Hartmann's solution) is most common and covers the first 24 h from time of injury.

> ### Parkland formula
>
> Fluid requirement = $2–4\,mL\ \%TBSA^{-1}\,kg^{-1}$ body weight.
>
> Total calculated fluid should be divided into two:
> - Half given in the first 8 h.
> - Half in the subsequent 16 h.
>
> Example: 20% burn in 70 kg patient:
> - Total ($4\,mL\ \%TBSA^{-1}\,kg^{-1}$) IV fluid 5600 mL for first 24 h.
> - Give half (2800 mL) in first 8 h and then half over 16 h.

▶ The value of these resuscitation fluid formulae has been challenged not least because of difficulty in getting an accurate early estimate of the burn area. The formula should guide the initial fluid resuscitation but must be adjusted based on monitoring and clinical judgement.
- Give blood to maintain the haemoglobin concentration at $8–10\,g\,dL^{-1}$.
- Clinical measures of adequate resuscitation include:
  - Urine output (aim: adult $0.5\,mL\,kg^{-1}h^{-1}$, child $1\,mL\,kg^{-1}h^{-1}$). In patients with myoglobinuria, aim for higher urine output and consider an osmotic diuretic (e.g. mannitol).
  - CVP.
  - Cardiac output monitoring—allows individualized fluid therapy.
- Early use of albumin and colloid in these patients remains controversial.

Disability (neurological)

Altered level of consciousness is always significant—from the burn itself, associated injuries or drugs.

Exposure

- Stop the burn—exposed clothing should be removed, residual chemicals brushed or rinsed off, and affected areas rinsed with large volumes of water, unless contraindicated due to causative agent.
- Avoid heat loss. After cleaning, cover burns with dry dressings. Use forced air warming blankets and a warmed environment.
- Cover burns to prevent infection.
- Early specialist debridement of full thickness burns is indicated.
- Antibiotics should not be given empirically and should be guided by a senior microbiologist.

Transfer

- Stabilize patients before any transfer to a burns centre.
- If progressive airway and breathing problems, intubate the trachea before transfer.
- Ensure experienced transfer team with appropriate portable equipment (see 📖 Transport and transfer, p.60).

Preoperative

- Ideally surgery should take place in a dedicated burns centre with a specialist team. Initial debridement and wound coverage should occur within the first 48 h.
- Thorough airway assessment and preparation for a difficult intubation essential (oedema and scarring to larynx and soft tissues can progress rapidly).
- Operating room and table should be warmed (to >27°C).
- Blood and blood products should be available (cross match 6–8 units)—debridement can cause substantial bleeding.
- Plan postoperative care (e.g. HDU/ICU/isolation room).
- Discuss surgical plan/positioning with surgeons—multiple positions may be needed for extensive burns.

Intraoperative

- Consider invasive monitoring (arterial and CVP). Positioning of lines, ECG stickers, BP cuffs may be difficult because of burn. Consider crocodile clips attached to surgical staples in three-lead pattern for ECG monitoring and ear probes on lip or nostril for pulse oximetry. NIBP can be measured even if burned skin below cuff if essential to do so but invasive monitoring is better. Monitor hourly urine output.
- RSI and tracheal intubation in acute situation—uncut tube to allow for significant facial swelling over first 24 h. Secure tube carefully—remember patient may need to be prone or lateral during surgery.
- Temperature measurement is mandatory, use forced air and fluid warmers to maintain normothermia.
- Procedures can be very stimulating. Consider high-dose opioids. Longer-acting drugs will be required postoperatively (PCA or infusion); avoid NSAIDs.
- Insert nasogastric or nasojejunal tube for postoperative nutrition.
- Extubation may be possible if burn does not involve face or airway, there is normothermia and acceptable gas exchange.

- If there is airway injury/oedema, postoperative ventilatory support will be needed. Extubate fully awake with demonstrable return of airway reflexes, and the presence of a cuff leak.

Choice of drugs

- Drug pharmacokinetics will change with the time from injury (initially poorly perfused with low drug clearance; later hyperdynamic state with high drug clearance). There may be an ↑ anaesthetic requirement in the hyperdynamic phase.
- Upregulation of extra-junctional acetylcholine receptors leads to potentially significant potassium rise with suxamethonium (greatest risk 48 h to 1 year).
- Rocuronium (1 mg kg^{-1}) can be used as an alternative to suxamethonium. Sugammadex should be available with this technique for rapid reversal of neuromuscular block if needed.
- ↑ dose and frequency of non-depolarizing blockers may be required. A nerve stimulator should be used.
- Significant protein loss will potentiate effect of highly protein-bound drugs (e.g. NSAIDs).
- Tolerance to analgesia may also occur.

Common operative procedures

- *Debridement* can result in discrete but significant blood loss (estimated 1 mL per cm^2). Check Hb intraoperatively and transfuse to maintain Hb 8–10 g dL^{-1}. Can be very painful as healthy tissue is dissected.
- *Change of dressings* may be far more involved than suggested by the name of the procedure. Discuss with surgeons—often involves extremes of position/multiple patient movements. If simple, it can be performed using ketamine, midazolam, or Entonox$^{®}$.
- *Skin grafting* occurs at several stages during burn care. Most pain is from harvesting skin from donor sites (bupivacaine with adrenaline to donor sites will reduce pain and bleeding).

Postoperative

- Needs to be in a high-care area, ideally in a specialist burns ICU or ward.
- Many patients will remain intubated and are transferred to ICU.
- Bronchoscopy/lavage may be useful to look for thermal damage/carbonaceous deposits
- Use a multimodal pain management—regular paracetamol, opioid infusions (e.g. morphine), and patient-controlled pumps. Opioid tolerance is common. Avoid NSAIDs where possible (renal risk, vulnerable gastric mucosa). Consider adjuvant for neuropathic pain (e.g. gabapentin, amitriptyline) and antidepressants if needed. Involve the pain team early.
- Patients will need psychological support.
- Patients will often have regular (up to daily) anaesthetics for dressing changes, grafting, and wound debridement. Ensure minimum breaks in nutrition and medication.

Further reading

Alvarado R, Chung KK, Cancio LC, et al. Burns resuscitation. *Burns* 2009; **35**:4–14.
Latenser BA. Critical care of the burn patient: the first 48 hours. *Crit Care Med* 2009; **37**:2819–26.
McCormack J, Oglesby A. Trauma and burns in children. *Anaesth Intensive Care Med* 2008; **10**:81–6.

Limb reimplantation

Key points
- Reimplantation of digits is a relatively common procedure.
- Advances in microsurgical techniques have improved outcome.
- Whole-limb reimplantation is possible.
- Patients commonly have coexisting injuries.
- Reimplantation procedures are usually prolonged.

Preoperative
- Patients should be resuscitated according to standard trauma guidelines and other injuries excluded. Bleeding following limb loss may be significant and may need to be controlled with tourniquets.
- Longer ischaemic times reduce chance of implant survival, but so does the presence of other injuries left untreated. Outcomes can be improved by keeping amputated tissue cool (pack in ice).
- Assess patient in a thorough and timely manner, protect the airway, gain IV access, and send bloods for routine tests and include crossmatch. Prior to injury patients are often young and fit.

Intraoperative
- The physiological goal is optimal perfusion/flow to revascularized tissue—high cardiac output in a vasodilated patient.
- The procedure is likely to be prolonged and may have several stages; bone and vascular repair followed by other structures.
- Factors increasing viscosity and reducing limb perfusion include hypothermia, ↑ haematocrit, age, and smoking.
- General anaesthesia is the most common technique—propofol and volatiles reduce SVR. Remifentanil gives excellent analgesia intraoperatively. Consider adding a regional block (improved perfusion, good analgesia), e.g. epidural for lower limb.
- Use invasive monitoring (arterial and CVP)—keep CVP >12 mmHg, MAP >75 mmHg, and urine output 1 mL kg^{-1} h^{-1}. Non-invasive cardiac output monitoring can be used to guide fluid therapy. Inotropes (usually dobutamine) may be necessary.
- Occasionally, despite adequate filling and inotropes, graft perfusion is poor. Elevation of MAP with low-dose vasoconstrictors may help—always discuss with surgeons and monitor closely for over-constriction.
- Reperfusion of a limb generates an acid and potassium load relative to the ischaemic time and proportion of limb reperfused. At the same time, circulating volume increases—BP may decrease significantly.
- Keep the patient warm, use peripheral and core temperature probes. Maintain a difference (core-peripheral) of <2°C. Warm fluid, use forced air warmer and a warming mattress—pressure area care is important—long procedure.
- Beware of concealed but significant blood loss (weigh swabs, check the haemoglobin concentration regularly). Aim for a haemoglobin concentration of 9–10 g dL^{-1} and a haematocrit of 0.3–0.4 (flow inversely proportional to viscosity).

Postoperative
- Meticulous postoperative care of the limb is vital to graft survival. After long procedures it is often better to keep the patient sedated and ventilated and transfer to ICU (aim for normal $PaCO_2$ and PaO_2).
- Care is directed at maximizing graft perfusion by minimizing oedema and venous congestion (judicious IV fluids, elevate limb, medical leaches, DVT prophylaxis, avoid constricting clothing/bandages), optimizing perfusion (MAP >75 mmHg or ±10% of normal if hypertensive), cardiac output monitoring, and urine output $1 \text{mL kg}^{-1}\text{h}^{-1}$, ideally without inotropes. If necessary dobutamine is preferred (inodilation).
- Ensure normothermia and minimize the core—peripheral temperature gradient to prevent peripheral vasoconstriction.
- Treat the consequences of reperfusion—SIRS response, myoglobinuria/renal dysfunction.

Soft tissue infections and abscesses

Key points
- Severe skin infections can progress rapidly.
- Immediate resuscitation, early surgery, and IV antibiotics are key treatments.
- Discuss antibiotic choice with microbiologist.
- Exclude and treat systemic infection.
- Ensure tissue samples taken at surgery for microbiology.

Background
- *Skin abscesses* are most commonly caused by *Staphylococcus aureus* in the community. They can be very painful. Incision and drainage of the abscess is usually curative. Beware—minor abscesses on appearance can be deep on exploration.
- *Diabetic peripheral neuropathy*, microvascular disease, and hyperglycaemia predispose diabetics to skin infections. Most commonly these involve the feet. Over half of diabetic foot infections are complicated by osteomyelitis and may need amputation.
- *Necrotizing fasciitis* is a rare, destructive, rapidly spreading infection (trunk and perineum commonest sites) of the deeper tissues requiring prompt recognition, aggressive debridement, and broad-spectrum IV antibiotics. Mortality is high (25%). It is usually caused by multiple (usually bowel) organisms (type I—synergistic gangrene) or group A streptococci (type II). Exotoxins are involved in tissue destruction. It presents with severe pain often following minor/unrecognized skin damage, overlying skin changes may be mild initially, progressing to widespread necrosis of skin, muscle, and deeper tissues.
- *Gas gangrene* occurs with deep infection with *Clostridium* bacteria. Gas-producing bacteria give the classic sign of crepitus to palpation of affected tissues. It may be spontaneous or follow penetration of contaminated materials (e.g. trauma, injecting of soiled drugs—IV drug user). It is life threatening and requires debridement or amputation.
- *Toxic shock syndromes* related to toxin produced by *Staphylococcus aureus* or Group A *Streptococcus*. The patient may have septic shock (tachycardia, hypotension, vasodilation) and multiorgan failure. Treatment involves removal of toxin (e.g. tampon, skin infection), IV antibiotics (addition of clindamycin may be synergistic in streptococcal toxic shock), resuscitation (fluids and inotropes), and early admission to ICU.

Perioperative
- Surgery for skin infections ranges from the common incision and drainage (I&D) of abscesses to the rarer massive debridement.
- Patients with abscesses are often otherwise fit, but may be obese or have underlying disease (e.g. diabetes, Crohn's disease). Few have signs of systemic infection. These cases are rarely emergencies and patients should be fully fasted. The initial incision is intensely stimulating requiring deep anaesthesia to prevent laryngospasm. Short-acting

opioids (e.g. alfentanil) can be useful. LA infiltration is often unhelpful (acidic inflamed tissue). Abscesses may be deeper or more involved than first expected. Pain is often improved with drainage, and regular paracetamol and weak opioid should suffice.

- Emergency debridement to remove necrotic tissue and halt the spread of infection is often associated with sepsis. Dissection should continue until viable skin is reached. Do not delay surgery. Involve senior surgical, anaesthetic, and microbiology staff early. Resuscitation should be ongoing, and antibiotics started as soon as possible. Follow the surviving sepsis care bundles. Patients will need invasive monitoring, large amounts of fluid, blood, and blood products, and vasopressors (see 📖 Septic shock, p.110). Involve the ICU team early. Consider keeping patient sedated and ventilated so can return to the operating room for further debridement once stabilized on ICU.

Obstetric Emergencies

Emergency Caesarean section

Key points
- Clear multidisciplinary communication is essential for optimal management of obstetric emergencies.
- Re-assess the degree of urgency. Category 1 Caesarean section (CS) may become category 2 with intrauterine fetal resuscitation and allow time for regional anaesthesia (RA).
- Review regularly and optimize indwelling epidurals so that they may be topped up if required for category 1 CS.
- Practice the failed intubation drill regularly and remember that mothers do not die of failed intubation but of failed oxygenation.

Background

Definition
The urgency of the CS, applied at the time of decision to operate, is categorized in Table 11.1.

Table 11.1 Categorization of degree of urgency of Caesarean section

Category	Definition
1	Immediate threat to life of woman or fetus
2	Maternal or fetal compromise; not immediately life-threatening
3	Needing early delivery but no maternal or fetal compromise
4	At a time to suit the woman and maternity team

Categories 1 and 2 are defined as emergency CS. The National Sentinel Caesarean Section Audit (NSCSA) report defined 30 min as a standard for decision-to-delivery interval for a category 1 CS. In some situations (e.g. major abruption) delivery must be achieved much sooner in order to avoid neonatal brain injury. Good multidisciplinary communication is essential to minimize delay.

Preoperative
Try to optimize the mother and fetus before anaesthesia. In the case of maternal collapse, resuscitation is based on ABC:
- Give high-flow oxygen provided delivery is not unduly delayed (see later in topic).
- Switch off the oxytocin infusion.
- Place the mother in the left-lateral position.
- Give fluid bolus—1 L crystalloid.
- Treat hypotension unresponsive to fluid bolus with a vasopressor.
- Consider tocolysis e.g. glyceryl trinitrate inhaler (2 puffs = 800 micrograms) or terbutaline 250 micrograms SC. Avoid if abruption suspected.

The aim is to optimize the fetal condition and decrease the urgency for delivery, to maximize the time to enable successful RA and reduce the necessity for GA.

Providing a high FiO_2 briefly will improve oxygen delivery to the hypoxic fetus during either RA or GA. However exposure to high FiO_2 for >10 min may produce adverse effects such as placental vasoconstriction, fetal acidosis, and lipid peroxidation.

Before undertaking anaesthesia for emergency CS, the anaesthetist should:
- Take a history of salient factors—previous anaesthetics or regional block, general health, medication, allergies, recent oral intake.
- Assess the obstetric status—indication for CS (maternal or fetal), category of emergency, previous obstetric history, known blood loss, coagulation status.
- Assess the airway.
- Check IV access—confirm cannulae secure and patent.
- Ensure the mother is in the left-lateral position/tilt before anaesthesia.
- Note the presence and effectiveness of any indwelling epidural.
- Explain further anaesthetic management and what to expect. Explain risks and gain informed consent for procedures required.
- Reassure the mother. She will be very anxious at this time of urgent preparation for delivery

Perioperative

RA is safer than GA for CS. The NSCSA report suggested that 54% of Category 1 CSs can be performed under RA. The Royal College of Anaesthetists standard is >85% RA for emergencies (combined grades 1–3) with <3% RA to GA conversion rate.

Anaesthetic options
- Epidural top-up if indwelling epidural working well.
- Spinal.
- GA.

The choice is influenced by the urgency, presence of an effective epidural, additional co-morbidities or coexisting factors such as haemorrhage, coagulopathy, body mass index, airway assessment findings, spinal examination. If there is no indwelling epidural, a GA may be the quickest in a category 1 CS situation. However, it is associated with most life-threatening complications for the mother. Unless contraindicated, single-shot spinal anaesthesia is appropriate for most mothers without an indwelling epidural who require a category 2 CS and may be suitable for category 1—the 'rapid sequence spinal'.

Epidural top-up
Before topping up:
- Review regularly mothers with indwelling epidurals to optimize the block and identify mothers with unusual blocks, e.g. high block.
- Identify inadequate epidurals, which should be replaced by spinal anaesthesia or GA for CS.
- Check existing block height, start fluid co-load.
- Prepare vasopressor.
- Continuous presence of the anaesthetist is essential once surgical top-up is initiated.

- The location of the epidural top-up of epidural is controversial. Topping-up commenced in the delivery room gains time to establish a surgical block and reduces the necessity for GA in a category 1 CS. However, maternal monitoring is suboptimal and there is a risk of high block and systemic toxicity. The distance from delivery room to the operating room may influence this practice.

Drugs for epidural block for CS:
- The most commonly used drugs are lidocaine 2%, bupivacaine 0.5%, and levobupivacaine 0.5%. These may be used alone or with adjuncts.
- Adrenaline 0.1 mL of 1 in 1000 adrenaline added to 20 mL LA solution results in adrenaline 1 in 200 000. If using lidocaine this is necessary to increase the maximum safe dose. It has a beneficial analgesic effect at spinal cord level.
- Sodium bicarbonate 8.4% 2 mL added to 20 mL of lidocaine.
- Opioids, e.g. fentanyl 100 micrograms or diamorphine 3 mg.

Lidocaine is the least toxic LA and when combined with bicarbonate and adrenaline, the onset time for surgical block is 50% of that for levobupivacaine. There is risk of drug error and it takes time to prepare the mixture, but many consider it the drug of choice.

Top-up for a working epidural—the practicalities:
- Will require 15–20 mL of 2% lidocaine or 0.5% levobupivacaine ± adjuvants:
  - Aspirate epidural catheter with 2-mL syringe.
  - Place mother in left-lateral position or initially sitting.
  - The need for a test dose and the time to wait following a test dose in patients with epidural analgesia already established is unknown and will depend on the drug used.
  - Inject bolus over 3 min.
  - Repeat BP measurement at 5-min intervals.
  - If top-up in delivery room, transfer to operating room after injecting 15 mL of LA.
  - Remain with the mother continuously.
  - Do not give top-up of concentrated LA in delivery room if epidural has been atypical or there is history of dural puncture.

On arrival in the operating room (all anaesthesia methods):
- Quickly recheck the anaesthetic machine.
- Position on operating table with 15° left tilt or pelvic wedge.
- Confirm presence of expert assistance and intubating trolley.
- Attach monitors (AAGBI Guidelines for Monitoring).
- Oxygen for fetal distress as previously described. See later in topic for preoxygenation before GA.
- Recheck IV cannula. Site additional wide-bore cannula if hypovolaemic.
- IV fluid warming system. Replace blood loss with crystalloid initially.
- Insert urinary catheter.
- Carry out rapid World Health Organization checklist.

When time allows, prior to delivery consider:
- TED (thromboembolus deterrent) stockings.
- Lower leg pneumatic compression device.

- Ranitidine 50 mg IV diluted to 20 mL given over 2 min and 10 mg IV metoclopramide.
- Give antibiotics as early as practicable to reduce chance of wound infection.

Regional block prior to skin incision:
- Test the block.
- A block to cold from T4 to S5 with loss of touch to T5 should avoid the need for supplement or conversion to GA.
- Sacral spread is important for pain-free surgery. S1 is easy to test at lateral border of foot.
- Should have dense motor block of legs if block is adequate.
- Document block level and state modality tested.

Breakthrough pain during RA:
- Administer Entonox® from the anaesthetic machine.
- If epidural, consider top-up with LA if total dose allows or add epidural fentanyl.
- Consider IV opioid, e.g. fentanyl 100 micrograms or alfentanil 0.5–1.0 mg.
- Offer GA and document this offer if declined.

Single-shot spinal

A spinal is useful for emergency CS in a mother without an indwelling epidural. They are generally reliable, provided there is no contraindication. Standard drug is 2.5 mL 0.5% heavy bupivacaine with 300 micrograms diamorphine or 25 micrograms fentanyl. In most cases this will produce a surgical block within 10–15 min.

Spinal anaesthesia for CS—the practicalities:
- Consider underestimated blood loss or concealed haemorrhage.
- Start pre-load with warmed fluids.
- Prepare phenylephrine for use either as an intermittent bolus or infusion.
- Position the mother either lateral or sitting. Consider use of the Oxford position with patient lateral with a wedge under upper thoracic spine to prevent extreme cephalad spread of heavy bupivacaine.
- Inject spinal using pencil point needle no higher than L3/4.
- Pre-empt hypotension with either immediate phenylephrine bolus of 50–100 micrograms or else by continuous infusion (e.g. 20 mL h^{-1} of phenylephrine 100 micrograms mL^{-1}). Phenylephrine is associated with less fetal acidosis and less maternal nausea and vomiting than ephedrine and is considered the vasopressor of choice.
- Maternal pallor and symptoms of nausea, shortness of breath and impending 'faint', will often precede measured hypotension.
- Where a recent epidural surgical top-up produces an inadequate block, a spinal may be considered. Beware misidentification of the epidural injectate as CSF. The usual dose of spinal may produce an unexpectedly high block in this situation, but a conservative dose may result in failed RA. The consensus is to reduce the dose by 20%.
- Some advocate' Rapid Sequence' spinal in category 1 CS to minimize delay.
- Test the block as previously described.

General anaesthesia
Indications for GA CS are:
- Maternal request.
- Contraindication to GA, e.g. hypovolaemia or coagulopathy.
- Lack of time to establish RA.
- Failed RA.

A survey suggested that failure of RA accounted for 10% GAs for CS.

Potential problems associated with GA for CS:
- The incidence of failed intubation is much greater than in the non-obstetric population (1:250 vs 1:2000). The reasons for the difference include full dentition, large breasts, fluid retention, application of cricoid pressure with lateral table tilt displacing larynx, inexperienced anaesthetist, and instruction to declare 'failed intubation' early. Maternal deaths occur because of failed oxygenation not failed intubation.
- Aspiration of stomach contents. Worse outcome from aspiration pneumonitis than in non-pregnant counterparts.
- Problems related to indication for GA, e.g. hypovolaemia, coagulopathies, cardiac, neurological.
- Potential for awareness.
- More postoperative pain and PONV.

GA for CS—the practicalities:
- Give 0.3M Na citrate 30 mL orally.
- Consider fetal heart Doppler, to reassess degree of urgency and enable possibility of RA.
- Ensure expert assistance and airway trolley to hand.
- Pre-oxygenate. At term, mothers have reduced FRC ($\downarrow$ 20–40%), and $\uparrow$ oxygen consumption ($\uparrow$ 35%). This shortens the time for denitrogenation but also reduces time from apnoea to hypoxaemia. The desired endpoint is to achieve $F_{ET}O_2 \geq 90\%$. This may be achieved following 2–3 min of tidal volume breathing or 8 deep breaths. Use high-flow oxygen and tight-fitting facemask with head-up table tilt. 30° head-up tilt will increase FRC and reduce the risk of reflux.
- Obtund hypertensive response to laryngoscopy in pre-eclampsia, (e.g. alfentanil 10 micrograms kg^{-1} ±10–20 mg labetalol). Ketamine may be considered in cases of hypovolaemic collapse.
- Ventilate the lungs with 50% oxygen in nitrous oxide with volatile anaesthetic. In the case of severe fetal distress the FiO_2 may be $\uparrow$ to 1.0. Maintain normocapnia.
- At least 0.75 MAC end-tidal vapour concentration (plus 50% nitrous oxide) is required for bispectral index <60.
- The obstetric anaesthetist should be familiar with and have rehearsed failed intubation drills. Rescue airway equipment such as ProSeal® LMA, Aintree® catheter, and cricothyroid cannulae should be available and familiar. When intubation fails but ventilation by facemask or other means is possible, a decision must be made as to whether to continue with GA or to wake the patient up. The choice will be influenced by the urgency of the surgery, the ease of maintaining the airway, experience of the anaesthetist, suitability and ease of anticipated RA. The fetal status may also guide management for the experienced anaesthetist.

- See failed intubation drill in 📖 Failed tracheal intubation, p.356.

After delivery under GA:
- Give analgesia, e.g. 10–20 mg morphine.
- Change gas flows to give 70% nitrous oxide in oxygen to minimize the concentration of volatile required to maintain anaesthesia and reduce the tocolytic effect of the volatile. Aim for 0.75 MAC volatile.
- Consider LA infiltration of wound, ilioinguinal block, or TAP block.
- Reverse neuromuscular block and extubate with mother in left-lateral position.

After delivery (all anaesthesia methods)
- Give slow bolus of 5 IU oxytocin. Half-life 4–10 min.
- If persistent uterine atony, consider infusion of 40 units of oxytocin over 4 h, ergometrine 500 micrograms IM, or prostaglandin, e.g. carboprost 250 micrograms IM or intramyometrial PRN every 15 min, up to 8 doses.

Postoperative
- Recover in an appropriately staffed recovery area until stable.
- Venous thromboembolism prophylaxis—↑ risk in emergencies. Hydrate, early mobilization, graduated compression stockings, low-molecular heparin. Venous thromboembolism (VTE) risk assessment and follow local guidelines.
- Consider postoperative analgesia—paracetamol, NSAID, oral opioid, epidural diamorphine 3 mg.

Further reading

Allam J, Malhotra S, Hemingway C, *et al.* Epidural lidocaine-bicarbonate-adrenaline vs levobupivacaine for emergency Caesarean section: a randomised controlled trial. *Anaesthesia* 2008; **63**:243–9.

Banks A, Levy D. General anaesthesia for operative obstetrics. *Anaesth Intens Care Med* 2007; **8**:317–19.

Kinsella SM, Girgirah K, Scrutton MJL. Rapid sequence spinal for category–1 urgency caesarean section: a case series. *Anaesthesia* 2010; **65**:664–9.

Lewis G. Saving Mother's Lives: Reviewing maternal deaths to make motherhood safer – 2006-08. The Eighth Report of the Confidential Enquiries into maternal Deaths in the United Kingdom. *BJOG* 2011; **118**(Suppl. 1):1–203.

Lucas DN, Yentis SM, Kinsella SM, *et al.* Urgency of Caesarean section: a new classification. *J R Soc Med* 2000; **93**:346–50.

National Institute of Health and Clinical Excellence. *Caesarean Section. Clinical Guideline.* London: RCOG Press, 2004, pp. 52–3.

Thomas J, Paranjothy S. Royal College of Obstetricians and Gynaecologists Clinical Effectiveness Support Unit. *The National Sentinel Caesarean Section Audit Report.* London: RCOG Press, 2001. Available at: ⚘ http://www.rcog.org.uk/resources/public/pdf/,scs_audit.pdf.

Emergency Caesarean section in mothers with valvular heart disease

Key points
- Mothers should be cared for in centres with expertise in managing high-risk valvular heart disease in pregnancy.
- Pulmonary hypertension is associated with mortality of 30–50% in pregnancy.
- Regular assessment by the same team is crucial.
- Multidisciplinary planning is essential and should be documented clearly.
- CS should be reserved for obstetric indications.
- Anticipate and make clearly documented plans for managing emergency Caesarean delivery or onset of other complications such as pre-eclampsia or haemorrhage.
- This group are at particular risk of VTE.

Background

Cardiac disease is the most common cause of maternal death (Centre for Maternal and Child Enquiries (CMACE) report 2011). Valvular heart disease may be congenital or acquired. Optimum pregnancy outcome depends upon accurate diagnosis and assessment of severity of the valvular disease. Mothers with high-risk lesions should be cared for in centres with expertise in the management of these conditions in pregnancy.

- Valvular disease is classified by the haemodynamic effect (stenosis vs regurgitation) and by the affected valve. Mechanical valves create challenges in the management of anticoagulation.
- In valvular heart disease, the normal haemodynamic changes of pregnancy can precipitate cardiac symptoms in previously stable women or exacerbate symptoms in those previously symptomatic.
- Baseline exercise tolerance is an important predictor of the ability to tolerate pregnancy.
- Ideally mothers with valvular disease will have had preconception optimization:
  - Exchange medication contraindicated in pregnancy (e.g. ACEIs) for those drugs known to be safer, e.g. beta-blockers and diuretics.
  - Percutaneous or surgical intervention if indicated.
  - Discuss risks and benefits of warfarin vs heparin. Warfarin is teratogenic in the 1st trimester but provides more effective anticoagulation if there is a high risk of embolism; heparin does not cross the placenta, so it is better for the fetus. Heparin is advised from week 36.

Antenatal care

Regular assessment throughout pregnancy by the same team is crucial.
- Increases in heart rate, blood volume, and cardiac output are poorly tolerated in mothers with left-sided obstructive lesions.
- The decrease in SVR of pregnancy improves forward flow in regurgitant lesions but following delivery, the increase in SVR and auto-transfusion from the uteroplacental bed may precipitate pulmonary oedema.

- Pulmonary hypertension is very high risk in pregnancy—the mortality is 30–50%.
- Deterioration may be due to infection, anaemia, arrhythmias, or bacterial endocarditis.
- Cardiac demand is minimized by bed rest and oxygen. VTE prophylaxis essential if bed rest is required.

Preoperative

Multidisciplinary planning is essential and should be documented clearly. Current consensus is that women with valvular disease are best managed with instrumental vaginal delivery with adequate pain control, to minimize expulsive efforts. Avoid caval compression and monitor according to the lesion and degree of cardiac risk. Early epidural placement is preferred, provided it is not contraindicated by coagulopathy.

CS should be reserved for obstetric indications. Make contingency plans in case emergency delivery is required or other complications, such as hae-morrhage or pre-eclampsia, ensue. Emergency CS delivery must always be anticipated and, if required, as much advance warning as possible be given to the anaesthetic team.

Intraoperative

The practical management of anaesthesia for emergency CS will depend upon several factors:
- The urgency for delivery.
- Presence of indwelling epidural and the efficacy of block.
- The underlying cardiac status of mother and ability to lie flat.
- Valve lesion: stenotic, regurgitant, presence of intracardiac shunt.
- Coagulation and volume status.
- Presence of other medical complications, including pre-eclampsia.
- Anticipated length of surgery.
- Anticipated requirement for DC cardioversion.
- Anticipated requirement for postoperative mechanical ventilation.
- Anticipated easy of intubation, feeding history, and the preference and skill of anaesthetist.

RA and GA have been described for most valvular lesions. Whatever method is used, anaesthesia must be smooth and titrated carefully, continuously monitoring the effects on maternal physiology whilst ensuring pain-free anaesthesia. Use invasive monitoring in symptomatic patients or if there are complications such as pre-eclamptic toxaemia (PET) and haemorrhage. The preferred technique for emergency CS in most cases is to use a well-functioning indwelling epidural.

Anaesthetic technique
Epidural
- Titrating the block with incremental boluses of LA to the desired level results in most stable cardiovascular status.
- Titrate level and give fluid guided by appropriate haemodynamic monitoring.
- Avoid prophylactic administration of ephedrine and arbitrary volume preload.
- Treat hypotension secondary to sympathetic block with phenylephrine.

Spinal
A spinal block may be tolerated in some well-compensated lesions.

Combined spinal epidural
A low-dose combined spinal epidural may provide a dense sacral block, enabling the epidural to be titrated for upper level. This is more stable haemodynamically, but provides a slower onset of surgical block than a spinal.

General anaesthesia
- Obtund the sympathetic response to laryngoscopy, suction, and extubation (opioid, beta-blockade, adequate depth of anaesthesia).
- Depending on the fasting status and perceived difficulty of intubation, consider TIVA with remifentanil/propofol and rocuronium.
- May need to avoid myocardial depression associated with volatile agents.

Considerations during delivery
- Anti-aspiration prophylaxis.
- Bacterial endocarditis—give prophylactic antibiotics according to current guidelines.
- Haemorrhage may be tolerated poorly if fixed cardiac output and compensation may be obtunded by drugs such as beta-blockers. It is difficult to estimate the blood loss if it is concealed (abruption) or mixed with liquor. Injudicious fluid therapy may precipitate pulmonary oedema.
- Anticoagulation—all patients with mechanical valves should be therapeutically anticoagulated using heparin from 36 weeks. Unfractionated heparin is easier to monitor and reverse at short notice at the time of delivery. According to the valve site and type, instructions for interrupting and recommencing anticoagulation must be documented clearly.
- The delivery of the placenta following vaginal or CS delivery is associated with an increase in the SVR and preload.
- Be prepared to treat new-onset dysrhythmias.
- VTE and other emboli. This group of patients is at particular risk of thrombosis. Beware additional risk if intracardiac R–L shunt and hence risk of cerebral or myocardial thrombotic or air embolism.
- Oxytocics:
  - A bolus dose of 5 units oxytocin can cause ↓ MAP 35%, ↓ SVR 50%, ↑ CO 50%, ↑ HR 20–30% and ↓ SVR 20–30%. It is dangerous if used in mothers with fixed cardiac output but this has to be balanced against the risk of uterine atony and blood loss, which is also tolerated poorly. Consider slow infusion of dilute drug, e.g. 10 units per hour for 4 h.
  - Ergometrine IV is associated with pulmonary vasoconstriction and hypertension, so IV administration is contraindicated.
  - Carboprost (PGF2α) is associated with hypertension, pulmonary oedema and is also contraindicated.
  - Consider prophylactic B-Lynch suture to avoid need for oxytocic drugs.

Postoperative

Provide post CS care in a HDU for a minimum of 72 h. Most cardiac deaths occur after delivery. Advise on contraception before discharge.

Further reading

Dob D.P, Yentis S.M. Practical management of the parturient with congenital heart disease. *Int J Obstet Anesth* 2006; **15**:137–44.

Kuczkowski K.M, van Zundert A. Anesthesia for pregnant women with valvular heart disease: state-of-the-art. *J Anesth* 2007; **21**:252–7.

Lewis G. Saving Mother's Lives: Reviewing maternal deaths to make motherhood safer – 2006–08. The Eighth Report of the Confidential Enquiries into maternal Deaths in the United Kingdom. *BJOG* 2011; **118**(Suppl. 1):1–203.

Lupton M, Oteng-Ntim E, Ayida A, et al. Cardiac disease in pregnancy. *Curr Opin Obstet Gynecol* 2002; **14**:137–43.

Stout K.K., Otto C.M. Pregnancy in women with valvular heart disease. *Heart* 2007; **93**:552–8.

Thilen U, Olsson SB. Pregnancy and heart disease: a review. *Eur J Obset Gynecol Reprod Biol* 1997; **75**:43–50.

Massive obstetric haemorrhage

Key points
- Obstetric haemorrhage is an important cause of maternal death.
- The aim of resuscitation is to maintain uterine blood flow and fetal oxygen delivery.
- Severe antepartum haemorrhage often mandates urgent delivery of the fetus by CS.
- There is no role for regional anaesthesia in a hypovolaemic patient or if there is ongoing severe haemorrhage.

Background
Obstetric haemorrhage remains a major cause of maternal mortality. In the 2006–2008 UK Confidential Enquiry into Maternal Deaths, 3.9 deaths per million maternities were directly attributable to haemorrhage.

Definitions
The definition of obstetric haemorrhage varies widely. Haemorrhage may be classified according to timing relative to delivery:
- Antepartum haemorrhage—after 24 weeks but before delivery of the baby.
- Primary postpartum haemorrhage (PPH)—within the first 24 h after delivery.
- Secondary PPH—from 24 h to 6 weeks postpartum.

Management of antepartum haemorrhage

Aetiology
In the antepartum period, the major causes of haemorrhage are:
- Placental abruption.
- Placenta praevia.
- Uterine rupture.
- Spontaneous abortion.
- Extra-uterine pregnancy.

Organizational considerations
Protocols for the management of massive obstetric haemorrhage should be available on all labour wards. These should be reviewed regularly and rehearsed.

In the case of massive obstetric haemorrhage, immediately mobilize the following multidisciplinary team members:
- Experienced midwifery staff.
- Initially 1st-line obstetric and anaesthetic staff who are trained in management of haemorrhage.
- Subsequently, consultant obstetrician and anaesthetist.
- Haematology consultant on-call.
- Blood transfusion service staff.
- Porters for delivery of specimens and blood.

Ideally, one team member should be identified to document accurately vital signs, timing of events, fluids and drugs infused, and urine output.

Resuscitation

The aim of resuscitation is to maintain normovolaemia and oxygen-carrying capabilities, and to maintain uterine blood flow and fetal oxygen delivery.

- Ensure left-lateral position with head down tilt to relieve aorto-caval compression and optimize venous return.
- Administer high-flow oxygen, provided delivery is anticipated promptly.
- Establish two large-bore IV cannulae (14 G) and send blood for baseline U&Es, FBC, clotting, and blood grouping.
- Order clotting products early, especially in placental abruption, which is associated with high risk of coagulopathy.
- Infuse up to 2000 mL of warmed IV crystalloid or colloid to restore circulating volume.
- Transfuse blood as required. In an emergency, uncrossmatched 'O RhD negative' blood should be available. When time allows, give group-specific or, ideally, crossmatched ABO and Rhesus compatible blood.
- Give 4 units of FFP for every 6 units of RBC. Think ahead: it takes time to defrost FFP.
- Transfuse platelets if count <50 × $10^9 L^{-1}$. Anticipate low platelet count after approximately two blood volumes have been replaced.
- Consider cryoprecipitate (2 packs) if fibrinogen <1 g L^{-1} or following discussion with senior haematologist.
- Keep the patient warm. Hypothermia exacerbates coagulopathy.

Treat the cause of the bleeding

- Severe antepartum haemorrhage often mandates urgent delivery of the fetus by CS. Surgery should not be delayed by resuscitation, as it may be the only definitive treatment to control the haemorrhage.
- In placental abruption with fetal distress, a category 1 CS is appropriate. However, if the fetus is dead and the mother stable, the mother can be allowed to deliver vaginally unless there are other indications for CS.
- In major placenta praevia, CS is normally required regardless of whether the fetus is viable.

Monitoring and investigation

Establish the following monitoring:

- Ensure continuous fetal cardiotocography.
- Full routine monitoring. Tachycardia is often the first and only sign of massive haemorrhage because healthy women can maintain a normal BP despite loss of up to 30% of their circulating blood volume.
- Measurement of hourly urine output is a useful guide to volume status.
- Near-patient tests such as haemoglobin analysis (e.g. Hemocue®) and thromboelastography may also be useful in guiding treatment.
- Consider insertion of an arterial and central venous catheter in complex cases.

Management of postpartum haemorrhage

The Royal College of Obstetricians and Gynaecologists suggest the following grading of PPH:

- Minor haemorrhage: 500–1000 mL estimated blood loss within 24 h of delivery.

- Moderate haemorrhage: 1000–2000 mL estimated blood loss within 24 h of delivery.
- Severe haemorrhage: >2000 mL estimated blood loss within 24 h of delivery.

Aetiology
- Uterine atony is the most common cause of PPH (70%).
- CS.
- Trauma to the genital tract.
- Retained placental tissue.
- Primary coagulation disorders (rare).

All causes of obstetric haemorrhage may be exacerbated by coagulopathy, which may be pregnancy-related, e.g. amniotic fluid embolism or placental abruption.

Management
Management of a patient with a massive PPH is largely the same as for an antepartum haemorrhage.

Mechanical and pharmacological management
Treatment of uterine atony includes:
- Bimanual uterine compression to stimulate contraction.
- Oxytocin 5 units intravenously. A repeated dose may be given if necessary.
- Ergometrine 0.5 mg IV or IM (contraindicated in hypertension).
- Oxytocin infusion IV (30–40 units in 500 mL at 125 mL h^{-1}).
- Carboprost 0.25 mg IM (or intramyometrial), repeated every 15 min up to maximum dose of 2 mg.
- Misoprostol 1000 micrograms rectally.

Surgical management
If haemorrhage is not controlled by mechanical and pharmacological measures, transfer the mother to the operating room promptly, for examination under anaesthesia.
- Remove retained placenta products or clots within the uterus.
- Repair severe genital tract trauma.
- Consider use of balloon tamponade: may be used following CS or vaginal delivery.
- Consider uterine haemostatic sutures such as the B-Lynch suture: requires hysterotomy for insertion so is most appropriate after CS.
- Consider bilateral ligation of the internal iliac or uterine arteries.
- Consider selective radiologically-controlled arterial occlusion or embolization. In elective CS where PPH can be anticipated (e.g. placenta percreta), uterine arterial balloons can be sited preoperatively.
- Hysterectomy—difficult decision but do not delay in life-threatening situation.

Choice of anaesthesia
- There is no role for RA in a hypovolaemic patient or if there is ongoing severe haemorrhage. A GA using a RSI is mandatory.
- Rarely, if there is haemodynamic stability and normal coagulation, a regional technique may be employed with care.

New adjuncts to aid management of massive obstetric haemorrhage

Cell salvage techniques

- Cell-salvaged blood incorporating leucocyte depletion filters has been used without complication in obstetric patients.
- Reduces risk of complications associated with autologous blood.
- Often accepted by Jehovah's Witnesses if it is set up in continuity with the patient's circulation.

Antifibrinolytics

Tranexamic acid may be considered in massive obstetric haemorrhage that has failed to respond to conventional treatment (1g IV every 4h for 12h).

Recombinant Factor VII

- Case reports suggest it may be useful in massive obstetric haemorrhage that has failed to respond to other measures but there is limited evidence.
- It must be used in conjunction with replacement of deficient clotting factors, RBCs, fibrinogen, and platelets.

Further reading

Allam J, Cox M, Yentis SM. Cell salvage in obstetrics. *Int J Obs Anesth* 2008; **17**:37–45.

Lewis G. Saving Mother's Lives: Reviewing maternal deaths to make motherhood safer – 2006–08. The Eighth Report of the Confidential Enquiries into maternal Deaths in the United Kingdom. *BJOG* 2011; **118**(Suppl. 1):1–203.

Stainsby, D, MacLennan, S, Hamilton, PJ. Management of massive blood loss: a template guideline. *Br J Anaesth* 2000; **85**:487–91.

The Royal College of Obstetricians and Gynaecologists. *Prevention and Management of Postpartum Haemorrhage*. London: RCOG Green-top Guideline No. 52, 2009.

Placenta praevia and placenta accreta

Key points
- Placenta praevia and placenta accreta can both cause massive haemorrhage.
- Use of RA may reduce blood loss and transfusion requirement compared with GA but GA is most appropriate if there is cardiovascular compromise.

Background—placenta praevia

Definitions
The placenta lies either wholly or partly in the lower segment of the uterus. Previously graded I–IV, now defined as:
- Major—placenta lies over the cervical os.
- Minor—placenta lies in the lower segment but not overlying the os.

Diagnosis
Suspect placenta praevia if:
- Painless vaginal bleeding.
- High presenting part.
- Abnormal lie.

Diagnosis of placenta praevia confirmed by:
- Transvaginal ultrasound.
- MRI if ultrasound has been unsatisfactory.

Problems associated with placenta praevia
Antenatal

Premature separation of the placenta from uterus may cause a rapid, exsanguinating haemorrhage. Admit following any significant bleed in 3rd trimester until delivery by CS.

Delivery
- The placenta may have to be incised to deliver the fetus, hence major haemorrhage must be anticipated.
- ↑risk of morbidly adherent placenta—placenta accreta.

Postnatal

Risk of PPH from poorly contracting lower segment.

Background—placenta accreta

Definitions
- Placenta accreta vera—placenta grows through the endometrium *to* the myometrium.
- Placenta increta—placenta grows *into* the myometrium.
- Placenta percreta—placenta grows *through* the myometrium to the uterine serosa and surrounding structures.

Risk of placenta accreta
- ↑ risk if anterior placenta praevia and previous CS.
- ↑ risk if short CS to conception interval.

- History of previous CS:
  - 1 previous CS increases risk to 25%.
  - >2 CS increases risk to 50%.

Diagnosis of placenta accreta
Confirmed by:
- Ultrasound.
- MRI.
- Colour flow Doppler.
- Power amplitude ultrasonic angiography.

Preoperative
Refer also to 🕮 Major obstetric haemorrhage, p.272.

Preparation and monitoring
- Two anaesthetists (one consultant), particularly if risk of placenta accreta.
- Immediate availability of 4 units group-specific blood.
- Immediate availability of O-negative blood at time of incision if group-specific blood unavailable.
- Two large-bore IV cannulae (14 G) *in situ*.
- Fluid warming device.
- Consider rapid infuser and cell salvage in cases with high risk of placenta accreta.
- Consider invasive arterial and central venous monitoring if active haemorrhage or risk of morbidly adherent placenta.

Intraoperative
Choice of anaesthesia
Recent evidence suggests a reduction in blood loss and transfusion requirement with RA compared to GA.

General anaesthesia
GA using RSI is most appropriate in situations with cardiovascular compromise.

Regional anaesthesia
- Can be used safely in placenta praevia if patient is normovolaemic and has low risk of accreta.
- Patient must be counselled about the risk of conversion to GA.
- Consider combined spinal epidural as procedure may be prolonged.

Management if continued haemorrhage
Pharmacological management
- Oxytocin 5 units intravenously followed by infusion of 30–40 units intravenously over 4 h to maintain contraction of thin-walled lower segment.
- Oxytocics as required, see oxytoxic ladder (🕮 Emergency Caesarean section, p.262).

Physical management
- Bimanual compression.
- Hydrostatic balloon catheterization or uterine packing.
- Intermittent aortic compression.

- B-Lynch suture.
- Hysterectomy may be required if placenta accreta/percreta.

Special considerations

- Consider preoperative placement of intrailiac or uterine arterial balloon catheters.
- Postoperative radiological embolization.

Further reading

Hong J-Y, Jee Y-S, Yoon H-J, *et al*. Comparison of general and epidural anaesthesia in elective caesarean section for placenta praevia totalis: Maternal haemodynamics, blood loss and neonatal outcome. *Int J Obstet Anaesth* 2003; **12**:12–16.

Pareskh N, Husanini SW, Russell IF. Caesarean section for placenta praevia: a retrospective study of anaesthetic management. *Br J Anaesth* 2000; **84**:725–30.

Retained placenta

Key points
- Retained placenta occurs in 2% of deliveries and is a significant cause of morbidity and mortality.
- If operative intervention is required, RA is recommended unless there is significant hypovolaemia.

Background

Definition
The placenta is deemed retained if not delivered within 60 min of birth of the fetus and occurs in 2% of deliveries worldwide.

Risk factors
- Previous retained placenta.
- Pre-term delivery.
- Induced labour.
- Multiparity.
- Previous uterine trauma.

Complications
Retained placenta is a significant cause of morbidity and mortality. Potential complications include:
- Primary PPH.
- Uterine inversion.
- Secondary PPH—usually due to infected retained products.
- Puerperal sepsis.

Types of retained placenta
There are three kinds of retained placenta:
- Simple adhesion (*placenta adherens*).
- Separated but '*trapped*' by closed os or hourglass constriction ring. ↑ incidence with prophylactic IV bolus of ergometrine, which causes simultaneous constriction of os at time of placental separation.
- Morbid adhesion—*placenta accreta*. Placenta becomes morbidly adherent because of absence or deficiency of *deciduas basalis* between villi and myometrium. This causes abnormal adherence of the placenta and prevents normal separation of placenta from the myometrium. Accreta associated with placenta praevia in 34–50% cases: poor blood supply in lower segment results in deficient development of *decidua basalis*.

Conservative management of simple retained placenta
- Oxytocic ladder (see 🕮 Emergency Caesarean section, p.262).
- Controlled cord traction.
- Breastfeed to stimulate release of endogenous oxytocin.
- Uterine massage to 'rub up' a contraction.
- Empty the bladder.
- Vary maternal position—encourage upright position.

- IV access and fluid as guided by vital signs. Send blood for group and screen. Tachycardia may be the only sign until significantly hypovolaemic.
- Wait up to 60 min if haemodynamically stable.
- If closed os or uterine constriction ring, consider tocolytic to relax uterine smooth muscle, e. g. glyceryl trinitrate 2 puffs sublingually (800 micrograms) or IV bolus 100–200 micrograms.
- Consider intraumbilical venous oxytocin injection (e.g. 30 units oxytocin in 30 mL 0.9% saline via neonatal nasogastric tube).

Operative management

- RA is recommended if not hypovolaemic. Either top-up indwelling epidural with 15 mL concentrated LA or use spinal 2.0–2.5 mL hyperbaric bupivacaine 0.5%. A T6 block to cold should ensure maternal comfort.
- GA if shocked: consider using ketamine. If closed os or constriction ring trapping the placenta, equipotent doses of all the volatile anaesthetic agents cause uterine relaxation in a dose-dependent manner.
- Give an appropriate antibiotic, e.g. co-amoxiclav 1.2 g.
- For management placenta accreta: see ⊞ Placenta praevia and placenta accreta, p.276.
- Post-delivery, oxytocin 40 units in 500 mL 0.9% saline over 4 h prevents uterine atony and PPH.

Further reading

Broadbent CR, Russell R. What height of block is needed for manual removal of placenta under spinal anaesthesia? *Int J Obstet Anesth* 1999; **8**:161–4.

Carroli G, Bergel E. Umbilical vein injection for management of retained placenta. *Cochrane Database Syst Rev* 2001; **4**:CD001337. Review. Update in: *Cochrane Database Syst Rev* 2011; **5**:CD001337.

Weeks A.D. The retained placenta. *Best Pract Res Clin Obstet Gynaecol* 2008; **22**:1103–17.

Ectopic pregnancy

Key points
- The incidence of ectopic pregnancy is 11 per 1000 reported pregnancies.
- Significant blood loss may be concealed.
- Surgeons should be prepared and scrubbed before anaesthesia is induced.

Background

Definition
- An ectopic pregnancy is one that implants outside the uterine cavity.
- Most occur in the Fallopian tubes: 2% may implant in the cervix, ovaries, or abdomen.
- In the UK, the incidence has ↑ over the past 20 years to 11 per 1000 reported pregnancies due to ↑ rates of chlamydial infection and assisted reproduction.
- According to the 8th Report of the Confidential Enquiries into Maternal Deaths in the United Kingdom, ectopic pregnancies remain the leading cause of death in the 1st trimester of pregnancy with a mortality rate of 16.9 per 100 000 ectopic pregnancies, generally due to massive haemorrhage.

Risk factors
- In patients using contraception (contraceptive failure)—intrauterine contraceptive device failure, uterotubal anomalies and endometriosis.
- In patients not using contraception (reproductive failure)—previous ectopic pregnancy, previous pelvic inflammatory disease, previous tubal surgery, smoking, use of assisted conception.
- <50% of ectopic pregnancies are associated with risk factors.

Management
Medical
In selected patients with haemodynamic stability and a serum human chorionic gonadotrophin (hCG) concentration <3000 IU L^{-1}, methotrexate (single dose 50 mg per m^2 IM) is as safe and efficient as a surgical approach, with favourable subsequent fertility:
- ≥15% will require >1 dose of methotrexate.
- <10% will require surgical intervention.

Surgical
Indications include haemodynamic instability, impending tubal rupture, contraindications to methotrexate (e.g. maternal immunocompromise, liver disease, and blood dyscrasias), coexisting uterine pregnancy, and failed medical management. The surgical approach may be laparoscopic or open laparotomy.

Salpingotomy versus salpingectomy
- If *healthy* contralateral Fallopian tube, there is little evidence to compare conservative with radical surgical treatment.
- Salpingotomy may be associated with a higher subsequent rate of intrauterine pregnancy compared with salpingectomy.
- If contralateral tubal *disease*, salpingotomy should be performed if future fertility is desired.

Preoperative

- Presenting symptoms may be atypical and non-specific. Significant blood loss may be concealed. Tachycardia may be the earliest indication of significant blood loss.
- At least one large-bore IV cannula should be sited prior to operating room. If significant haemorrhage, start hypotensive resuscitation (aiming for a MAP 40–80 mmHg) to minimize blood loss but improve tissue oxygenation.
- Ensure FBC, group and screen, or preparation of group-specific blood/ crossmatched blood, ± clotting screen are requested on admission. Consider early preparation of coagulation factors if anticipating excessive blood loss.
- Discuss with surgeon the ultrasound findings and location of abnormal pregnancy.
- Cornual or interstitial pregnancies (2–4% of ectopic pregnancies, 2–2.5% mortality rate) are associated with a higher risk of major haemorrhage.
- If anticipating major haemorrhage, consider use of intraoperative cell salvage.

Intraoperative

- RSI with surgeons scrubbed and immediately available to start surgery if mother compromised.
- Ensure IV fluids are warmed. Hypothermia exacerbates coagulopathy.
- Treat haemorrhage as required. If massive haemorrhage, replace platelets and clotting factors. Check fibrinogen and calcium levels and request input of a senior haematologist.
- Consider use of invasive monitoring.

Special considerations

Laparoscopy versus laparotomy

- A laparoscopic approach is suitable in the haemodynamically stable patient, and is associated with less blood loss and fewer hospital days.
- In the haemodynamically unstable patient, an open surgical approach generally allows control of blood loss most promptly.
- The final choice of surgical technique will depend upon the skill and experience of the surgeon.

Heterotropic pregnancy

- This is a simultaneous intra- and extrauterine pregnancy. The incidence is 0.6–2.5 per 10 000 pregnancies.
- It is more common in patients undergoing assisted reproductive techniques.
- Intrauterine pregnancy may proceed uneventfully following surgical management of ectopic pregnancy. Use drugs safe in pregnancy until surgical findings confirmed.

Further reading

Lewis G. Saving Mother's Lives: Reviewing maternal deaths to make motherhood safer – 2006–08. The Eighth Report of the Confidential Enquiries into Maternal Deaths in the United Kingdom. *BJOG* 2011; **118**(Suppl. 1):1–203. Available at: ℘ http://onlinelibrary.wiley.com/doi/10.1111/bjo.2011.118.issue-s1/issuetoc.

Royal College of Obstetricians and Gynaecologists. *The Management of Tubal Pregnancy*. London: RCOG, Guideline No. 21, 2004. Available at: ℘ http://www.rcog.org.uk.

Pregnancy-induced hypertension, pre-eclampsia, and eclampsia

Key points
- Hypertension is associated with maternal and fetal morbidity and mortality.
- In the UK in 2006–8 there were 19 deaths from pre-eclamptic toxaemia (PET) or eclampsia.
- A very high BP may cause intracranial haemorrhage (ICH).
- The tissue oedema associated with PET causes airway narrowing and increases the risk of failed intubation.

Background
- Hypertension is the most common medical problem encountered during pregnancy and is associated with both maternal and fetal morbidity and mortality.
- Pre-eclampsia is a systemic disorder and the aetiology is complex and not completely understood.
- Risk factors include:
  - Age >40 years.
  - Nulliparity.
  - Previous or family history of pre-eclampsia.
  - Multiple pregnancy.
  - Pre-existing medical co-morbidities (e.g. insulin dependent diabetes, hypertension, antiphospholipid syndrome).

Definitions
- *Hypertension*—sustained SBP >140 mmHg or DBP >90 mmHg.
- *Chronic hypertension*—hypertension that existed before pregnancy or before 20 weeks' gestation. May develop superimposed pre-eclampsia.
- *Pregnancy-induced hypertension*—new onset of hypertension, without proteinuria after 20 weeks' gestation.
- *Pre-eclampsia (PET)*—multi-system disorder involving pregnancy-induced hypertension and significant proteinuria (>300 mg 24 h^{-1} or 2+ on urine dipstick). It occurs in up to 10% of pregnancies.
- *Severe pre-eclampsia*—incidence 5 per 1000 pregnancies in UK. Diagnosis requires at least 1 of the following:
  - Sustained SBP >160 mmHg or DBP >110 mmHg.
  - Proteinuria >5g 24 h^{-1} or 3+ on urine dipstick.
  - Oliguria <500mL 24 h^{-1}.
  - Pulmonary oedema.
  - Upper abdominal pain.
  - Impaired liver function tests.
  - Thrombocytopenia <100 x 10^9 L^{-1}.
  - Neurological disturbances.
- *Eclampsia*—incidence 27.5 per 100 000 pregnancies in UK. Defined as convulsions that arise from PET, although signs of pre-eclampsia may not be present until after seizures. May occur in pregnancy or early puerperium.

Mortality from pre-eclampsia or eclampsia

Maternal mortality continues to decrease. In the last Confidential Enquiry into Maternal and Child Health in the UK 2006–8, the mortality rate of PET or eclampsia was 0.83 per 100 000 pregnancies (19 deaths), secondary to:

- ICH—9 deaths (indicates failure of antihypertensive therapy).
- Anoxia following cardiac arrest in association with eclamptic seizures—5 deaths.
- Hepatic—rupture, failure/necrosis and 'other'—5 deaths.

Pre-eclampsia

Prevention

Low-dose aspirin initiated before 16 weeks' gestation in women at risk for PET.

Definitive treatment

Delivery of placenta—symptom resolution begins within 24–48 h.

Antihypertensive therapy

Aim to control BP <150/80–90 mmHg. High SBP may cause ICH. Normalizing BP may cause placental hypoperfusion.

1st-line treatment

- Labetalol 200 mg PO (decreases BP in 30 min, repeat dose if required in 1 h).
- Alternative 1st-line treatments include methyldopa and nifedipine.

Rapid control of severe hypertension

- Labetalol 20 mg IV over 2 min (decreases BP in 5 min; repeat dose every 10 min; max. dose 300 mg).
- Hydralazine 5 mg IV (decreases BP in 20 min; repeat dose every 20 min; max. dose 20 mg).
- Nifedipine 10 mg PO every 15–30 min. Avoid sublingual nifedipine—can cause rapid reduction in placental perfusion.
- In resistant cases, infusions of glyceryl trinitrate may be required (10–200 micrograms min^{-1} infusion in 0.5% glucose or 0.9% saline, 100 micrograms mL^{-1})
- Automated BP monitoring systems underestimate systolic pressure in PET.
- Consider use of invasive arterial monitoring in severe cases.

Magnesium

- Magnesium prophylaxis is given to patients with severe PET to reduce risk of eclampsia.
- Give 4 g loading dose over 10–15 min followed by infusion of 1 g h^{-1} continued for 24 h following delivery or after last fit, in eclampsia.

Fluid management

- In severe PET, fluid overload can cause pulmonary oedema and ARDS, which has been a significant cause of maternal death in the past.
- Restrict total fluids to 85 mL h^{-1}. Careful recording of fluid balance is essential.

- There is no evidence for use of diuretics in antepartum or intrapartum period. Postpartum course of furosemide may normalize BP more rapidly and reduce need for anti-hypertensive treatment.
- CVP monitoring rarely required unless complex (i.e. PET associated with haemorrhage). CVP may correlate poorly with left heart filling pressures; aim for CVP ≤4 mmHg to minimize risk of pulmonary oedema.

Regional anaesthesia in pre-eclampsia

- Epidural analgesia should control excessive surges in BP during painful contractions and may subsequently be used if CS required, provided not contraindicated by coagulopathy.
- Preload before RA is not required because ↑ sensitivity to catecholamines and vasopressors reduces the risk of hypotension. Treat promptly with vasopressor if hypotension does occur. Fluid restrict as discussed previously.

Investigation of clotting

- In pregnancy-induced hypertension without proteinuria, a platelet count is not routinely required.
- In pre-eclampsia, a platelet count is mandatory, ideally performed just before block placement. The lowest acceptable platelet count for safe RA is uncertain.
- In severe PET, send clotting screen with FBC to avoid unnecessary delay.
- Common general guidelines are:
  - Platelet count >100 × 10^9 L^{-1}—RA acceptable.
  - Platelet count 80–100 × 10^9 L^{-1}—perform clotting screen, proceed if normal
  - Platelet count 70–80 × 10^9 L^{-1}—opinion varies. A clotting screen is required and refer to local protocol. Consider rate of platelet fall and possibility of platelet dysfunction.
  - Consider risks and benefits. Most UK obstetric units consider platelet count of 80 × 10^9 L^{-1} as lowest acceptable limit, but this is based on limited evidence.
- Check platelet count and clotting screen prior to *removal* of epidural catheter.

General anaesthesia in pre-eclampsia

- GA is indicated for CS if there is significant thrombocytopenia or coagulopathy or if inadequate time to establish regional block for Category 1 CS.
- Failed intubation is more common in the obstetric population compared with non-pregnancy (1 in 250 vs 1 in 2000). This may be compounded in PET because tissue oedema causes airway narrowing. Oedema and engorgement of nasal airways may also make awake fibreoptic intubation more difficult.
- Attenuate the hypertensive response to laryngoscopy. An excessively high BP may cause ICH. Methods to reduce BP pre-induction include:
  - Magnesium sulphate 30 mg kg^{-1} (if not already loaded) ± alfentanil 7.5 micrograms kg^{-1}.
  - Esmolol 1 mg kg^{-1} IV.
  - Labetalol 10–20 mg IV over 2 min.

- Consider treatment before extubation.
- Effective postoperative multimodal analgesia is required. Consider bilateral TAP blocks ± PCA. Avoid NSAIDs because they may cause renal impairment and platelet dysfunction.

3rd stage of labour
- Use 5 units oxytocin IM or IV (given slowly).
- If uterine atony, consider further oxytocin bolus or infusion of 10 units h^{-1} for 4 h.
- Avoid ergometrine or syntometrine because they may exacerbate hypertension.
- Consider physical measures to treat uterine atony, e.g. balloon tamponade or B-Lynch suture.

Eclampsia
- Eclampsia usually occurs in association with signs or symptoms of pre-eclampsia, although these may not be evident until after convulsions have occurred.
- ~40% of seizures occur in each of the antepartum and postpartum periods. 20% occur intrapartum.
- Management is aimed at immediate control of convulsions and secondary prevention of further convulsions.
- Eclampsia in the antenatal period is not an indication for a Category 1 CS in the absence of acute fetal distress. BP control and loading with magnesium should precede delivery.

Immediate management
- Airway, breathing, circulation—remember left-lateral tilt.
- Load with magnesium sulphate 4 g IV over 5 min.

Secondary prevention
Maintenance infusion of magnesium sulphate 1 g h^{-1} IV for 24 h after last seizure.

Recurrent seizures
- Give further bolus of magnesium sulphate 2–4 g IV or increase infusion rate to 1.5–2.0 g h^{-1}. Magnesium levels may be monitored clinically (i.e. loss of deep tendon reflexes and respiratory depression). Caution in oliguria (magnesium renally excreted) and check blood levels to avoid toxicity.
- If convulsion persists, consider single dose of diazepam.
- If continuing convulsions, consider intubation with thiopental and transfer to ICU.

HELLP syndrome
- HELLP syndrome is a form of severe pre-eclampsia/eclampsia and the term is an abbreviation of the main findings: Haemolytic anaemia, Elevated Liver enzymes and Low Platelet count.
- It occurs in ~20% of patients with pre-eclampsia/eclampsia.
- It rarely presents before the 3rd trimester. 1/3 of cases present in postnatal period.

- Features include:
  - Evidence of haemolysis—falling Hb concentration without evidence of bleeding, elevated lactate dehydrogenase, elevated bilirubin.
  - Elevated liver function tests. Epigastric pain is present in 90% of cases of HELLP. May be associated with nausea and vomiting. Significant pathology (hepatic haemorrhage and rupture) can precede the thrombocytopenia.
  - Low platelets.
- Partial HELLP may occur (ELLP, HEL, EL, LP).
- Morbidity may be associated with other major organ involvement including:
  - Neurological—cerebral haemorrhage, cerebral oedema, and hypertensive encephalopathy.
  - Haematological—DIC.
  - Renal—acute tubular necrosis, acute renal failure.
  - Cardiopulmonary—pulmonary oedema, ARDS, myocardial ischaemia, and cardiac arrest.
  - Hepatic—catastrophic complications are rare (e.g. liver haemorrhage/rupture).
  - Infection and sepsis.

Management of HELLP syndrome

- Definitive treatment is delivery of the placenta. Corticosteroids do not reduce maternal or neonatal complications.
- The mode and timing of delivery is influenced by gestational age, maternal and fetal condition. Severe HELLP syndrome will require an urgent CS.
- Coagulopathy is likely to contraindicate the use of RA.
- There is a high risk of PPH. Transfuse blood products as required.
- Other management is largely supportive and should be undertaken on a HDU/ICU. Recovery can be expected to begin within 24–48 h following delivery of the placenta.

Further reading

Duley L, Matar HE, Almerie MQ, *et al.* Alternative magnesium sulphate regimens for women with pre-eclampsia and eclampsia. *Cochrane Database Syst Rev* 2010; **4**(8).

Lewis G. Saving Mother's Lives: Reviewing maternal deaths to make motherhood safer – 2006–08. The Eighth Report of the Confidential Enquiries into Maternal Deaths in the United Kingdom. *BJOG* 2011; **118**(Suppl. 1):1–203. Available at: http://onlinelibrary.wiley.com/doi/10.1111/bjo.2011.118.issue-s1/issuetoc.

Martin JN, Rose CH, Briery CM. Understanding and managing HELLP syndrome: the integral role of aggressive glucocorticoids for mother and child. *Am J Obstet Gynecol* 2006; **195**:914–34.

National Institute for Health and Clinical Excellence. *Hypertension in pregnancy: the management of hypertensive disorders during pregnancy.* London: NICE, 2010. Available at: http://www.nice.org.uk.

Royal College of Obstetricians and Gynaecologists. The Management of Severe Pre-eclampsia/Eclampsia. London: ROCG, 2006. Available at: http://www.rcog.org.uk.

Urological Emergencies

Ureteric obstruction

Key points
- Most cases are treated initially by X-ray-guided percutaneous nephrostomy insertion with a LA.
- Some patients need endoscopic ureteric stent insertion with GA.
- Patients can have severe sepsis or develop sepsis after treatment.

Background
- Ureteric obstruction can be caused by stones, blood clot, tumour, or extrinsic compression. Acute treatment is to decompress the obstructed hydronephrotic kidney by percutaneous nephrostomy insertion (tube insertion into pelvis of kidney using a Seldinger technique usually under LA) with definitive relief of obstruction at a later date. This can include endoscopic stent insertion and ureteroscopy and laser fragmentation of stone under GA.
- If the urine above the obstruction is infected, the patient will often be septic and may have renal failure. In this case, urgent nephrostomy is needed in addition to IV antibiotics.
▶ Patients with urosepsis may present with non-specific signs of shock and abdominal pain.

Preoperative
- Early goal-directed therapy for sepsis including invasive monitoring, fluid resuscitation, and vasopressors as needed.
- Give IV antibiotics preprocedure, based on urine or blood culture and microbiology advice. Empirical therapy should include a combination of an aminoglycoside (gentamicin 3–5 mg kg^{-1} IV) with a fluoroquinolone (ciprofloxacin 400 mg IV) or extended spectrum penicillin and beta-lactamase inhibitor (co-amoxiclav 1.2 g IV) according to local policy.
- Nephrostomy is undertaken in prone or 3/4 lateral position in a dedicated fluoroscopy suite (often distant from operating room complex). Ensure anaesthetic facilities and trained assistant available. Patients may require just monitoring (most common), analgesia/sedation, or GA.

Intraoperative
- Instrumentation of the infected collection can precipitate marked haemodynamic instability—fluids, inotropes/vasopressors may be required.
- Send for culture any urine/pus aspirated from the collecting system. Significant bleeding occurs in 1–3% of procedures.
- Even with LA infiltration, pain during the procedure is common. Incremental fentanyl (0.5–1 micrograms kg^{-1}) may be necessary.
- If GA, tracheal intubation and controlled ventilation for prone positioning will be necessary.

Postoperative
- Consider HDU/ICU care for patients with sepsis.
- Continue IV antibiotics.
- Hourly urine output and renal function monitoring.

Testicular torsion

Background
- Most common between 12–18 years, but can occur at any age. Malrotation of the spermatic cord causes strangulation of the testicular blood supply and infarction associated with severe testicular pain. Diagnosis is clinical but can be confirmed using colour Doppler ultrasonography to assess testicular blood flow.
- Derotation within 4–6 h of the onset of symptoms is associated with a high chance of preserving testicular function. Surgery will involve manual derotation or orchidectomy depending upon the viability of the testis. Fixation of the contralateral testis will also be undertaken.

Preoperative
- Although co-morbid conditions are uncommon, this will often be the patient's first anaesthetic. Record any allergies and enquire specifically about any family history of idiosyncratic reactions to anaesthesia.
- Surgery is most commonly performed under GA. Where contraindications to GA exist, subarachnoid or caudal blockade may be considered, accepting a sensory level at or above T10. Anaesthetic technique should not cause unnecessary delays to surgery.

Intraoperative
- A RSI and tracheal intubation is appropriate. The pain associated with a torted testicle is likely to cause delayed gastric emptying. The patient must be considered to have a full stomach regardless of the timing of last oral intake.
- Beware of vagal responses. Torsion or traction of the spermatic cord stimulates vagal afferents. Adequate anaesthesia decreases risk. Ask the surgeon to stop if excessive bradycardia and treat with glycopyrronium or atropine if necessary.
- Opioid analgesia (e.g. fentanyl 1–2 micrograms kg^{-1}) and infiltration of LA at the end of the procedure will provide analgesia.

Postoperative
Patients will often be suitable for discharge on the day of surgery. Regular oral analgesia (paracetamol, NSAID ± weak opioid) will usually suffice.

Fournier's gangrene

Key points
- This fulminant necrotizing fasciitis progresses rapidly with 30–50% mortality.
- The most important prognostic factor is the time to surgery.
- Early, aggressive, and repeated surgical debridement is the key treatment.

Background
- Fournier's gangrene is a fulminant necrotizing fasciitis (see 📖 Soft tissue infections and abscesses, p.258) of the perineal, genital, or perianal regions. It is more common in men. Associations include diabetes, alcoholism, and immunosuppression. A mixed infection spreads along fascial planes at up to 3 cm h^{-1} to involve the genitals, anterior abdominal wall, and retroperitoneum. Thrombosis of perforating vessels results in rapid ischaemia/infarction overlying skin. Systemic symptoms are often out of proportion to the visible signs of infection.
- Treatment includes resuscitation, and broad-spectrum IV antibiotics and most importantly rapid and aggressive surgical debridement of the affected areas.
- Surgery involves extensive debridement of the skin; wounds will be left open for subsequent re-exploration. Exploration of the retroperitoneum will necessitate laparotomy and urinary/faecal diversion may be needed to avoid further soiling of wounds.

Preoperative
- Although preoperative haemodynamic optimization is desirable, this should not delay surgical debridement. All other measures are of secondary importance.
- Take samples for blood culture. Analysis of an ABG sample will be useful to identify acidosis and assess adequacy of resuscitation.
- Blood loss will be significant. Crossmatch at least 4–6 units.
- Give a combination of broad-spectrum IV antibiotics as soon as diagnosis suspected. Aerobic and anaerobic cover will be required. Discuss with a microbiologist.
- Consider early goal directed therapy for sepsis (see 📖 Septic shock, p.110).

Intraoperative
- Anticipate cardiovascular collapse on induction. Prepare inotropes and vasopressors ready for immediate use (e.g. ephedrine, metaraminol and adrenaline 10 micrograms mL^{-1}).
- RSI and tracheal intubation is necessary.
- Insert central venous catheter and arterial line for invasive monitoring.
- Insidious blood loss will be considerable. Transfuse as required.
- Monitor and preserve normal body temperature as far as is practicable.

Postoperative
- The extent of surgical injury, sepsis, and the necessity for repeated examinations under anaesthesia often make extubation impractical.

- Transfer the patient to ICU for ongoing haemodynamic and ventilatory support.
- Postoperative multiple organ failure is common—consider early renal replacement therapy.
- On average, patients will return to the operating room for wound inspection and further debridement three times.
- The benefit of hyperbaric oxygen therapy is unproven and its use impractical in most centres.

Further reading

Thwaini A, Khan A, Malik A, et al. Fournier's gangrene and its emergency management. *Postgrad Med J* 2006; **82**:516–19.

Renal transplantation

Key points
- There is usually several hours' warning beforehand.
- Patients have multiple co-morbidities as well as chronic renal failure.
- Need to optimize haemodynamic status to ensure best chance of graft survival.
- IV access can be difficult.
- Drug pharmacokinetics are altered in renal failure and then variable depending on graft function postoperatively.
- Patients are immunosuppressed—need for meticulous infection control.

Background
- Kidneys come from donors with brainstem death (see 📖 Anaesthesia for organ retrieval, p.244), circulatory death (non-heart beating donors), or from live donors. Live kidney donation is an elective procedure.
- Patient and graft survival after kidney transplant depends on ischaemic time of kidney, maintenance of kidney perfusion, blood and HLA matching, patient compliance with immunosuppression, cause of renal failure, age of recipient, co-morbidities, and surgical factors.
- Recipients are assessed before going on the transplant waiting list. This should involve renal physicians, surgeons, and anaesthetists. Patients often understate any health problems in order to get a transplant. The time between assessment and surgery is variable and patients may have developed new health problems. Patients are routinely screened for HIV, CMV, hepatitis B and C infections, and should have preoperative investigations available (chest X-ray, ECG, echocardiography, and exercise test if indicated).
- Surgery (right iliac fossa incision) involves anastomosis of the donor renal artery and vein to recipient external (usually) iliac vessels, and ureter to the recipient bladder with a ureteric stent inserted. This usually takes about 2–3 h and is not usually associated with a significant blood loss.

Preoperative
- The transplant coordinator informs the anaesthetic team when an organ is available and a suitable recipient has been identified. The time when surgery takes place is therefore variable.
- During the preoperative visit ascertain the cause of the patient's renal failure, assess effects of chronic renal failure, check for comorbidities (diabetes and heart disease common), and determine the location of AV fistulae. Have a plan for venous access—patients often have poor veins (including central veins) due to multiple previous line insertions.

- Ensure blood results available—K^+ <6 mmol L^{-1} is acceptable, chronic anaemia is common. Check coagulation.
- Involve a senior anaesthetist. Patients usually spend a long time on the transplant waiting list and there is a shortage of donated organs. There is a pressure to do these cases even when the patient's condition or preoperative work-up is suboptimal.
- Recipients usually have preoperative renal dialysis as this improves transplant outcomes. This, coupled with preoperative fasting, will usually make the patient dehydrated.
- Patients are often on several cardiac drugs—consider withholding antihypertensives preoperatively (e.g. ACEIs, long-acting calcium channel blockers) to decrease incidence of intra- and postoperative hypotension.

Intraoperative

- Protect functioning fistulae with soft padding and use alternative sites to position NIBP cuff and IV cannula.
- Avoid cannulating veins in the forearm and do not site an arterial line unless absolutely necessary—these vessels may be needed for subsequent AV fistula formation.
- IV induction with propofol, fentanyl, and atracurium, intubate trachea and ventilate, and maintain anaesthesia with volatile or propofol (TIVA is the simplest technique). Monitor muscle relaxation; use fluid and patient warmers to avoid hypothermia.
- A central venous catheter for monitoring and drug infusions is inserted after induction of anaesthesia. Use an ultrasound scanner and take care with dilator insertion (do not push too far into the vein) during Seldinger insertion in patients who have had numerous previous central venous catheters—they may have vein stenosis.
- Avoid suxamethonium, especially if K^+ >5.5 mmol L^{-1}, or neuropathies as there is risk of severe hyperkalaemia. Non-depolarizing muscle relaxants can have a prolonged action in renal failure; atracurium is preferred.
- Clearance of morphine and its metabolite morphine-6-glucuronide is prolonged in renal failure. Use fentanyl, IV paracetamol, and TAP block or LA infiltration by the surgeons for analgesia.
- Avoid nephrotoxic drugs (e.g. NSAIDs).
- Maintain 'normal' BP using fluid and small doses of vasopressors (e.g. metaraminol). Non-invasive cardiac output monitoring may also be useful. The target intraoperative CVP is usually 8–12 mmHg.
- Hartmann's solution is preferred to 0.9% sodium chloride. Starch solutions are avoided as they may decrease graft survival.
- Use local protocols for administration of immunosuppressants, steroids, antibiotics, heparin, and diuretics (e.g. mannitol) during surgery.
- Patients can be extubated at the end of surgery.

Postoperative

- The patient will need monitoring in HDU/transplant ward setting to ensure they are warm, well hydrated, and for assessment of transplant function.
- The transplant kidney may not function immediately (especially if from a donor after circulatory death). Sometimes it can take several days. Urine output does not indicate graft function. Monitor U&Es. Some patients may need haemodialysis if delayed transplant function.
- Consider a vasopressor or inotrope infusion (e.g. metaraminol, noradrenaline, or dobutamine) if the patient is hypotensive postoperatively despite fluid bolus and no evidence of bleeding. Discuss with renal physicians and surgeons (patient may need ultrasound/Doppler of kidney to assess patency of vascular anastomoses and renal perfusion).
- Renal vein thrombosis can occur in up to 5% patients. It is prevented with routine thromboprophylaxis. Routine Doppler examination helps diagnosis.
- When adequately filled, give fluid at a rate equal to the previous hour's urine output plus 50 mL per hour. Give orally or Hartmann's IV (or 0.9% sodium chloride if K^+ a problem).
- Use fentanyl PCA (e.g. 20 micrograms bolus, 5-min lockout, no background) and regular paracetamol for postoperative analgesia. Tramadol or hydromorphone can also be used.
- Early postoperative complications include vascular and ureteric disruption. Surgical re-exploration may be needed. In case of bleeding reverse heparin and consider desmopressin 0.3 micrograms kg^{-1} IV over 20 min.
- Patients may need blood transfusion if chronic anaemia, evidence of myocardial ischaemia, or haemodilution caused by plasma volume expansion to improve graft function. Ensure appropriate blood given (cytomegalovirus status).
- Patient's regular drugs need review as dosage requirements may be different post transplant. The renal team should do this.

Further reading

Rabey P. Anaesthesia for renal transplantation. *Br J Anaesth CEPD Rev* 2001; **1**(1):24–7.

Paediatric Emergencies

Pain relief in children

Key points

- There are many different pain assessment tools depending on the developmental stage and clinical setting.
- Try to use a multimodal treatment plan because this may enable use of lower doses of drugs and consequently fewer side effects.

Pain assessment

When assessing pain in infants and children a useful approach is QUESTT:

- *Q*uestion the child.
- *U*se a pain rating scale.
- *E*valuate the behavioural and physiological changes.
- *S*ecure parents involvement.
- *T*ake cause of pain into account.
- *T*ake action and evaluate results.

Self-reporting of pain is the preferred approach but this is not possible in the very young or cognitively impaired child. Instead, pain assessment is based on observation of behaviour and physiology. There are many different pain assessment tools depending on the developmental stage of the child and the clinical setting (acute procedural pain, postoperative pain, chronic pain); examples include:

- Numeric Rating Scale Visual Analogue Scale (VAS) (age 6–18 years).
- Wong–Baker FACES Pain Rating Scale (age 3–18 years).
- Face Legs Activity Cry and Consolability (FLACC) observational pain tool (aged 1 month upwards), see Table 13.1.

Pain management

See the Association of Paediatric Anaesthetists of Great Britain and Ireland (APAGBI) website for excellent guidelines on pain management in children.

Pharmacological treatment

- A multimodal treatment plan uses combinations of drugs that act at different parts of the pain pathway and may enable use of lower doses of drugs and, consequently, fewer side effects.
- Drugs include non-opioid analgesics, opioids and local anaesthetics and their adjuncts.
- The World Health Organization ladder for cancer pain provides a plan for treating mild, moderate, and severe pain (Fig. 13.1).

Table 13.1 FLACC pain tool

Score	0	1	2
Face	No particular expression or smile	Occasional grimace or frown; withdrawn or disinterested	Constant grimace or frown; frequent/constant quivering chin, clenched jaw
Legs	Normal position or relaxed	Uneasy, restless, tense	Kicking or legs drawn up
Activity	Lying quietly, normal position, moves easily	Squirming, shifting back and forth, tense	Arched, rigid or jerking
Cry	No cry (awake or asleep)	Moans or whimpers; occasional complaint	Crying steadily, screams or sobs, frequent complaint
Consolability	Content, relaxed	Reassured by occasional touching, hugging or being talked to, distractible	Difficult to console or comfort

Reproduced with permission from the World Health Organization. Available at http://www.who.int/cancer/palliative/painladder/en. (Accessed 23rd February 2012).

• Opioid-strong ±		
• Regional blockade • Ketamine	• Opioid—mild	
• Non-opioids • Paracetamol/NSAIDs	• Non opioids • Paracetamol/NSAIDs	• Non-opioids • Paracetamol/NSAIDs
Severe pain	**Moderate pain**	**Mild pain**

Fig 13.1 World Health Organization pain ladder. Reproduced by permission of Hodder Education. R. Bingham (2007) *Hatch and Sumner's Textbook of Paediatric Anaesthesia* (3rd edn), p. 493.

Non opioid analgesics: paracetamol

- The dosing regimen for oral paracetamol is given in Table 13.2.
- Outside the neonatal period rectal absorption of paracetamol is erratic.
- Parenteral administration is a more reliable method (Table 13.3).
- Paracetamol is used widely and has few side effects within the normal dose range; the maximum daily dose is safe for short-term use.
- Risk factors for hepatotoxicity include:
  - Children <2 years of age.
  - Children taking liver enzyme-inducing drugs.
  - Malnourished children (including children who have not eaten for several days).

Table 13.2 Paracetamol by mouth

	Single dose (mg kg^{-1})	Dosing regimen	Maximum daily dose (mg kg^{-1})
28–32 weeks PMA	20	10–15 mg kg^{-1} 8–12 h	30
>32 weeks PMA	20	10–15 mg kg^{-1} 6–8 h	60
1–3 months	20	15–20 mg kg^{-1} 6–8 h	60
>3 months	20	20 mg kg^{-1} 6 h	90

PMA, postmenstrual age.

Table 13.3 Intravenous doses of paracetamol

	Dosing regime	Maximum daily dose
Neonate	7.5 mg kg^{-1} 4–6 h	30 mg kg^{-1} day^{-1}
Child (<10 kg)	7.5 mg kg^{-1} 4–6 h	30 mg kg^{-1} day^{-1}
Child (10–50 kg)	15 mg kg^{-1} 4–6 h	60 mg kg^{-1} day^{-1}
Child (>50 kg)	1 g 4–6 h	4 g

Non-opioid analgesics: non-steroidal anti-inflammatory drugs

- Children tolerate NSAIDs better than adults and GI effects are less common. A proton pump inhibitor or H$_2$-receptor antagonist may be used if there is a risk of ulceration.
- Avoid NSAIDs in children with severe acute asthma and asthma patients with a history of a previous reaction.
- There are no convincing human data that demonstrate delayed bone healing and NSAIDs should not be withheld in children with bone fractures.
- NSAIDs should be used with caution in children with renal or hepatic impairment or a history of bleeding diathesis.

- *Ibuprofen* has fewer side effects than other NSAIDs; dose 5–10 mg kg^{-1} 6 h to maximum of 30 mg kg^{-1} day^{-1} but not exceeding 2400 mg. Repeated doses for analgesia are not recommended <3 months of age.
- *Diclofenac* is available in both enteral and parenteral forms; dose (age >6 months) 1 mg kg^{-1} 8 h (max. 150 mg day^{-1}) PO/PR/IV.
- *Ketorolac* has a higher incidence of side effects including bleeding.
- *Aspirin* and aspirin containing products are avoided in children because of the risk of Reyes syndrome.

Opioids

Opioids are indicated for moderate to severe pain (Table 13.4).

Weak opioids:

- *Codeine* is a prodrug. It is converted to morphine by the cytochrome P450 enzyme CYP2D6. There is developmental and genetic variation with this system, which may lead to ineffective analgesia or unexpected overdose.
- *Tramadol* is a weak opioid that binds to mu opioid receptors as well as blocking serotonin and noradrenaline reuptake.

Strong opioids:

Morphine is the most common opioid used in acute severe pain.

- Adequate analgesic concentrations of morphine can be achieved using regular oral morphine or more commonly by a morphine infusion, nurse-controlled analgesia (NCA), or patient-controlled analgesia (PCA).
- Intermittent dosing leads to periods of inadequate analgesia and/or side effects from plasma concentrations that are too high.
- IM injections are painful and usually avoided in children.
- Morphine doses should take into account the changes in pharmacokinetics in the developing infant.
- Premature and term neonates have immature hepatic and renal systems with consequent ↓ metabolism and elimination of drugs.
- Neonates and infants <3 months of age are also at greater risk of respiratory depression because the ventilatory responses to hypoxaemia and hypercapnia are immature.

Diamorphine is more lipid soluble than morphine and therefore has a faster onset of action. It is gaining popularity for use in emergency departments using the intranasal route. Dose (child over 10 kg): 100 micrograms kg^{-1} (max. 10 mg).

Fentanyl is very lipid soluble and can also be delivered by the transmucosal (fentanyl 'lollipops') and transdermal route (fentanyl patches). It has no active metabolites and can be used in a PCA as an alternative to morphine (e.g. in patients with renal failure).

Patient-controlled analgesia/nurse-controlled analgesia/morphine infusions
Recommended IV loading doses and infusions of morphine for acute pain are given in Tables 13.5 and 13.6.

Table 13.4 Commonly used opioids

Drug	Potency relative to morphine	Oral dose >6 months (unless stated)	Intravenous dose >6 months (unless stated)
Morphine	1	**Neonate:** 80 mg kg⁻¹ 6 h **Child:** 200–400 micrograms kg⁻¹ 4 h	See below
Codeine	0.1	0.5–1 mg kg⁻¹ 6 h	Not recommended
Tramadol	0.1	>1 year 1–2 mg kg⁻¹ 6 h	>1 year 1–2 micrograms kg⁻¹ 6 h
Fentanyl	50–100	NA	**Bolus:** 0.5–1 micrograms kg⁻¹ **Infusion:** 0.5–2 micrograms kg⁻¹ h⁻¹
Oxycodone	1–1.5	>1 month 100–200 micrograms kg⁻¹ (max. 5 mg) 4–6 h	NA
Hydromorphone	5	40–80 micrograms kg⁻¹ 4 h	20 micrograms kg⁻¹ 2–4 h

Table 13.5 Intravenous loading of morphine dose for acute pain

Age	Increments	Total dose
Preterm neonate	5 micrograms kg^{-1} at 5-min intervals	Up to 25 micrograms kg^{-1}
Term neonate	10 micrograms kg^{-1} at 5-min intervals	Up to 50 micrograms kg^{-1}
1–3 months	20 micrograms kg^{-1} at 5-min intervals	Up to 100 micrograms kg^{-1}
>3 months	50 micrograms kg^{-1} at 5-min intervals	Up to 100–200 micrograms kg^{-1}

Table 13.6 Morphine infusion (based on protocol from Bristol Royal Hospital for Children (BRHC))

0–1 months:	**Maximum** of 5 micrograms kg^{-1} h^{-1}
1–3 months:	**Maximum** of 10 micrograms kg^{-1} h^{-1}
Over 3 months:	**Maximum** of 40 micrograms kg^{-1} h^{-1}

NCA:
- For use in small babies and older children who are unable to use PCA, e.g. child with cerebral palsy (Table 13.7).
- Provides a constant background infusion and allows the nurse looking after the patient to give a bolus dose for breakthrough pain or minor procedures.

Table 13.7 NCA (Bristol Royal Hospital for Children protocol): morphine 1 mg kg^{-1} in 50 mL 0.9% saline (concentration of 20 micrograms kg^{-1} mL^{-1})

	Term – 1 month	1–3 months	>3 months
Background	5 micrograms kg^{-1} h^{-1}	10 micrograms kg^{-1} h^{-1}	10–20 micrograms kg^{-1} h^{-1}
Bolus	5 micrograms kg^{-1}	10–20 micrograms kg^{-1}	10–20 micrograms kg^{-1}
Lockout	20 min	20 min	20 min
2-h maximum	**25 micrograms kg^{-1} 2 h^{-1}**	**50 micrograms kg^{-1} 2 h^{-1}**	**200 micrograms kg^{-1} 2 h^{-1}**

PCA:

Suitable for children who are able to understand the PCA instructions (around 6 years and older) and can activate the PCA device. Dosing regimes for morphine and fentanyl by PCA are given in Tables 13.8 and 13.9.

Table 13.8 Morphine 1 mg kg^{-1} in 50 mL 0.9% saline (concentration of 20 micrograms kg^{-1} mL^{-1})

	<50 kg	>50 kg
Background[a]	6 micrograms kg^{-1} h^{-1} (i.e. 0.3 mL h^{-1}) on 1st–2nd postoperative day	0.3 mL h^{-1} on 1st–2nd postoperative day
Bolus	1 mL (i.e. 20 micrograms kg^{-1}) over 1 min	1 mL over 1 min
Lockout	5 min	5 min
2-h maximum	200 micrograms kg^{-1} 2 h^{-1}	12 mL

[a]Background infusion: a low background infusion may improve sleep pattern and improve pain scores without increasing side effects. Consider for the initial postoperative period in children having major surgery, or in medical patients with severe pain, e.g. mucositis in children receiving chemotherapy.

Table 13.9 Fentanyl PCA (Bristol Royal Hospital for Children). Dose 50 micrograms kg^{-1} fentanyl made up to 50 mL with 0.9% saline (maximum 50 kg—use undiluted fentanyl)

Dose	0.5 mL
Lockout interval	5 min
Background infusion	0.5 mL on 1st–2nd postoperative day (1 mL h^{-1} =1 microgram kg^{-1} h^{-1})
2 hour maximum	6 mL

- Opioid side effects include: respiratory depression (especially neonates and infants <3 months), nausea and vomiting, pruritus, urinary retention, and dysphoria.
- All children having opioid infusions should be monitored using: pulse and BP, respiratory rate and depth, sedation level, pain assessment and, in young infants, apnoea monitoring, and pulse oximetry.

Ketamine
- Ketamine potentiates opioid-induced analgesia as well having an opioid-sparing effect; it can be used as a co-analgesic with morphine.
- The Bristol Royal Hospital for Children protocol is: ketamine 1 mg kg^{-1} combined with morphine 1 mg kg^{-1} made up to 50 mL with 0.9% saline (initially start at normal PCA settings).

Local anaesthetics
- Amide LAs (bupivacaine, levobupivacaine, ropivacaine, lidocaine) are commonly used for local infiltration and RA techniques (Table 13.10).
- They are metabolized by the liver (reduced in neonates) and plasma bound to α_1 acid glycoprotein and albumin (reduced in neonates).

- Cardiac toxicity of LAs is heart-rate dependent.
- Neonates and young infants are therefore more likely to accumulate LA and are more susceptible to cardiac toxicity.
- Consider levobupivacaine in infants and blocks requiring high infusion rates.

Table 13.10 Suggested maximum doses of bupivacaine and levobupivacaine

Single bolus injection	Maximum dosage
Neonates	$2\,mg\,kg^{-1}$
Children	$2.5\,mg\,kg^{-1}$
Continuous infusion	**Maximum infusion rate**
Neonates	$0.2\,mg\,kg^{-1}\,h^{-1}$
Children	$0.4\,mg\,kg^{-1}\,h^{-1}$

Adjuncts to LAs for epidural and caudal routes comprise:
- Opioids:
  - Fentanyl: lipophilic drugs bind to receptors in the substantia gelatinosa of spinal cord adjacent to catheter; there is less rostral spread.
  - Morphine: hydrophilic drugs have more rostral spread with ↑ risk of respiratory depression; they can be used in lumbar epidural for thoracic upper abdominal surgery.
  - Complications of epidural opioid: pruritus, nausea and vomiting, urinary retention, and respiratory depression; all can be treated with naloxone as central opioid effects.
- Clonidine:
  - Dose—single bolus: $1-2$ micrograms kg^{-1}; infusion: $0.08-0.2$ micrograms $kg^{-1}\,h^{-1}$.
  - Approximately doubles the duration of analgesia following a single-shot caudal block.
  - Side effects—sedation, dose-related hypotension and bradycardia; there have been case reports of apnoea and respiratory depression in neonates.
- Ketamine (preservative free):
  - Dose $0.5-1\,mg\,kg^{-1}$.
  - Approximately trebles the duration of analgesia following a single-shot caudal block.
  - Case reports of neurotoxicity with ketamine preparations containing preservative.

Nitrous oxide
- A mixture of 50% oxygen and 50% nitrous oxide (Entonox®) may be used for analgesia and is self-administered with demand flow system.
- Usually suitable for children aged 5 years and over.
- Used for procedural pain e.g. fracture manipulation, drain removal.

Glucose
- There is evidence that the use of oral glucose solution helps relieve pain in neonates during painful procedures. This phenomenon appears to decrease with age.
- The dose, given 2 min before procedure is glucose 30% oral solution, 0.5 mL for preterm neonates and 1 mL for term neonates.

Non-pharmacological methods
- The patient should be looked after in a child-friendly environment with close involvement of parents.
- Techniques include diversion/distraction, play therapy, hypnosis, cuddling/massage, relaxation, and guided imagery.

Further reading

Association of Paediatric Anaesthetists of Great Britain and Ireland. *Good Practice in Postoperative and Procedural Pain*. London: APAGBI, 2009. Available at: ℬ http://www.apagbi.org.uk/sites/apagbi.org.uk/files/APA%20Guideline%20part%201.pdf.

British Medical Association and the Royal Pharmaceutical Society of Great Britain. *British National Formulary*. UK: BMJ Publishing Group. Latest edition (62nd) 2011.

Hockenberry MJ, Wilson D. *Wong's Essentials of Pediatric Nursing*, 8th edn. St. Louis, MO: Elsevier-Mosby, 2008.

The Royal College of Nursing. *The recognition and assessment of acute pain in children*. London: RCN, 2009. Available at: ℬ http://www.rcn.org.uk/childrenspainguideline.

Airway emergencies in children

Key points
- Airway emergencies in children are generally caused by anaphylaxis, choking, airway infection, or a mediastinal mass.
- Ideally, the airway should be secured in the operating room or the intensive care unit (ICU).
- Senior anaesthetists and ENT surgeon(s) must be involved early.

Background
There are four major categories of airway emergencies in children:
- Anaphylaxis.
- Choking and inhaled foreign body (see 📖 Inhaled foreign body, p.332).
- Infection of oropharynx, larynx or trachea, specifically:
  - Retropharyngeal abscess.
  - Epiglottitis.
  - Croup or bacterial tracheitis.
- Anterior mediastinal mass ± SVC obstruction.

Most airway emergencies in children require:
- The presence of a consultant ENT surgeon.
- A calm environment to minimize distress to the child.
- Administration of 100% oxygen and, where possible, secure IV access.
- Transfer of the child to operating room or ICU for definitive airway management (if possible).
- A difficult intubation trolley nearby.
- Clear communication between *all* staff regarding management plan and individual responsibilities.
- Most children will require discussion with the regional paediatric intensive care unit (PICU) for ongoing care.

Specific management
Anaphylaxis
The presenting symptoms and signs can include:
- Airway and breathing problems, e.g. stridor, shortness of breath, wheeze.
- Cardiovascular collapse.
- Skin changes, e.g. urticara.

Specific management
- Administer 100% oxygen and secure IV access.
- Give adrenaline 0.15–0.5 mg IM, or 1 microgram kg^{-1} IV by slow titration to effect (see 📖 Anaphylaxis, p.374).
- Intubate if impending airway failure:
  - May require smaller tracheal tube than predicted by age.
  - Induction may precipitate cardiovascular collapse, so fluid bolus and resuscitation drugs should be prepared.
- Consider fluid bolus if cardiovascular collapse (20 mL kg^{-1} crystalloid).
- If marked bronchospasm, give nebulized salbutamol.

- Consider IV infusion of adrenaline ± salbutamol depending on degree of cardiovascular collapse and bronchospasm.
- Hydrocortisone and chlorphenamine (minimal effect in acute phase but may reduce incidence of late relapse) (Table 13.11).

Table 13.11 Dosing regimes for chlorphenamine and hydrocortisone

	<6 months	6 months–6 years	6–12 years	>12 years
Chlorphenamine (IM or slow IV)	250 micrograms kg^{-1}	2.5 mg	5 mg	10 mg
Hydrocortisone (IM or slow IV)	25 mg	50 mg	100 mg	200 mg

Inhaled foreign body
- Most common in children aged 1–3 years.
- Presentation varies depending on location, size, and chronicity of the foreign body.
- New onset cough, wheeze, or stridor in young child is suspicious.
- Further management is discussed in 🕮 Inhaled foreign body, p.332.

Infection: retropharyngeal abscess
The symptoms and signs include:
- Fever, sore throat, torticollis, neck pain.
- ± pharyngeal bulge (23%).
- ± drooling (10%).
- Inflammation extending to surrounding tissue can cause anatomical distortion, making glottis hard to visualize or even locate. Be prepared for an emergency tracheostomy. Aim to secure airway without rupturing abscess and soiling the airway with pus.

Specific management
- If stridor present—cautious inhalational induction with sevoflurane (or halothane) in 100% oxygen. Gentle CPAP may help maintain airway patency.
- A cuffed tube will prevent soiling of lungs from spontaneous rupture or surgical drainage.
- Give broad-spectrum antibiotics e.g. cefotaxime and metronidazole (most deep neck infections contain beta-lactamase producing organisms and most abscesses contain anaerobes).
- Depending on degree of preoperative airway compromise, transfer to PICU may be required.

Infection: epiglottitis
The presenting symptoms and signs include:
- Rapid-onset fever and drooling (often <12 h).
- May appear toxic.
- Stridor is a late sign.
- May adopt characteristic posture sitting forward, neck extended.

Induction will take longer than usual due to severe airway obstruction. Inflammation can make glottis very difficult to visualize. Look for air bubbles from the glottic opening. Use a bougie and railroad a tracheal tube over it. Be prepared for an emergency tracheostomy.

Specific management

- Cautious inhalational induction with sevoflurane (or halothane) in 100% oxygen. Gentle CPAP may help maintain airway patency.
- May require a tracheal tube at least one whole size smaller than predicted by age.
- Give broad-spectrum antibiotics, e.g. cefotaxime.
- Will require admission to PICU usually for 48 h.

Infection: viral laryngo-tracheitis (croup) and bacterial tracheitis

The presenting symptoms and signs include:

- *Croup*: barking cough, stridor, mild pyrexia.
- *Bacterial tracheitis*: productive cough, stridor, appears toxic.

Management of croup

- Dexamethasone 150 micrograms kg^{-1} (more effective than prednisolone 1 mg kg^{-1}).
- Nebulized adrenaline 0.1 mL kg^{-1} of 1:1000 adrenaline (max. 5 mL: if volume <2 mL dilute with 0.9% saline). Often very effective and alleviates need for intubation. Is *not* associated with 'rebound' deterioration but effects may last only for a few hours. Repeat as required.
- Inhalation induction with sevoflurane (or halothane) in 100% oxygen. Maintenance of spontaneous ventilation until the airway is secured is still recommended because there may be coexisting problems such as tracheal stenosis or compression. Gentle CPAP may help maintain airway patency.
- May require smaller tracheal tube than predicted by age.
- Antibiotics not usually required (infection usually viral in origin).
- Will require transfer to PICU.

Management of bacterial tracheitis

- Glucocorticoids and nebulized adrenaline are unlikely to be effective.
- If the diagnosis is in doubt, inhalational induction is recommended. However, if there are copious secretions and productive coughing this may be difficult and rapid sequence intubation may be preferable.
- Presence of ENT surgeon may be required for immediate bronchoscopy and bronchial toilet if secretions are copious and tenacious.
- Give broad-spectrum antibiotics including anti-staphylococcal therapy, e.g. cefotaxime and flucloxacillin.
- Will require transfer to PICU.

Anterior mediastinal mass ± SVC obstruction

The presenting symptoms and signs include:
- Sudden-onset wheeze or stridor in older child (i.e. inhaled foreign body unlikely).
- Minimal signs of infection.

Acute leukaemia with anterior mediastinal mass or lymphoma can cause tracheal deviation and compression ± SVC obstruction and present in this way.

Immediate management
- Seek PICU and oncological/haematological advice.
- Do not give steroids except under oncological guidance (as may precipitate tumour lysis syndrome).
- Avoid intubation unless airway compromise critical, and transfer (with senior anaesthetist and resuscitation equipment) as soon as possible to tertiary paediatric centre.
- If SVC obstruction suspected, site IV cannula in lower limb.

Other causes of upper airway obstruction in children

Many causes of upper airway obstruction present to a tertiary paediatric centre but are not generally considered 'airway emergencies'. Examples include:
- Laryngo/tracheamalacia.
- Vocal cord palsy.
- Respiratory papillomatosis.
- Subglottic pathology (cysts, haemangioma, stenosis).
- Laryngeal clefts.
- Intubation injury.

Further reading

Bruce IA, Rothera MP. Upper airway obstruction in children. *Pediatric Anesthesia* [Special Issue: The Pediatric Airway] 2009; **19**(Suppl. 1):88–99.

Jenkins IA, Saunders M. Infections of the airway. *Pediatric Anesthesia* [Special Issue: The Pediatric Airway] 2009; **19**(Suppl. 1):118–30.

Major trauma in children

Key points
- Trauma is the leading cause of death in children aged 1–14 years.
- The primary survey and resuscitation of children follows the well-established airway, breathing, circulation, disability, and exposure (ABCDE) approach.
- Signs of shock are less obvious in children.

Background
- Trauma is the leading cause of death in children aged 1–14 years and half of all cases involve multiple organs or body regions.
- Blunt trauma is more common; penetrating trauma is more lethal.
- Blunt trauma impacts airway and breathing more than the circulation because neuroventilatory derangements are five times more common than haemodynamic derangements. However, haemodynamic derangements (bleeding and shock) are twice as lethal.

Primary responsibilities for the anaesthetist
- Secure and maintain the airway, oxygenation, and ventilation.
- Ensure adequate circulating volume with appropriate blood and fluid replacement.
- Maintain body temperature.
- Prepare to transport the child from the ED to the operating room, CT scanner or PICU.

Specific management
Resuscitation and primary survey
ABCDE (airway, breathing, circulation, disability, exposure) approach.
- Airway:
  - Administer 100% oxygen and stabilize cervical spine.
  - Intubate the trachea if required (record GCS score and pupil responses first).
- Breathing:
  - Evaluate rate and depth of breathing.
  - Exclude or treat immediately life-threatening chest injury, e.g. tension pneumothorax, haemothorax, flail chest, penetrating chest wound.
- Circulation:
  - Evaluate heart rate, capillary refill time (CRT), and BP for signs of shock.
  - Establish IV/IO access (preferably two large-bore IV cannulae).
  - Draw blood for crossmatch, routine haematology/biochemistry.
  - Control active haemorrhage and look for concealed haemorrhage (e.g. in cavities of thorax, abdomen, retroperitoneum, pelvis, long bones, and head in infants).
  - Treat shock with fluid bolus $10 \, \text{mL} \, \text{kg}^{-1}$ isotonic crystalloid. Repeat four times; if no response, obtain surgical opinion. Transfuse blood after $40 \, \text{mL} \, \text{kg}^{-1}$ of crystalloid.

- If no signs of active or concealed haemorrhage, consider spinal transection as cause of shock.
- Disability:
  - Record GCS and pupil responses (should do this before intubation).
  - Continue to record pupil responses every half an hour.
  - Look for signs of life-threatening head or spinal injury.
  - Consider the need for analgesia if the child is awake or analgesia and sedation if the child is intubated and ventilated.
- Radiology:
  - Chest and pelvis.
  - Imaging of the cervical spine is also important but since a normal X-ray does not exclude cervical spine ± cord injury a CT scan is usually required if suspicious.
  - Consider an abdominal ultrasound scan if suspicious of abdominal injury.

Additional information
- Airway:
  - Always assume a full stomach and perform a RSI with cricoid pressure.
  - Insert an orogastric tube as gastric distension common and may compromise ventilation.
- Breathing:
  - Beware—even with preoxygenation, children desaturate quicker than adults because of a relatively smaller functional residual capacity and greater oxygen consumption.
  - Children are more likely to develop respiratory failure than are adults with an equivalent injury.
- Circulation:
  - Signs of shock are less obvious in children.
  - Tachycardia may be the only sign. Suspect hypovolaemia if heart rate >140 min^{-1} in infant, >100 min^{-1} in older child.
  - CRT is measured centrally but is unreliable in presence of hypothermia.
  - Hypotension is a late sign. The BP may be normal despite 25–35% loss of total blood volume.

Secondary survey
- 'SAMPLE' history (symptoms, allergies, medications, last meal, events of injury).
- Head-to-toe exposure and assessment for any other injuries.
- Maintain body temperature. Children lose heat rapidly because they have a larger body surface area, reduced subcutaneous tissue, and ↑ minute ventilation with associated heat of vapourization.
- Consider arterial access, blood gas analysis, and urinary catheterization.

Prepare for transfer from the resuscitation room—the result of the secondary survey determines the destination (radiology department, operating room, PICU).

Special considerations in major trauma

Head injury

- Early CT scan of head and neck, early consultation with paediatric neurosurgical centre.
- Continue with cervical spine immobilization.
- Avoid hypercarbia—ventilate to achieve normocapnia.
- Avoid hypotension.
- Maintain a CPP of at least 50 mmHg.
- Position with 30° head-up tilt.
- Control seizures—consider IV phenytoin 20 mg kg^{-1}.
- Control temperature—prevent excessive hypothermia or any hyperthermia.

Thoracoabdominal injury

- Significant lung contusions may occur in the absence of rib fractures because a child's soft ribs are less likely to fracture. Lung contusions cause shunting and respiratory distress, which may develop several hours after admission and will require oxygen therapy ± intubation and positive pressure ventilation.
- Ruptured diaphragm is more common in children than adults and may be overlooked as respiratory distress is usually not severe.
- Injury to the heart and great vessels less common in children due to the greater elasticity and mobility of mediastinal structures.
- Be aware of hypotension on opening the abdomen in the child with intra-abdominal bleeding.
- Avoid nitrous oxide as it may distend air-containing spaces, e.g. pneumothorax, tracheal bronchial injury, bowel injury.

Massive transfusion

- Beware citrate toxicity, hypocalcaemia, and hyperkalaemia in infants after massive transfusion. Monitor ionized calcium and potassium.
- After transfusion of 50% total blood volume, give FFP and consider the need for platelets and cryoprecipitate.
- Prevent hypothermia, using warmed fluids and body warming devices.

Burns and scalds

- Facial burns and/or inhalational injury imply risk of airway compromise—intubate early.
- Circumferential burns to the thorax may compromise breathing.
- Hypovolaemia from burns occurs late. If shocked, look for concealed haemorrhage.
- Burns require extra fluid (in addition to maintenance):
  - Additional fluid (mL) = % burn × weight (kg) × 4 (Parkland formula).
  - Give half in first 8 h, remainder over 16 h (calculating from time of burn injury).
  - Assess adequacy of fluid replacement by urine output (aim: 1 mL kg^{-1} h^{-1}).
- Prevent hypothermia (burnt children lose heat rapidly).
- Administer analgesia.
- Transfer to a specialist centre if burn is: >5% surface area; 'special area' e.g. face, hands, feet, perineum; circumferential burn, inhalation, chemical or electrical injury.

Child protection
- Trauma comprises both accidental and non-accidental injury (child abuse).
- All cases of major trauma in children (regardless of cause) should be reported to the hospital child protection team.

Useful formulae
Useful formulae for resuscitation of the injured child are given in Table 13.12.

Table 13.12 Formulae for resuscitation of the injured child

Airway/breathing	Circulation	Other
Tracheal tube (TT) size: age/4 + 4	Total blood volume = 70–80 mL kg^{-1}	Weight = (age + 4) × 2
TT insertion depth in cm to the lips: age/2 + 12	Tachycardia: Heart rate >140 (infant) Heart rate >100 (other children)	Orogastric tube (OGT) size: 2 × size of TT (e.g. size 4 TT, size 8 OGT)
	Estimate of SBP: 70 mmHg + (2 × age)	Urinary catheter size: 2 × size of TT (e.g. size 4 TT, size 8 catheter)

Useful intravenous drug doses
Intubation
- Suxamethonium: 1–2 mg kg^{-1} (± atropine 10–20 micrograms kg^{-1}).
- Ketamine: 2 mg kg^{-1}.
- Fentanyl: 2–5 micrograms kg^{-1}.

Sedation for transport to CT scan or PICU
- Morphine infusion: 1 mg kg^{-1} in 50 mL gives 1 mL h^{-1} = 20 micrograms kg^{-1} h^{-1}. Infuse at 1–3 mL h^{-1}.
- Midazolam infusion: 5 mg kg^{-1} in 50 mL gives 1 mL h^{-1} = 100 micrograms kg^{-1} h^{-1}. Infuse at 1–3 mL h^{-1}.
- Vecuronium infusion: 3 mg kg^{-1} in 50 mL gives 1 mL h^{-1} = 60 micrograms kg^{-1} h^{-1}. Infuse at 1–3 mL h^{-1}.

Other
10% calcium gluconate 0.5 mL kg^{-1} IV (to treat hypocalcaemia or hyperkalaemia in massive transfusion).

Further reading
Advanced Life Support Group. *Advanced Paediatric Life Support: The Practical Approach* (4th edn), 2005. New York: John Wiley & Sons (Wiley-Blackwell).

Nichol DG (ed). *Rogers Textbook of Pediatric Intensive Care* (4th edn). Philadelphia, PA: Lippincott Williams & Wilkins, 2008.

Steward DJ, Lerman J (eds). Trauma including acute burns and scalds. In: *Manual of Pediatric Anesthesia* (5th edn). Philadelphia, PA: Churchill Livingston, 2001.

Pyloric stenosis

Key points
- Pyloric stenosis is a medical and not a surgical emergency.
- The incidence is approximately 1:400 with multifactorial aetiology (genetic and environmental). It affects mostly first-born males and is more common in the offspring of affected parents.
- Presentation is typically with projectile vomiting in a well, hungry baby.
- The metabolic picture is a hypochloraemic, hypokalaemic, hyponatraemic metabolic alkalosis, although most present with only a mild imbalance.
- Hypovolaemia and biochemical abnormalities must be corrected before surgery.
- Death is rare.

Background
Clinical presentation and diagnosis
- Pyloric stenosis usually presents between the 3rd and 5th weeks of life in otherwise well, full-term babies.
- It is characterized by non-bilious projectile vomiting, which may become blood stained.
- Infants are initially hungry between feeds but fail to gain weight and may become lethargic and dehydrated.
- There may be mild jaundice from starvation-induced glucuronyl transferase deficiency.
- Associated abnormalities occur in <20% of cases (cardiac, renal, intestinal).
- Clinical diagnosis—gastric peristaltic waves may be seen with a test feed and the presence of an olive-shaped mass to the right of the umbilicus is diagnostic (better felt with the stomach empty).
- Ultrasound scan may be required if the clinical picture is uncertain.

Pathophysiology
- Hydrogen, potassium, sodium, and chloride ions are lost from the stomach.
- The high plasma bicarbonate concentration overwhelms the reabsorptive capacity of the proximal convoluted tubule and bicarbonate is lost in the urine (pH >7).
- Secondary hyperaldosteronism from hypovolaemia results in Na^+ and H_2O retention and further K^+ loss. H^+ in the glomerular filtrate is also exchanged for K^+ in an attempt to normalize pH. There is an extracellular to intracellular shift of K^+ due to alkalosis. The net result is reduced total body K^+, although plasma K^+ may be normal.
- Reduced K^+ forces Na^+ to exchange with H^+ instead of K^+ in the distal tubules leading to paradoxical aciduria.
- Only when Cl^- status is restored, is there enough in the glomerular filtrate to allow tubular exchange with bicarbonate and excretion of bicarbonate to produce an alkaline urine and restoration of pH.
- Correction of K^+ and Cl^- is necessary to achieve correction of alkalaemia.

Preoperative

- Keep nil by mouth, give IV fluids, and insert a nasogastric tube and keep on free drainage with regular aspiration.
- Correct dehydration and metabolic imbalance over 24–48 h.
- Severe dehydration (15%) requires a 20-mL kg^{-1} bolus of 0.9% saline (0.9%) or colloid followed by reassessment.
- For mild-to-moderate dehydration the deficit is added to normal maintenance requirements as 5% glucose 0.45% saline with KCl 10 mmol 500 mL (often run at 6–8 mL kg^{-1} h^{-1}).
- Replace nasogastric losses with an equal volume of 0.9% saline.
- Therapy is guided by regular assessment of capillary gases.
- Surgery does not take place until electrolytes are in the normal range.
- Uncorrected alkalosis can cause dysrhythmias and postoperative apnoeas.

Intraoperative

- Induce anaesthesia in a warm operating room with full monitoring and warming devices.
- Aspirate the nasogastric tube in the prone, supine, and left and right lateral positions (4-quadrant aspiration).
- Induction may be gaseous or IV. Effective preoxygenation of babies can be difficult and cricoid pressure may distort laryngeal anatomy, while non-depolarizing neuromuscular blocking drugs have a rapid onset in neonates because of their high cardiac output.
- A reasonable choice of induction is oxygen and sevoflurane followed by neuromuscular blockade with atracurium (0.5 mg kg^{-1}).
- Maintain anaesthesia with oxygen, air, and volatile of choice (unlike nitrous oxide, nitrogen in air splints alveoli and reduces atelectasis).
- Provide analgesia with paracetamol (20–30 mg kg^{-1} PR or 10 mg kg^{-1} IV) and LA infiltration by the surgeon (bupivacaine 0.25%) at the end of the procedure, supplemented with intraoperative opioids (fentanyl 1 microgram kg^{-1}) if necessary.
- Skin incision may be right hypochondrial or periumbilical, but the procedure is increasingly performed laparoscopically.
- Surgery involves a longitudinal incision of the 'pyloric tumour' to the level of the mucosa (Ramstedt's pyloromyotomy).
- The anaesthetist may be asked to inject air through the nasogastric tube to check the pyloric mucosa is intact.
- If surgery has been less than an hour, reverse neuromuscular blockade at the end of procedure and extubate the baby awake.

Postoperative

- Remove nasogastric tube but continue IV fluids until feeding, generally within 6–12 h.
- Give regular paracetamol postoperatively (max. 40 mg kg^{-1} 24 h^{-1} IV, 60 mg kg^{-1} 24 h^{-1} PO or PR).
- Apnoea monitoring for up to 24 h (minimum 6 h).
- Vomiting may not settle immediately.
- Complications rare: mucosal perforation and wound infection.

Further reading

Fell D, Chelliah S. Infantile pyloric stenosis. *Br J Anaesth CEPD Rev* 2001; **1**:85–8.

Congenital diaphragmatic hernia

Key points

- Congenital diaphragmatic hernia (CDH) is a defect in the diaphragm that usually develops early in gestation and is associated with extrusion of intra-abdominal organs into the thoracic cavity.
- The incidence is 1:2000 to 1:5000 live births ('hidden incidence' of termination, stillborn, or immediate death).
- 85–90% of defects are posterolateral through the foramen of Bochdalek, of which 75–80% are left-sided. Hernias through the foramen of Morgagni (anteromedial), and paraoesophageal hernias, make up the remainder.
- It is not a surgical emergency and morbidity and mortality have improved with immediate stabilization of the neonate, delayed surgery, and avoidance of ventilator-induced lung injury.
- Mortality is 30–50% and related to the degree of pulmonary hypoplasia.

Background

Pathophysiology

- There is failure of lung and diaphragm development, with a reduced number of airways and pulmonary arteries. Diaphragmatic closure normally occurs by 9–10 weeks of gestation. If closure is delayed, or if there is premature return of intestines into the abdomen before obliteration of the pleuroperitoneal canals, the midgut can herniate into the thoracic cavity.
- The degree of pulmonary hypoplasia depends on the gestational age at the time of herniation.
- Herniation through the left foramen of Bochdalek may include stomach, left kidney, and parts of the colon and liver.
- Mediastinal shift can cause compression of the contralateral lung.
- Pulmonary vasculature is immature and there is abnormal muscularization with exaggerated responses to hypoxaemia and acidosis.
- There is also an imbalance of endogenous pulmonary vasoconstrictors and vasodilators, leading to pulmonary hypertension and right-to-left shunt.
- There may be associated left ventricular dysfunction.

Associated congenital anomalies

- Cardiac anomalies are present in ~20% (especially patent ductus arteriosus (PDA) and hypoplastic left heart).
- Chromosomal (trisomy 13/18/21).
- GI tract-malrotation common.
- Associated syndromes: Fryns, Goldenhar, Beckwith–Wiedemann, Cantrell's pentalogy (exomphalos, diaphragmatic hernia, sternal defect, intracardiac defects, and ectopia cordis).

Antenatal diagnosis and management

- Antenatal ultrasound scan at 20 weeks may show polyhydramnios, intrathoracic gastric bubble, and mediastinal shift.
- Low lung-to-head ratio and presence of liver herniation may correlate with poor outcome despite maximum care.
- Antenatal diagnosis enables referral to a specialist centre with neonatal facilities.
- Fetoscopic tracheal plugging is an experimental *in utero* technique attempting to improve the growth of hypoplastic lungs by causing airway expansion from accumulation of surfactant-rich fluid. There is insufficient evidence currently to demonstrate improved survival after fetoscopic surgery compared with standard postnatal management.

Clinical presentation

- Respiratory distress in the first 24h, with classic triad of cyanosis, dyspnoea, and apparent dextrocardia.
- Examination reveals a bulging chest/scaphoid abdomen, ↓ breath sounds, and bowel sounds in the chest.
- Chest X-ray shows apparent dextrocardia with bowel in the left chest if there is a left-sided hernia.
- Can occasionally present late with a small hernia.

Classification (Wiseman and MacPherson 1977)

- Group 1—early herniation during bronchial branching results in severe pulmonary hypoplasia and death.
- Group 2—herniation during distal bronchial branching results in unilateral hypoplasia. Prognosis depends on balance between ductal and vascular resistances.
- Group 3—
  - Late herniation with adequate lung development.
  - Respiratory distress with air swallowing.
- Group 4—postnatal herniation with normal lungs.

Postnatal management

- The aim is to maintain oxygenation and lung perfusion with minimal barotrauma.
- Lung compliance often worsens after surgery so a period of cardiorespiratory stabilization is necessary to improve hypoxia and acidosis, reduce right-to-left shunt and improve pulmonary perfusion.
- Preoperative stabilization from the time of birth is associated with improved lung compliance and better outcome.
- Significant co-morbidities should be identified and optimized.
- Early intubation and decompression of the stomach with a nasogastric tube (with avoidance of mask ventilation) are important to prevent further distension of the viscera.
- Care is needed with ventilation because hypoplastic lungs are more likely to rupture. High ventilatory pressures can also cause release of vasoactive mediators resulting in pulmonary vasoconstriction and worsening hypertension.

- Pre-emptive high-frequency oscillatory ventilation (HFOV) may be started early or considered when conventional ventilation requires high peak inspiratory pressures (e.g. >25 cmH$_2$O).
- Pulmonary hypertension can be treated with inhaled nitric oxide and IV epoprostenol. The evidence for nitric oxide alone is limited but it may have a synergistic effect if given with epoprostenol.
- Inotropes (dopamine or dobutamine) may be necessary to support the circulation and minimize right-to-left shunt.
- Surgery is ideally delayed until the baby has been stable on conventional ventilation with inspired O$_2$ concentrations <50% and minimal inotropes for 24h. This may not be possible and surgery may need to be performed on the special care baby unit while on HFOV.
- Poor prognostic indicators include the need for immediate intubation, infants born at <33 weeks' gestation, weight <1kg, P(A–a)O$_2$ difference >500mmHg (67 kPa), PIP >40 cmH$_2$O, and arterial pH <7.0.

Extracorporeal membrane oxygenation

- Considered in babies >35 weeks and >2kg who have severe disease refractory to medical therapy.
- Used for stabilization before surgery or as rescue postoperatively.
- The alveolar–arterial difference in partial pressure of oxygen [P(A–a) O$_2$ difference] and oxygen index (FiO$_2$ × MAP/PaO$_2$) are used as severity indices.
- Most commonly a circuit is established between the internal jugular vein and the common carotid artery.
- Improves survival rates for those with a high risk of mortality but may not improve survival for others.
- Complications include bleeding, intracranial haemorrhage, and sepsis.

Intraoperative

- The surgical approach is classically transabdominal with primary repair or patching if the defect is large. Reduction of viscera may initially worsen lung compliance and primary closure of the abdomen may not be possible. A chimney prosthesis or silastic pouch can be applied or abdominal closure performed with a patch.
- Insert a central venous line (avoiding lower extremities if concern of IVC compression after reduction, but beware the risk of pneumothorax with an internal jugular).
- An arterial line is useful, preferably right radial, for regular pre-ductal gas sampling.
- Echocardiography can be used to document flow characteristics and cardiac function.
- The anaesthetic technique is generally a low-dose volatile/high-dose opioid (fentanyl or a remifentanil infusion) with muscle relaxation to reduce the pulmonary vascular response to surgical stress.
- Avoid nitrous oxide because of diffusion into the viscera and worsening lung compliance.
- Maintenance fluids should contain glucose, and third space and blood loss replaced with 0.9% saline, colloid, or blood as necessary.

- Sudden deterioration and desaturation after a 'honeymoon period' may be caused by a pulmonary hypertensive crisis with right-to-left shunt and should be treated with 100% oxygen and hyperventilation, analgesia and adequate anaesthesia. However, it may also be caused by a pneumothorax, which must be treated appropriately.
- Do not attempt to 're-inflate' the hypoplastic lung as there is a high risk of pneumothorax of the other lung.
- Avoid hypothermia as this increases pulmonary vascular resistance and oxygen consumption and may worsen acidosis.
- Babies usually remain ventilated and postoperative analgesia can be provided with a morphine infusion (10–20 micrograms $kg^{-1}h^{-1}$).
- A thoracic epidural may assist weaning (inserted via lumbar or caudal route) in babies without significant pulmonary disease.

Postoperative

- Respiratory function is often worse postoperatively and continued treatment of pulmonary hypertension necessary.
- Outcome depends on the severity of pulmonary hypoplasia and degree of pulmonary hypertension.
- Long-term complications include reactive airways disease, chronic lung disease, gastro-oesophageal reflux, neurodevelopmental delay, and sensorineural hearing loss.

Further reading

Brett CM, Davis PJ, Bikhazi G Anesthesia for Neonates and Premature Infants. In Motoyama EK, Davis PJ (eds) *Smith's Anesthesia for Infants and Children* (7th edn). Philadelphia, PA: Mosby, 2006, pp.545–50.

Exomphalos and gastroschisis

Key points

- Exomphalos and gastroschisis are distinct clinical entities that present with herniation of abdominal contents at birth.
- The incidence is 1:5000 to 1:10 000 live births (incidence of exomphalos decreasing and gastroschisis increasing).
- The diagnosis is made usually by antenatal ultrasound scan, enabling planned delivery and prompt surgery in a tertiary centre.
- Herniated organs may have an impaired blood supply and there may be associated intestinal obstruction.
- Major fluid and heat loss, as well as sepsis, are perioperative concerns.
- Repair may be primary or staged depending on the ease with which contents are returned to the abdomen.
- Outcome is good, and depends on associated defects in exomphalos and the state of the bowel in gastroschisis.

Background

Exomphalos

- An embryonic central abdominal wall defect allowing herniation of abdominal viscera into the umbilical cord.
- The embryonic intestine develops during the 6th week of gestation and migrates through the umbilical ring into the cord. The intestine then returns to the abdominal cavity by the 10th to 12th week. Failure of the gut to return results in exomphalos.
- It is often associated with non-rotation or malrotation of the intestine and may contain other organs, e.g. liver and spleen.
- Herniated viscera are covered with a membranous sac and the bowel is usually healthy.
- Exomphalos is associated with other abnormalities:
  - Chromosomal trisomies.
  - Cardiac—Fallot's tetralogy and atrial septal defect.
  - Bladder or cloacal extrophy.
  - GI—imperforate anus, intestinal atresia, malrotation.
  - Other midline abnormalities-vertebral, myelomeningocele, cleft palate.
  - Beckwith–Wiedemann syndrome (macroglossia, gigantism, and pancreatic islet cell hyperplasia).
  - Cantrell's pentalogy (exomphalos, diaphragmatic hernia, sternal defect, intracardiac defects and ectopia cordis).

Gastroschisis

- Abdominal wall defect, usually to the right of the umbilical cord.
- Development is suggested to result from occlusion of the omphalomesenteric artery during gestation; other organs are usually not involved.
- Herniated intestines are not protected by a membrane and may be inflamed, oedematous, and thickened from exposure to amniotic fluid in utero. Stenosis, ischaemia, and perforation of the bowel may develop.

- There may be other gut abnormalities (intestinal atresias common) but few associated anomalies.
- Associated with low maternal age, maternal smoking, and aspirin.
- Both defects are associated with prematurity and intrauterine growth retardation, but the latter is more common in gastroschisis.

Diagnosis and initial management

- The diagnosis is made by antenatal ultrasound scan.
- Antenatal diagnosis allows planned delivery in a centre with neonatal and surgical expertise.
- Those with exomphalos are investigated for other anomalies.
- Neonates with gastroschisis may benefit from early delivery to limit bowel damage.
- Priorities involve minimizing fluid and heat loss, preventing gut ischaemia and sepsis, and decompressing gastric contents.
- Careful positioning of the baby may be necessary to avoid compromising gut perfusion.
- If there is no sac or it has ruptured, the bowel is covered with a sterile waterproof bowel bag. Otherwise a sterile dressing is applied.
- A nasogastric tube is inserted and broad-spectrum antibiotics commenced.
- Neonates with gastroschisis or ruptured exomphalos need surgery within hours due to risk of fluid and heat loss.
- Those with unruptured exomphalos can be operated on electively.
- In some centres it is routine to apply a silo without GA immediately after the baby is born. The bowel is reduced gradually over several days followed by definitive closure of the defect under GA.

Preoperative

- Large volumes of fluid may be needed (0.9% saline and 4.5% human albumin solution (HAS)) to prevent hypovolaemia and metabolic acidosis caused by extensive losses into the bowel. Electrolyte imbalance may occur as a result of large volume replacement and significant haemodilution may require blood transfusion. Maintenance fluids should contain glucose.
- Adequacy of fluid replacement should be assessed by monitoring capillary refill, core–peripheral temperature gradient, urine output, and acid–base status.
- Investigations should include FBC, electrolytes, glucose, acid–base status, and crossmatch.
- Babies with exomphalos require echocardiography and investigation of other abnormalities.

Intraoperative

- Usual neonatal precautions should be taken to keep the baby warm (warm operating room, warming mattress, warming blanket, plastic drapes, warm humidified anaesthetic gases, warmed fluids).
- Apply full monitoring (pulse oximeter, ECG, and NIBP) before induction.
- Aspirate the nasogastric tube.

- IV or inhalational induction (sevoflurane) may be appropriate followed by a non-depolarizing neuromuscular blocker (e.g. 0.5–1 mg kg^{-1} atracurium) and intubation.
- RSI may be performed but preoxygenation can be difficult and the effect of atracurium in neonates is rapid.
- Maintain anaesthesia with oxygen, air, and a volatile; avoid nitrous oxide because of the risk of worsening bowel distension.
- Insert two IV lines for volume and replacement (consider siting in arms as abdominal distension on reduction may impair venous return from legs).
- Consider an arterial line for large defects or if significant comorbidity.
- Intraoperative analgesia can be provided with fentanyl (5–10 micrograms kg^{-1}) or a remifentanil infusion, followed by a morphine infusion (10–20 micrograms kg^{-1} h^{-1}) for postoperative analgesia if the baby is to remain ventilated.
- Epidural or caudal analgesia should be considered, with smaller doses of IV fentanyl (1–2 micrograms kg^{-1}) intraoperatively, if the baby is likely to be extubated. Provide postoperative analgesia with a low-dose morphine infusion (5–10 micrograms kg^{-1} h^{-1}) if a regional procedure has not been performed.
- Fluid loss into third space may be large (20 mL kg^{-1} h^{-1} while bowel is exposed)—replace with 0.9% saline or 4.5% HAS, and blood as indicated.
- If there is associated intestinal atresia, a limited bowel resection, ideally with end-to-end anastomosis, may be needed. Once the bowel has been checked and managed as appropriate, it is returned to the abdominal cavity.
- During return of the bowel, intra-abdominal pressure increases, so it is important to monitor for reduction in lung compliance (↑ airway pressures/↓ tidal volumes).
- IVC compression may be caused by raised intra-abdominal pressure, leading to reduced cardiac output which may be indicated by weak peripheral pulses and reduced urine output. Reduced cardiac output may lead to tissue hypoperfusion with intestinal ischaemia and renal failure.
- An increase in intragastric pressure >20 mmHg and increases in CVP of >4 mmHg have been associated with failure to achieve successful primary closure.
- If primary closure is not possible a silastic pouch is formed to contain the bowel and closure is delayed until the bowel has been reduced gradually over several days.
- Insert a central line or percutaneous feeding line if parenteral nutrition is likely to be needed.
- If the defect is small and there is no cardiorespiratory compromise, the baby may be extubated once neuromuscular blockade is reversed.
- The bowel often becomes more oedematous over 48–72 h making abdominal distension worse after primary closure.

Postoperative

- Unless the defect is small, the baby usually remains paralysed and ventilated on the special care baby unit for several days until abdominal distension has resolved.
- If primary closure was not possible, the baby remains ventilated while the bowel is gradually returned to the abdominal cavity over several days. The baby can then return to the operating room for closure of the abdomen.
- Morphine infusion is continued. The addition of regular paracetamol (IV or PR) will have a morphine-sparing effect, which may be important in those with an ileus.
- The baby is monitored for signs of raised intra-abdominal pressure (reduced urine output and metabolic acidosis).
- Fluid balance must be carefully maintained and inotropes may be necessary.
- Prolonged ileus is common, especially in babies with gastroschisis and large exomphalos defects, and parenteral nutrition may be required for several weeks.
- Complications include: sepsis, abdominal wall breakdown, adhesions, necrotizing enterocolitis, renal failure, short-gut syndrome (if a large proportion of small bowel is resected) and gastro-oesophageal reflux.

Outcome

- Mortality and morbidity have ↓ due to improvements in surgery and neonatal care.
- Mortality is higher with exomphalos (30–50%) because of associated anomalies.
- Prognosis is good in those without cardiac or respiratory abnormalities.

Further reading

Poddar R, Hartley L. Exomphalos and gastroschisis. *Br J Anaesth CEACCP* 2009; **9**:48–51.

Oesophageal atresia and tracheo-oesophageal fistula

Key points
- The incidence of oesophageal atresia and tracheo-oesophageal fistula (TOF) is 1:3000 to 1:4000 live births.
- There are five major types although there are many anatomical variations.
- In 85% there is a blind oesophageal pouch with a fistula between the distal oesophagus and trachea, usually close to the carina.
- Up to 30% occur in premature or low birth weight (<2 kg) neonates.
- 30–50% have associated congenital abnormalities.
- Surgical repair is usually via a right thoracotomy with ligation of the fistula and primary end-to-end anastomosis of the oesophagus.
- The main anaesthetic concerns are avoiding ventilation through the fistula into the stomach before the fistula is ligated, and maintaining adequate oxygenation and ventilation during the procedure.
- Mortality depends on the severity of underlying lung disease and associated anomalies.
- Survival is >90% in otherwise healthy full-term neonates.

Background

Embryology
- The trachea and oesophagus develop from the foregut in the first 4–5 weeks of gestation.
- Anomalies of the tracheobronchial tree occur in almost 50% of patients with TOF, e.g. ectopic right upper bronchus, congenital bronchial or tracheal stenosis, and tracheal web. Anomalies are more common with isolated oesophageal atresia and least with the H type fistula.
- Duodenal or ileal atresia, malrotation and imperforate anus are common associated GI abnormalities.

Associated anomalies
- Cardiac—ventricular septal defect, atrial septal defect, patent ductus arteriosus, Fallot's tetralogy, coarctation.
- Airway—tracheomalacia, tracheal stenosis, laryngeal cleft.
- GI tract, genitourinary tract, and renal.
- VATER—vertebral, anorectal, tracheo-oesophageal fistula, oesophageal atresia, radial and/or renal.
- VACTERL—as VATER plus cardiac and limb.
- CHARGE—coloboma, heart defects, choanal atresia, retarded development and growth, genital hypoplasia, ear abnormalities.

Clinical presentation
- Most cases are diagnosed antenatally by ultrasound scan (polyhydramnios).
- Suspect in a 'mucousy' neonate with a history of maternal polyhydramnios.
- Coughing, choking, and cyanosis with initial feeds.

- Confirmed by inability to pass an orogastric tube which can be seen coiled in the upper oesophageal pouch on chest X-ray.
- Gas can be seen in the stomach and small intestine in the presence of a fistula but not in isolated oesophageal atresia.
- Barium swallow should not be performed due to risk of aspiration.
- The H type may present later with recurrent chest infections.

Types of tracheo-oesophageal fistula

The types and relative incidence of TOFs are depicted in Fig. 13.2.

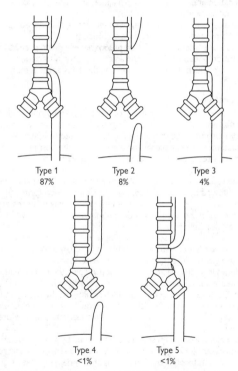

Fig. 13.2 Types of tracheo-oesophageal fistula. Reproduced by permission of Hodder Education. Bingham R, Lloyd-Thomas, Sury M (eds). *Hatch and Sumner's Textbook of Paediatric Anaesthesia* (3rd edn), p.493.

Preoperative

- The timing of surgery depends on the clinical condition and anatomical defect, and is usually performed in the first few days.
- Nil by mouth, IV fluids, and broad-spectrum antibiotics.
- Nurse head-up (to prevent gastro-oesophageal reflux), with a Replogle tube on continuous suction to aspirate secretions and prevent aspiration into lungs.
- Routine blood tests—FBC, U&E, glucose, blood gases, and crossmatch.
- Chest X-ray should be performed to determine the presence of consolidation and/or cardiac abnormalities, and renal ultrasound performed as indicated.
- Echocardiography preoperatively to determine position of aorta before thoracotomy, and to check for cardiac conditions.
- Some neonates require ventilation preoperatively (from prematurity or aspiration pneumonitis) which can cause gastric distension by ventilation through the fistula. Surgery in these instances is more urgent.

Intraoperative

- In most cases the procedure is performed as a primary one-stage repair via a right thoracotomy, although a right-sided aortic arch will require a left thoracotomy. An extrapleural approach is used to ligate the fistula and anastomose the proximal and distal ends of the oesophagus.
- In some centres the procedure may now be performed thoracoscopically.
- A staged repair with formation of a gastrostomy and division of the fistula followed by delayed oesophageal reconstruction (primary anastomosis or a jejunal or colonic interposition) may be necessary if the two ends of the oesophagus do not meet, and in those with low birth weight, respiratory compromise or other anomalies.
- A 'long gap' is usually associated with pure oesophageal atresia.
- The aim of induction is to avoid ventilating through the fistula, which may cause gastric distension and worsen ventilation.
- Techniques include inhalational induction keeping the baby breathing spontaneously until the airway is secured with a tracheal tube (TT), RSI avoiding positive pressure mask ventilation until the TT has isolated the fistula, or inhalational or IV induction followed by a non-depolarizing neuromuscular blocking drug with gentle manual ventilation before intubation.
- Inhalational induction with sevoflurane followed by a non-depolarizing neuromuscular blocking drug (e.g. atracurium 0.5–1 mg kg^{-1}) and gentle hand ventilation through the facemask is appropriate in most cases. It is good practice to ensure bilateral ventilation is possible, without inflating the stomach too much, before giving a non-depolarizing drug. If manual ventilation results in gastric distension a 'deep' intubation should be considered and the baby kept breathing spontaneously until the TT has isolated the fistula.
- The surgeon may wish to perform a rigid bronchoscopy before intubation to confirm position of the fistula. This should be done before muscle relaxant is given and anaesthesia maintained via the side

arm of the bronchoscope. The surgeon may also scope the oesophagus to look for an upper pouch fistula.

- If the fistula is near the carina it may be appropriate to deliberately insert the TT endobronchially, then slowly withdraw it until bilateral breath sounds are heard, confirming tracheal placement. It is then secured firmly.
- Gastric distension may be reduced by rotating the tube so the bevel is facing away from the fistula.
- Devices such as Fogarty catheters can be used to occlude a large fistula where ventilation may be a problem and where there is a risk of aspiration of gastric fluid into the lungs. The catheter is inserted through a fibreoptic bronchoscope and inflated after passing through the fistula tract.
- An arterial line may be inserted to monitor BP and blood gases.
- Anaesthesia is maintained with oxygen, air, and volatile (desflurane, sevoflurane, or isoflurane); nitrous oxide is avoided to prevent gastric distension. The 'nitrogen splinting' effect of air also reduces alveolar collapse.
- Rarely, the leak through the fistula causes severe gastric distension and ventilation problems that may be controlled by the surgeon placing a ligature around the gastro-oesophageal junction when the chest is open.
- Confirm the position of the TT each time the baby is moved.
- Surgical manipulation may cause lung or tracheal compression and hypoxia as well as reducing cardiac output from compression of major vessels, so good communication between anaesthetist and surgeon is essential.
- Manual ventilation may be preferred until the fistula is ligated to help detect changes in pulmonary compliance.
- The fistula can be confused with a bronchus so it is important to make sure both lungs can be ventilated when the fistula is clamped, before it is ligated.
- Once the fistula is ligated, the surgeon locates the upper pouch with the help of the anaesthetist gently advancing the Replogle tube or nasogastric tube to bring the blind end into view.
- Primary anastomosis is usually possible and the Replogle or nasogastric tube replaced with a 'trans-anastomotic' nasogastric tube before the proximal and distal ends of the oesophagus are brought together. This can be used as a stent and for enteral feeding later.
- Analgesia is provided with fentanyl (1–3 micrograms kg^{-1}) and IV paracetamol (10 mg kg^{-1}) intraoperatively and a low-dose morphine infusion (5–10 micrograms kg^{-1} h^{-1}) or thoracic epidural (placed from a caudal or lumbar space) for postoperative analgesia. Intercostal nerve blocks may be placed by the surgeon at the end of the procedure as an alternative to an epidural.
- Higher doses of fentanyl (5–10 micrograms kg^{-1}) or morphine (0.1–0.2 mg kg^{-1}) can be used followed by a morphine infusion postoperatively (10–20 micrograms kg^{-1} h^{-1}) if the baby is to remain ventilated.
- The lungs should be re-inflated under direct vision before the chest is closed.

Postoperative

- Some advocate continuing postoperative ventilation for up to 5 days to rest the anastomosis and avoid the risk of anastomotic damage in the event of urgent reintubation. However, in well babies where the anastomosis is not under tension, early extubation is increasingly encouraged.
- Feeding via the trans-anastomotic tube is usually started within the first few days and oral feeding commenced soon after, once the anastomosis has been checked with contrast.
- Postoperative suctioning must be proximal to the anastomosis.
- All babies should be cared for in a HDU.
- Anastomotic leak may cause mediastinitis and sepsis.
- Common chronic complications include:
  - Oesophageal dysmotility with reflux.
  - Oesophageal strictures and tracheomalacia.
  - 'Tracheal pouch' at site of fistula repair (difficult ventilation during subsequent anaesthetics may be caused by the TT sitting in pouch).

Further reading

Bingham R, Lloyd-Thomas, Sury M (eds). *Hatch and Sumner's Textbook of Paediatric Anaesthesia* (3rd edn). London: Hodder Arnold, 2008, pp. 492–4.

Inhaled foreign body

Key points
- Foreign body aspiration is common and can be life threatening.
- A history of choking may be present.
- Early diagnosis and treatment decrease morbidity; delayed diagnosis may result in pneumonia and increases morbidity.
- The gold standard for managing foreign body aspiration is removal via rigid bronchoscopy.
- An experienced anaesthetist and surgeon must be involved.

Background
- Foreign body aspiration is most common between the ages of 1–3 years because small children are prone to putting objects in their mouths.
- Organic products, especially peanuts, are often inhaled and these can cause airway hyper-reactivity and a pneumonitis. The absence of molar teeth prevents adequate chewing and there is a tendency to be distracted, resulting in inhalation and aspiration.
- Some foreign bodies lodge in the larynx or trachea and the child may die at home, but most are found in the proximal airways. Small sharp objects may lodge in the subglottic area.
- If an object is small enough to pass through the vocal cords, it generally does not cause complete tracheal obstruction.
- Coins more commonly end up in the upper oesophagus but oesophageal foreign bodies may cause respiratory distress if they compress the trachea.
- The presentation is often one of acute upper airway obstruction in a child with a history of choking. There may be stridor, cough, or a wheeze depending on where the foreign body is lodged. These initial symptoms may be missed if the episode was not witnessed.
- Aspiration may present days later with fever and a chest infection, or months later with atypical respiratory symptoms. Late diagnosis is associated with a higher complication rate.
- Auscultation may reveal ↓ air entry or wheeze on the affected side, but may be normal.
- Chest X-ray may be helpful in identifying and localizing the foreign body, although they are usually not radio-opaque and, therefore, cannot be seen. However, inspiratory and expiratory films may demonstrate air trapping on the affected side in expiration. Collapse or a pneumothorax may be present.
- Do not obtain a chest X-ray if the child is stridulous and there is a strong suspicion of foreign body aspiration.
- Fluoroscopy or flexible bronchoscopy may be performed if there is clinical suspicion with a normal chest X-ray.
- Inhalational induction and rigid bronchoscopy in the spontaneously breathing child is the technique of choice for removal if there is any concern of foreign body dislodgement.

Preoperative

- A history of aspiration should be sought and the patient examined for signs of respiratory distress (tachypnoea, tachycardia, agitation).
- If time allows, the child should be fasted before anaesthesia.
- Treat symptoms as indicated, e.g. wheeze, pneumonia.
- If there is respiratory distress or hypoxia, immediate bronchoscopy is needed despite the presence of a 'full stomach.'
- Avoid any manoeuvre that may distress the child and result in complete upper airway obstruction.
- Oral atropine (20–40 micrograms kg^{-1} to max. 900 micrograms) may be given to dry secretions and to protect against bradycardia from instrumentation of the airway.
- Avoid sedative premedication if there is any concern about potential upper airway obstruction.

Intraoperative

- The procedure requires an experienced paediatric anaesthetist and ENT surgeon.
- If the child is not distressed it may be possible to secure IV access before induction.
- The surgeon must check that the necessary equipment and attachments are present and working and the anaesthetist must ensure that it is possible to connect the breathing system to the side arm of the rigid bronchoscope (e.g. Storz).
- Positive pressure ventilation with paralysis does provide optimal oxygenation and an immobile airway but when the bronchoscope is in a lobe of a lung, the remainder of that lung and the other lung are not oxygenated or ventilated. Maintaining spontaneous ventilation should prevent the foreign body being pushed distally, and also allows the child to entrain gases from around the bronchoscope to oxygenate the remainder of the lungs when the scope is in a distal bronchus. However, anaesthesia needs to be 'deep' to tolerate instrumentation.
- A volatile induction with sevoflurane in 100% oxygen is the method of choice and IV access is secured, if not already, when the child is 'deep.'
- If the child has respiratory distress or is at risk of gastric aspiration he/ she can be placed in the 'sitting up' position during induction.
- Avoid nitrous oxide if there is any concern about gas trapping.
- Induction may be prolonged if there is significant airway obstruction; gentle CPAP may help overcome obstruction.
- Intravenous glycopyrronium bromide (5–10 micrograms kg^{-1}) may be given for its anticholinergic effect if oral atropine was not given preoperatively.
- Do not allow airway instrumentation until the child is in a deep plane of anaesthesia (assessed by pupil size and position, respiratory pattern, heart rate, and BP).
- If the object is visible and accessible via a laryngoscope, attempts should be made to remove it, taking care not to push it further into the airway. Blind finger sweeps must not be performed as further impaction may occur.

- If bronchoscopy is required, the vocal cords should be anaesthetized with LA spray (usually lidocaine up to $4\,mg\,kg^{-1}$) to help prevent coughing before insertion of the rigid bronchoscope.
- The anaesthetic Ayre's T piece is attached to the side-arm of the bronchoscope to maintain anaesthesia.
- Sometimes the surgeon may need to remove and reinsert the scope several times, interrupting delivery of gases via the side arm. Anaesthesia can be maintained in these situations by placing oxygen tubing in the nose and connecting it to the anaesthetic common gas outlet via the fresh gas tube of the Ayre's T piece.
- Maintenance of anaesthesia is generally with sevoflurane as it is less irritant than isoflurane; however, because of its rapid offset, it can be difficult to maintain an adequate depth of anaesthesia and supplementation with small increments of propofol ($0.5–1\,mg\,kg^{-1}$) may be necessary.
- Too light a plane of anaesthesia may cause coughing and breath-holding, while too deep a plane may lead to hypoventilation and apnoea. In these situations gentle manual ventilation may be necessary despite the concern that the foreign body could be dislodged further.
- It is particularly important to prevent the child coughing during attempted removal of the object with the grasping forceps.
- If, during extraction, the foreign body obstructs the subglottis or trachea, push it distally into a bronchus to enable ventilation through the healthy lung. Failure to retrieve a distal object may require thoracotomy.
- The bronchoscope may need to be removed together with the foreign body and forceps if it is too big to pass through the scope, in which case the bronchoscope should then be reinserted to examine the airway.
- Once the foreign body has been removed and the trachea and bronchi examined by the surgeon for trauma or other foreign bodies, the bronchoscope is withdrawn and the facemask applied by the anaesthetist.
- At the end of the procedure, if spontaneous ventilation is adequate, anaesthesia is discontinued and the child is placed sitting up or in the left lateral position. If spontaneous ventilation is inadequate, it may be necessary to support ventilation through the facemask until the child's respiratory effort improves. Deterioration may require intubation until the child emerges from anaesthesia and is then extubated awake.
- Dexamethasone IV ($0.25\,mg\,kg^{-1}$) is often given to reduce airway oedema.
- If oesophagoscopy is required, the child should be paralysed and intubated for the procedure.

Postoperative

- Most children will be extubated and returned to the ward.
- Admission to HDU may be necessary if there is ongoing respiratory distress or stridor.
- If there is significant airway oedema with respiratory distress or hypoxia, keep the child intubated and ventilated in the PICU.

- Dexamethasone may be continued for 24 h or more (0.1 mg kg^{-1} IV 6–8-hourly).
- Nebulized adrenaline (0.4 mg kg^{-1} of 1:1000) may relieve stridor but the effects lasts only 2–3 h and it may need to be given regularly.
- Continue IV maintenance fluids until drinking.
- Consider physiotherapy, bronchodilators and antibiotics as indicated.
- A repeat chest X-ray should be performed postoperatively to look for pneumothorax, pneumomediastinum, or alveolar collapse.

Complications of inhaled foreign body

- Hypoxia and cerebral insult from prolonged obstruction.
- Tracheitis, bronchitis, and atelectasis from inflammatory reaction.
- Pneumonia from inflammatory secretions.
- Pneumomediastinum and pneumothorax (extension of trapped air from alveolar rupture).

Complications of bronchoscopy

- Hypoxia and hypercarbia.
- Failure to remove the foreign body (may require thoracotomy).
- Loss of airway requiring tracheostomy.
- Laryngeal, tracheal, or bronchial trauma or perforation.
- Oesophageal perforation from rigid oesophagoscopy.

Choking protocol

- See the most recent Resuscitation Council (UK) guidelines (𝄞 http://www.resus.org.uk) for the latest treatment recommendations.
- Used if a known foreign body is obstructing the glottis and causing acute airway obstruction:
  - Encourage coughing if able and do not intervene unless the cough becomes ineffective.
  - If cough becomes ineffective and the child is conscious, perform five back blows followed by five chest/abdominal thrusts, then reassess and repeat.
  - Abdominal thrusts may cause intra-abdominal injury in infants, therefore alternate back blows and chest thrusts are recommended.
  - If the child is unconscious, open the airway and perform five rescue breaths followed by CPR (15:2) and check for a foreign body.
  - Failure to ventilate may necessitate emergency cricothyroidotomy for oxygenation and ventilation while the foreign body is being removed. Depending on the residual laryngeal or subglottic injury, the child may then require intubation for a period of time or a long-term tracheostomy.

Further reading

Zur KB, Litman RS. Pediatric airway foreign body retrieval: surgical and anaesthetic perspectives. *Pediatric Anesthesia* [Special Issue: The Pediatric Airway] 2009; **19**(Suppl. 1):109–17.

Ophthalmic Emergencies

Monica Baird

Penetrating eye injury

Key points
- A penetrating eye injury may warrant emergency surgery in an unfasted patient—discuss timing of surgery with surgeon.
- There is a risk of loss of vitreous during the induction of anaesthesia and during positioning—intraocular pressure (IOP) control is important.
- Penetrating eye injury may be associated with trauma, assault, alcohol, and recreational drug use.
- IOP control in children can be difficult—eye rubbing, crying, breath holding, and screaming increase IOP and risk extrusion of intraocular contents.

Background
- Penetrating eye injuries are uncommon. Patients require emergency surgery for removal of retained material and closure of the globe. Rarely, severe trauma can require enucleation of the eye.
- The mechanism of injury varies. Non-occupational injuries can be related to alcohol or recreational drug use.
- Uncooperative children may require preoperative sedation to protect the eye from rubbing.
- Consider delaying surgery until patient fasted—liaise with the surgeon to establish urgency.

Preoperative
- A patient with a penetrating eye injury may require GA and surgery in the presence of a full stomach.
- It may be possible, for a small eye injury in a cooperative patient, to close the globe either using LA drops or a low-volume LA eye block.
- Injury may have been associated with alcohol or recreational drug use. Plan for related complications during anaesthesia.
- Following enucleation postoperative pain can be severe and long-term phantom pain can occur. In non-vomiting patients, a preoperative dose of 75 mg pregabalin or 300 mg gabapentin may reduce the incidence of phantom pain.
- Ensure any other injuries are also dealt with.

Intraoperative
- Use an eye shield to protect the eye during induction of anaesthesia. Avoid external pressure on eye with mask during pre-oxygenation.
- If the patient is not fasted, they will require a RSI followed by immediate tracheal intubation. Suxamethonium is usually the safest muscle relaxant to use for RSI because of its rapid onset and short duration of action. Suxamethonium raises IOP and presents a theoretical risk of vitreous extrusion. Evidence of this occurring is lacking and the decision to use suxamethonium is a matter for clinical judgement. Alternatively, rocuronium 1 mg kg^{-1} provides good intubating conditions equally rapidly. Sugammadex enables rapid reversal of rocuronium if required, but is expensive.

- Propofol is the ideal induction drug because it produces a greater reduction in IOP than thiopental. Avoid ketamine, which increases IOP, and etomidate, which causes postoperative vomiting.
- Consider modifying the pressor and IOP response to intubation further with fentanyl 1 micrograms kg^{-1}, alfentanil 10 micrograms kg^{-1}, or lidocaine 1 mg kg^{-1}.
- Intubate as smoothly as possible to minimize the rise in IOP. A south-facing pre-formed tracheal tube will allow optimal surgical access to the operative field. This is not a case for an inexperienced trainee.
- Following intubation of the trachea, the patient should receive a non-depolarizing muscle relaxant to prevent coughing or straining.
- Consider emptying the patient's stomach using an orogastric tube after the induction of anaesthesia if the patient has been drinking alcohol for a prolonged period.
- There is a risk of bradycardia in response to surgical traction on the eye (oculocardiac reflex). Release of traction should terminate the bradycardia. Atropine must be drawn up and at hand in case bradycardia occurs. Prophylactic glycopyrronium 100–200 micrograms IV can be given.
- Give analgesia intraoperatively as appropriate; postoperative pain may be managed with paracetamol and a NSAID.
  Be guided by the extent of the initial injury and consequent surgery.
- Antibiotics and steroids may be requested for patients undergoing enucleation of the eye.
- It is important that nausea and vomiting are avoided postoperatively; dexamethasone 4 mg after induction, and ondansetron 4 mg or cyclizine 50 mg before recovery from anaesthesia, are appropriate anti-emetics.

Postoperative
- Aim for a smooth extubation.
- Recover the patient in a slight head-up position to prevent an avoidable postoperative rise in IOP.
- Pay attention to postoperative analgesia, particularly if the patient has undergone enucleation of the eye.

Further reading
Wilson A, Soar J. Anaesthesia for emergency eye surgery. *Update Anaesth* 2000; **11**:46–50. (http://update.anaesthesiologists.org/).

Retinal detachment

Key points
- Retinal detachment surgery is normally carried out during daytime hours; patients can therefore be fasted before their surgery.
- A LA block such as sub-Tenon's can be used alone or in combination with GA for retinal detachment surgery.
- Retinal surgery can take a long time.
- Retrobulbar and peribulbar blocks are relatively contraindicated.

Background
- Retinal detachment is becoming more common as the population ages. Most detachments occur in patients between 40–70 years of age.
- Retinal surgery is increasingly specialized within ophthalmology and senior anaesthetic support may be needed to ensure that these patients receive timely care from a surgeon with the appropriate skills.
- Surgery is often prolonged and may be carried out in almost complete darkness. The anaesthetist needs access to adequate illumination.

Preoperative
- Some patients need repeated surgery for detachment and this can result in significant preoperative anxiety. Consider a benzodiazepine premedication.
- Older patients can have significant co-morbidities. Investigate these and managed as optimally as possible within the time available.
- Discussion with the surgeon is useful to establish the best anaesthetic approach. If a low IOP is not desirable, controlled ventilation should be avoided and a supraglottic airway chosen.

Intraoperative
- Surgery for retinal detachment may be intermittently highly stimulating and a sub-Tenon's block makes management of anaesthetic depth and analgesia safer and more straightforward. If the patient has had retinal detachment surgery before, discuss with the surgeon the location of any baffles as these may make it more difficult to carry out a sub-Tenon's block.
- Retrobulbar and peribulbar blocks are relatively contraindicated as the axial length is usually high in patients with retinal detachment and perforation of the globe can occur during injection.
- As surgery can be prolonged, appropriate IV replacement fluids should be provided.
- Conduct of anaesthesia is uncomplicated and dependant on the type of airway used and whether GA is combined with sub-Tenon's anaesthesia. The airway should not intrude on the operation site and a flexible supraglottic airway or a south-facing oral tracheal tube should be used whenever possible.
- Avoid using nitrous oxide. A bubble of gas is often introduced into the globe and this will expand if nitrous oxide is present. A technique using either oxygen, air and volatile or oxygen, air and a propofol infusion is appropriate.

- At the end of the surgery, the ophthalmologist may need to examine the other eye or carry out stimulating checks on the operated eye. Avoid waking the patient too soon.
- Give antiemetic prophylaxis (e.g. dexamethasone and ondansetron).

Postoperative

- Pain should be mild to moderate after surgery for retinal detachment, and absent if a sub-Tenon's block has been performed.
- Paracetamol may be the only analgesia required. Avoid NSAIDs unless they have been agreed with the surgeon, as they may increase postoperative bleeding.
- The patient may need to be recovered in a particular head position, to ensure that the gas bubble is in the correct location in the eye.

Anaesthesia for Emergency Radiological Procedures

Computed tomography

Key points
- Compared with the operating room, the radiology department is complex, with radiological hazards, moving equipment, and limited access to the patient.
- The radiology department is frequently distant from sources of help, and additional emergency equipment such as a difficult intubation trolley may not be immediately available.
- Patients may be potentially very unstable with life-threatening disease. Although patients should be stabilized before being moved to radiology the risk of deterioration is always present.
- Anaesthesia and transfers should be undertaken only by experienced anaesthetists who are familiar with the environment and the equipment, and who can deal with any patient-related complications.

Background
Anaesthesia may be required for CT for children intolerant of the process, or for adults for both diagnostic and therapeutic procedures. Patients include the victims of trauma, those with altered mental status, and the critically ill. Advances in interventional procedures now mean that patients with severe haemorrhage may attend the radiology department for embolization. Additional considerations should always include the adverse effects of contrast media (e.g. allergic reactions, nephrotoxicity, volume effects in small children).

Prescan
▶Do not embark on anaesthesia or patient transfer until you are completely familiar with the layout of the radiology department, the equipment provided, including the machines, monitoring equipment and oxygen supply, the location of additional anaesthetic equipment, and the location of the resuscitation equipment. You must know the location of all routine and emergency drugs, and who to call if you need help. If you are likely to be responsible for managing emergency patients in the radiology department you must ensure familiarity with the surroundings before you need to transfer a patient there.
- The usual standards for monitoring and the requirements for trained assistance apply. If an anaesthetic machine is to be used, complete standard AAGBI checks before induction.
- If possible, plan for induction of anaesthesia in a location outside of the radiology department (e.g. operating room, ED, or ICU), then transfer the patient with full monitoring to the radiology department when stable. Although this factors in the risks of transfer, help, drugs, and equipment will all be more readily available in these other locations.
- Given the relatively high-risk environment, ensure that undertaking the scan is really in the patient's best interests.
- Undertake a thorough preoperative assessment:
  - Identify a history of contrast reactions. Radio-contrast media cause hypersensitivity reactions in up to 3% of patients; the most severe occur within minutes of injection.

- Trauma—understand the mechanism and the injuries identified to appreciate sources of instability that may manifest in the CT scanner. Anticipate airway difficulties, pneumothoraces, haemorrhage, and intracranial lesions, and use spinal precautions. Haemodynamic instability may warrant going directly to the operating room without a scan; if you consider this, discuss it urgently with the surgical team.
- Intensive care or surgical patients—assess organ function, the mode of ventilation, and the previous ABG values. The presence of renal dysfunction should warrant a discussion of the benefits and risks of contrast media. Prophylactic therapy with N-acetylcysteine probably does not reduce the adverse effects on renal function. Understand the reason for the scan and anticipate the effect of laying the patient fully supine.
- Patients may attend the radiology department to control bleeding by embolization. Know the current platelet, Hb, and clotting profile and what products have been given so far. You will need an arterial line and large-bore IV access, but do not delay definitive care for insertion of central lines. Pre-empt transfusion requirements by ordering products early. Prepare equipment for warming the patient and fluids. Ensure the massive transfusion policy is available and establish with the surgeons/radiologists a plan for failed embolization.
- Prepare drugs and infusions such as sedation and vasopressors.
- Ensure a patent peripheral cannula is available for the infusion of contrast media.

During the scan

- All emergency patients should be intubated following a RSI with cricoid pressure.
- Ideally the scanner should have an anaesthetic machine, monitoring and set up for dealing with ventilated patients. If this is not the case, ventilate the patient's lungs with a transport ventilator that you are familiar with.
- Anaesthesia is usually maintained intravenously; IV access must be secure and visible, additional ports or cannula should be available if further infusions are required or for the injection of contrast media.
- If the patient is breathing spontaneously via tracheal or tracheostomy tube, consider converting to a fully controlled mode, which will normally provide better control of blood gases during transport and, by enabling a pause in breathing, will improve the quality of the scan.
- When in the scanning room, connect the ventilator to the wall oxygen supply and connect monitors and pumps to mains power as soon as possible.
- Transfer the patient to the scanner table, being careful not to disconnect infusion lines, and monitoring equipment. It is often easiest to place the pumps and the monitor on the scanning table so that they move with the patient.
- Before transfer, ensure that adequate help is available to transfer the patient safely, particularly a trauma patient who may require log rolling and cervical spine stabilization.
- Time spent in this difficult environment should be kept to a minimum by ensuring that before leaving a better-supported area, all non-essential infusions have been removed, thought has been given to how pumps

and monitoring will be transferred, and that a spare set of anaesthetic drugs has been drawn up and is immediately to hand.

- Do a 'dummy run' of the patient into and out of the scanner to ensure no tension develops on tubing, wires, and lines, and that no part of the patient will contact the inner sides of the scanner.
- Ensure any cannula into which contrast is to be injected is patent and flushes easily. Extravasated contrast is toxic to tissues.
- It is best to maintain neuromuscular blockade.
- Ensure the monitor is visible from the control room at all times. Watch carefully the ventilator parameters, the FiO_2, the vital signs, and the capnograph. Abort the scan if you have any concerns.
- If asked to pause the ventilation, you must be in the scanner room and be wearing appropriate radiological protection. Restart ventilation as soon as possible—do not get distracted!
- Interventional procedures may warrant patient warming and monitoring of temperature and urine output, particularly in cases of haemorrhage.

Postscan

- Ideally, make sure the scan is reviewed by a radiologist whilst you are preparing to leave the scanner so you can plan the next course of action (e.g. go to the operating room, stay for further imaging, and draining of collection). Do not wait for the scan to be formally reported, however; return to the most sensible place of safety (the ED, operating room, or ICU) without delay.
- Reconnect all equipment to mains power as soon as possible.
- If reconnecting to a different ventilator and monitor ensure they work before departing.

Further reading

Hopkins R, Peden C, Gandhi S (eds). *Radiology for Anaesthesia and Intensive Care* (2nd edn). Cambridge: Cambridge University Press, 2009.

The Royal College of Anaesthetists. *Guidance on the provision of anaesthetic care in the non theatre environment.* Revised 2011 Royal College of Anaesthetists Guidance for Anaesthetic Services. Available at: ℘ http://www.rcoa.ac.uk/docs/GPAS-ANTE.pdf.

The Royal College of Obstetricians and Gynaecologists. *The role of emergency and elective interventional radiology in postpartum haemorrhage* (Good Practice No. 6). Available at: ℘ http://www.rcog.org.uk/womens-health/clinical-guidance/role-emergency-and-elective-interventional-radiology-postpartum-haem.

The Royal College of Radiologists. *Safe Sedation, Analgesia and Anaesthesia within the Radiology Department.* 2003. Available at: ℘ http://www.rcr.ac.uk/publications.aspx?PageID=310.

Thiele H, Hildebrand L, Schirdewahn C, *et al.* Impact of high-dose N-acetylcysteine versus placebo on contrast-induced nephropathy and myocardial reperfusion injury in unselected patients with ST-segment elevation myocardial infarction undergoing primary percutaneous coronary intervention. The LIPSIA-N-ACC (Prospective, Single-Blind, Placebo-Controlled, Randomized Leipzig Immediate Percutaneous Coronary Intervention Acute Myocardial Infarction N-ACC) Trial. *J Am Coll Cardiol* 2010; **55**:2201–9.

Magnetic resonance imaging

Key points
- The MRI suite is a very challenging environment in which to provide anaesthesia.
- It is likely to involve using relatively unfamiliar, MRI-compatible equipment.
- Access to and visibility of the patient is restricted.

Background
Providing anaesthesia within the MRI suite can be a complex process:
- It involves working in a remote location in the presence of a strong magnetic field (0.2–4 Tesla), varying gradient magnetic fields, and rapidly changing radiofrequency fields. The magnetic field is also present when not scanning.
- Help may not be immediately available, the patient may not be visible in the magnet, and access to them may be limited for prolonged periods.
- Because of these unique problems you must have been trained and educated in the potential hazards of patient management in this environment before you take a patient to the MR suite.

Indications for MRI requiring general anaesthesia
- Urgent MRI is becoming more common for suspected spinal cord or cauda equina compression and investigation of acute neurological conditions.
- Patients may be transferred from ICU, or rarely ED, already intubated and ventilated.
- If the patient requires induction of anaesthesia this should be undertaken in the closest anaesthetic room, which will ideally be adjacent to the MRI suite, and then transferred into the scanning room.
- Although indications for urgent MRI are increasing, there are relatively few indications for an emergency MRI scan under GA.
- The MRI suite is not a safe place for an unstable patient, particularly one requiring inotropes, because infusions may need to be discontinued temporarily. When out of hours, always ask: 'Is this scan necessary now?'.

Equipment
- Anaesthetic and monitoring equipment used in the MR environment must be certified as MR safe and/or MR conditional (safe only under certain specified conditions in the MR environment) and may therefore be specifically designed for MR and unfamiliar to you.
- Conditional equipment must be used only under the conditions specified, which will relate to the strength of the main magnetic field, the radiofrequency field strength, and the strength and rate of change of the time of varying gradient magnetic fields used for spatial information.
- Before starting anaesthesia or patient transfer, check the equipment in both the induction area and the MRI suite. Remove all monitoring and anaesthetic equipment that is not MR safe or conditional before entering the magnet area; the patient may, necessarily, be briefly unmonitored.

- It is hazardous and completely unacceptable to use standard monitoring in MR; currents can be induced in leads causing burns, and radiofrequency interference can render the scans uninterpretable.
- Standard infusion pumps cannot be taken within the 30-gauss line (a measure of magnetic field strength); the radiographers should be able to define this for you.
- Ideally, standard pumps should not be used within the scanning room at all; there is significant potential for malfunction. Only absolutely essential infusions should be continued and the pumps must either be MR safe or kept outside the 30-gauss line necessitating long infusion lines.
- Whenever possible, maintain anaesthesia with volatile agents delivered either through an MR safe anaesthetic machine in the magnet room or via a long circuit from a machine outside the magnetic field.
- Infusion lines and pumps may be passed through screened ports into the scanning room and this may require temporary cessation of infusions.

Preparation

▶ Do not embark on anaesthesia until you are completely familiar with the processes and equipment used in the MRI suite. You must understand the anaesthetic machine and ventilator and the MR monitoring equipment. You must know the location of additional anaesthetic and resuscitation equipment. Ensure access to all routine and emergency drugs, and know who to call for help.

- GA may be required because the patient is a child; in the urgent or emergency situation, this is likely to mean that the case is complex. Seek the assistance of an experienced paediatric anaesthetist.
- Ensure that you, the patient, and your trained assistant have no contraindications to entering the MRI scanning room. All patients and staff must complete a safety and exclusion questionnaire before entering the magnetic field. Remove all ferromagnetic items, such as bleeps or pens from pockets.
- Enquire about previous allergic reactions to the contrast media used in MRI. Patients with renal impairment are at risk of developing nephrogenic systemic fibrosis, a rare, potentially life-threatening condition caused by the contrast media.
- With your assistant and the radiographer, construct a plan for the management of the patient should they deteriorate. Emergency procedures are difficult to perform in the scanning room because of the high magnetic field. The plan should involve moving the patient out of the magnetic field to the nearby anaesthetic room. Do not shut down the magnetic field: this is not without hazard and should be done only if a patient or staff member is trapped or injured by a ferromagnetic object hurtling on to the magnet (injuries with ferromagnetic cylinders and patient trolleys have been reported).
- Rationalize all pumps and infusions to those absolutely necessary. Remove any PA catheter: the current induced by the scanning process can melt the thermistor.
- IV cannulae, arterial and central lines are MRI compatible. Standard ECG electrodes, their skin connectors, and standard non-invasive BP cuffs and oxygen saturation probes are not: change them for MR safe components before the patient is moved into the magnet room.

Induction of anaesthesia and transfer into the magnet

- Induction of anaesthesia usually occurs in an anaesthetic room outside the 5-gauss line adjacent to the scanning room (where standard anaesthetic and monitoring equipment is safe to use). When the patient is stable, remove all non-MR safe, or compatible monitoring equipment and transfer to the scanning room on an MRI compatible tilting trolley.
- Monitoring within the scanning room is undertaken with specifically designed MR compatible equipment, which transmits the physiological data to a monitor in the control room. Usual standards for monitoring apply, although the quality of some of the monitoring, particularly the ECG trace and pulse oximetry, may be compromised by the changing gradient magnetic fields and radiofrequency currents. Do not prolong patient time in the scanner in an attempt to obtain the perfect trace. $ETCO_2$ and NIBP are not subject to interference and should always be used.
- Complete the standard checks published by the AAGBI.
- It is usual for a MRI compatible anaesthetic machine with vaporizers to be used with an MR compatible ventilator, or a Penlon Nuffield ventilator and a long Mapleson D circuit or T-piece for children. There is usually only pipeline oxygen attached to the anaesthetic machine. Standard cylinders are highly ferromagnetic and very dangerous in the magnet area. Aluminium cylinders can be sourced but are not used commonly. Ensure suction is immediately available.
- It is possible to maintain anaesthesia using TIVA, but the pumps must remain outside the 30-gauss line, with extra long extension lines to the patient. A port cut in the magnet room screened wall between the scanning and the control room will facilitate this. Essential additional infusions are delivered in the same manner. Ensure the pump pressure deliverable is high enough to overcome the additional resistance of the long extension sets. For convenience and safety, inhalational anaesthesia from the machine in the scanning room is preferable.
- The ferromagnetic spring in the pilot balloon of the tracheal or tracheostomy tube is permitted in the scanning room, but should be taped away from the area to be scanned. If a patient is safe to be managed with a LMA, use an MR compatible LMA.
- Fit the patient with ear defenders and tape the eyes.
- Do a 'dummy run' of the patient into and out of the scanner, to ensure that no tension develops on the tubing, wires, or lines when the patient is maximally entered into the MRI scanner.
- Minimize heat loss by wrapping the patient in blankets (long scanning time).
- Ensure an appropriate $ETCO_2$, ET_{agent}, and if undergoing IPPV, adequate muscle relaxation, before leaving the scanning room.
- Monitor the patient from the scanning room. Do not hesitate to abort the scan if the patient develops signs of instability; liaise with the radiographer.
- Be aware that the length of the capnograph tubing factors in a delay in display of ~20 s. The ECG may be prone to interference and or distortion, which may mimic hyperkalaemia.
- Observe the patient carefully for contrast reactions during and immediately after injection of contrast.

Postscan

- When the scan is complete, provide 100% O_2 for at least 3 min whilst transferring the patient back onto the MRI compatible trolley. When stable, disconnect all monitoring and retreat to the nearby anaesthetic room.
- Here, reconnect to 100% O_2 ensuring ventilation and re-establish the ECG, BP, SpO_2, and capnograph.
- Once stability is established, you may either allow the patient to wake up using standard procedures, or maintain anaesthesia for transfer to another critical care area.
- Non-essential infusions may be recommenced.

Further reading

Association of Anaesthetists of Great Britain and Ireland. *MRI – Provision of anaesthetic services in magnetic resonance units*. London: AAGBI, 2002. Available at: ℘ http://www.aagbi.org/publications/guidelines/docs/mri02.pdf.

Association of Anaesthetists of Great Britain and Ireland. *MRI update – Provision of anaesthetic services in magnetic resonance units*. London: AAGBI, 2010. Available at: ℘ http://www.aagbi.org/publications/guidelines/docs/mri02.pdf.

Hopkins R, Peden C, Gandhi S (eds). *Radiology for Anaesthesia and Intensive Care* (2nd edn). Cambridge: Cambridge University Press, 2009.

Peden CJ, Twigg SJ. Anaesthesia for magnetic resonance imaging. *Contin Educ Anaesth Crit Care Pain* 2003; **3**:97–101.

Endovascular stenting

Key points

- This procedure requires angiography and is therefore frequently performed in the radiology department with all the problems of anaesthesia outside the operating room.
- Patients are likely to have severe co-morbidities associated with vascular disease, particularly coronary artery disease, renal dysfunction, and diabetes.
- Endovascular stenting can be performed with LA plus sedation and monitored anaesthesia care, spinal, epidural, or GA. Consider the potential complications of neuraxial block in a patient who will be heparinized during the procedure.
- Clear protocols and team training to manage complications are essential. Ensure availability of all equipment necessary to convert to an open procedure with GA and to manage aneurysm rupture, which will be particularly catastrophic in an isolated setting.
- Consider spinal cord protection and monitoring of spinal cord function for certain high-risk patients undergoing thoracic or thoracoabdominal endovascular stenting.

Background

- In the last decade there has been a dramatic increase in the number of vascular procedures performed with stents.
- The endovascular approach for aortic aneurysm repair avoids a major abdominal incision and results in significantly less blood loss and overall complications than an open repair; consequently, patient recovery is faster and hospital stay shorter (see ▯ Emergency abdominal aortic aneurysm repair, p.180).
- The stent creates a seal above and below the aneurysm sac, and excludes it from the blood flow and the distending pressure which otherwise would cause rupture. If the seal is not optimal, blood can flow around the graft into the sac causing an endoleak.
- To be eligible for this approach, the patient must have an aneurysm with a morphology that can be stented. Distal artery access must also be of sufficient calibre to allow stent and operator access.
- The stent consists of a fine metal framework covered by a Dacron® graft. Initially most stents were for infrarenal aneurysms but stent development has become increasingly sophisticated, enabling many more patients to undergo an endovascular procedure.
- This procedure has been performed urgently for dissecting aneurysms; however, stent availability may be a restricting factor in this setting.

Preparation

- As always, good communication is the key to patient safety.
- Discuss the procedural plan with the surgical and radiological team and clarify the area to be stented; for thoracic stenting hypotension and spinal cord protection may be necessary.

- Determine the potential length of the procedure (it can be 2 h or more in a complex stenting): this may influence the choice of anaesthesia.
- The team should have a plan formulated to deal with catastrophic complications and should be immediately able to locate equipment such as rapid infusion devices if needed.

Anaesthesia care

- Anaesthesia care for this procedure aims to maintain patient comfort, provide haemodynamic stability, facilitate stent placement with hypotension if needed, and to prevent or manage complications.
- If LA is used this is usually supplemented by sedation as the patient must remain immobile and supine on a hard angiography table during a relatively long procedure; patients can become quite restless toward the end of the procedure. Propofol and or remifentanil infusions are frequently used to supplement LA.
- GA and spinal and or epidural anaesthesia have also been widely used for this procedure. Neuroaxial procedures have been performed on many patients, subsequently fully heparinized, without complication.
- The choice of technique should be based on the standard practice for this team, adjusted on the basis of patient factors, including the urgency of the procedure.
- Attach standard monitoring. Insert an arterial line, usually radial, for direct arterial pressure monitoring and blood gas sampling. Large-bore IV access is essential; in the urgent patient or the more complex procedure, CVP and cardiac output monitoring may be appropriate.
- Record the patient's temperature and hourly urine output. Ensure that the patient does not become dehydrated, because renal function is likely to be compromised by the use of radiographic contrast during angiography and any periods of hypotension during stent deployment.
- Access is usually made via the femoral vessels and the patient is heparinized before stent placement. Ensure that the heparin is injected into a fast-running drip and time is given for circulation before stent introduction.
- Unlike open aortic aneurysm surgery, there is no cross-clamping. The critical time in this procedure is during stent placement, the graft must not move during deployment as it cannot be repositioned.
- The anaesthetist may be asked to drop the BP while the balloon is inflated on the stent and the device deployed, during abdominal aortic aneurysm repair a mean pressure of 60–70 mmHg should be low enough, and this is usually achieved by a bolus of propofol, ↑ remifentanil, or ↑ volatile agents. Thoracic graft placement is more critical and may require use of a hypotensive agent to drop the MAP to 50 mmHg; glyceryl trinitrate infusion, sodium nitroprusside, esmolol, and adenosine have all been described to achieve the brief period of greater hypotension required.
- Blood loss is not usually significant; however, it may not be obvious and can be retroperitoneal. Check the Hb concentration in the immediate postoperative period.
- At the end of the procedure, transfer the patient to a fully staffed recovery area for continued monitoring.

Complications

- Conversion to an open procedure occurs in 1–3% of cases.
- Other serious complications include damage to the ilio-femoral vessels, embolization of atheroma, adverse reaction to contrast media, device occlusion, migration and endoleak, and neurological deficit from occlusion of vessels.

Prevention of spinal cord injury

- Paraplegia is reported in 0–12% of patients. Patients at particular risk of spinal cord injury are those undergoing thoracic or thoraco-abdominal stent placement, those with symptomatic spinal ischaemia, previous thoracic aortic stenting, and ↑ length of the graft.
- Graft placement can occlude, or critically lower, perfusion pressure to the intercostal arteries, the artery of Adamkiewicz, and the arch vessels with the origin of the anterior spinal artery, resulting in spinal cord ischaemia.
- Strategies to prevent this disastrous complication include avoiding hypotension during the procedure, except when requested by the surgical and radiological team for stent placement, and increasing spinal cord perfusion pressure using CSF pressure monitoring and drainage. CSF pressure should be kept at or below 15 mmHg; of course, CSF drainage is not without its own complications.
- Monitoring with evoked potentials has been shown to demonstrate altered spinal cord perfusion when CSF pressure exceeded 15 mmHg; corrective action produced recovery of intraoperative evoked potentials.

Further reading

Chollet-Rivier M. Placement of aortic endoprosthesis. *Curr Opin Anesthesiol* 2000; **13**:409–13.

Davies MJ, Arhanghelschi I, Grauer R, *et al.* Anaesthesia for endoluminal repair of abdominal aortic enurysms. *Anaesth Intensive Care* 2002; **30**:66–70.

Lineberger CK, Robertson KM. Vascular stenting. *Curr Opin Anesthesiol* 2002; **15**:37–44.

Steib A, Collange C. Anaesthesia for other endovascular stenting. *Curr Opin Anesthesiol* 2008; **21**:519–22.

Weigang E, Hartert M, Siegenthaler MP, *et al.* Perioperative management to improve neurologic outcome in thoracic or thoracoabdominal aortic stent-grafting. *Ann Thorac Surg* 2006; **82**:1679–87.

Anaesthetic Emergencies

Failed tracheal intubation

Key points
- Failure to intubate is relatively rare. The threat to life is from failure to oxygenate, not failure to intubate.
- Competence with the emergency drill and in the use of all available kit is essential—never use a device for the first time in a life-threatening situation.

Background

The incidence of failed intubation is low (0.05%). Thorough preoperative airway assessment will never identify all of these. Three important points to remember are:
▶ Failure to oxygenate causes death, not failure to intubate.
▶ Tracheal intubation must be confirmed, in all situations, with capnography.
- A 'can't intubate, can't ventilate' (CICV) situation can occur in any scenario.

There are two main unanticipated difficult intubation scenarios in non-obstetric adults:
- Unanticipated difficult intubation for an elective patient, non-RSI.
- Unanticipated difficult intubation for a RSI.

The Difficult Airway Society (DAS) has developed the standard UK guidelines for these scenarios.

Unanticipated difficult intubation in an adult patient (non-rapid sequence induction)

The DAS flowchart of an Unanticipated difficult intubation in an adult patient is shown in Fig. 16.1.

Plan A: initial tracheal intubation plan

Call for help early in any situation.
- Optimize:
  - Positioning: extend head with flexed neck, ramp with pillows may help.
  - Muscle relaxation: deep enough? No cough on laryngoscopy.
  - Backward, upward, rightward pressure (BURP)/external laryngeal pressure. Manipulate the thyroid cartilage with own hand to get the best view *then* ask assistant to hold in place.
- Bougie:
  - Gum elastic bougie or an alternative plastic bougie.
  - Confirm tracheal placement: (a) clicks: bougie on tracheal cartilage; (b) hold up likely to be carina.
  - Railroad tracheal tube with care; 90° anticlockwise rotation aids smooth placement.
- Alternative laryngoscopes:
  - Initially try a different size Macintosh blade (3 or 4).
  - Short handle—easier with obese or large-chested patients.

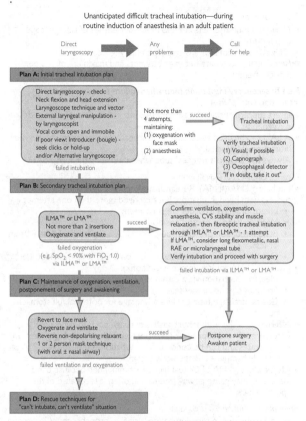

Unanticipated difficult tracheal intubation—during
routine induction of anaesthesia in an adult patient

Direct
laryngoscopy → Any
problems → Call
for help

Plan A: Initial tracheal intubation plan

Direct laryngoscopy - check:
Neck flexion and head extension
Laryngoscope technique and vector
External laryngeal manipulation -
by laryngoscopist
Vocal cords open and immobile
If poor view: Introducer (bougie) -
seek clicks or hold-up
and/or Alternative laryngoscope

Not more than
4 attempts,
maintaining:
(1) oxygenation with
face mask
(2) anaesthesia

— succeed → Tracheal intubation

Verify tracheal intubation
(1) Visual, if possible
(2) Capnograph
(3) Oesophageal detector
"If in doubt, take it out"

failed intubation

Plan B: Secondary tracheal intubation plan

ILMA™ or LMA™
Not more than 2 insertions
Oxygenate and ventilate

— succeed →

Confirm: ventilation, oxygenation,
anaesthesia, CVS stability and muscle
relaxation - then fibreoptic tracheal intubation
through IMLA™ or LMA™ - 1 attempt
If LMA™, consider long flexometallic, nasal
RAE or microlaryngeal tube
Verify intubation and proceed with surgery

failed oxygenation
(e.g. SpO$_2$ < 90% with FiO$_2$ 1.0)
via ILMA™ or LMA™

failed intubation via ILMA™ or LMA™

**Plan C: Maintenance of oxygenation, ventilation,
postponement of surgery and awakening**

Revert to face mask
Oxygenate and ventilate
Reverse non-depolarising relaxant
1 or 2 person mask technique
(with oral ± nasal airway)

— succeed →

Postpone surgery
Awaken patient

failed ventilation and oxygenation

**Plan D: Rescue techniques for
"can't intubate, can't ventilate" situation**

Fig. 16.1 Unanticipated difficult tracheal intubation during routine induction of
anaesthesia in adult patient. Reproduced with permission from the Difficult Airway
Society, Difficult Airway Society Guidelines 2004.

- Alternative blades—McCoy flexible tip, straight (Miller or
  Henderson), polio.
- Videolaryngoscopes are evolving rapidly and can significantly
  improve the laryngoscopic view. Storz C-MAC® and McGrath®
  use Macintosh blades. Usually need stylet and angled tube end to
  manipulate through cords.
- Indirect laryngoscopes have inbuilt channels to guide the tracheal tube.
  Intubation observed through an integral prism viewer, e.g. Airtraq®.

Plan A summary
- Maximum four attempts at intubation (four entries of laryngoscope into mouth).
- Only two attempts for any one type of laryngoscope.
▶Remember: oxygenate between attempts and maximum of 30 s per airway attempt.

Plan B: secondary intubation plan when failure to secure tracheal intubation with plan A
- Insert supraglottic airway device (SAD) to maintain ventilation and oxygenation.
- A SAD can be used as conduit for tracheal tube placement, fibreoptic intubation (FOI) ideal.
- Always use an uncut tracheal tube when intubating through a SAD.

A range of SADs are available:
- Intubating LMA (ILMA). Research suggests first option in Plan B. 92% success with blind intubation, but may need more then one attempt.
  - Needs practice to order steps correctly.
  - Maintain head in neutral position.
  - Blind intubation or FOI through the LMA using tracheal tube 8.0 mm or less.
  - Can leave LMA in place after intubation or remove with a 'pusher'.
- Pro-Seal® LMA (pLMA, Intavent Orthofix).
  - Ideal for intubation via a catheter exchange technique.
  - Provides a good airway seal.
  - Gastric drainage tube definite advantage for potential full stomach patients.
- Alternative SADs with inbuilt gastric drainage ports include: i-gel® (Intersurgical) and Supreme® LMA (Intavent). Both have high insertion success rates and can be conduits for intubation, although the sLMA is potentially hampered by the bowl design.
- Classic LMA (cLMA): FOI technique recommended because blind intubation may cause airway trauma and often fails because of the aperture bars.

Fibreoptic intubation via a conduit
The technique for direct intubation using a bronchoscope/fibrescope comprises:
- The SAD (left in place after intubation) or Berman airway is used as a conduit.
- Pre-load appropriate size *uncut* tracheal tube onto the bronchoscope.
- Tracheal tube railroaded over the bronchoscope when tracheal intubation confirmed.

The technique for using Aintree Intubation Catheter® (AIC) (Cook Medical) comprises:
- Insert SAD and ventilate patient's lungs.
- Preload AIC onto a bronchoscope and pass through a fibrescope adapter attached to the SAD, allowing continued ventilation.
- Railroad AIC over the bronchoscope and through the trachea.

- Two options now available:
  - Oxygenate through the AIC (via 15 mm Rapi-fit® adapter with anaesthetic circuit or jet ventilate (e.g. Manujet®) via luer lock adaptor supplied.
  - Intubate with 7.0 mm tracheal tube (or larger as AIC 6.5 mm external diameter) railroaded over AIC. Remove AIC and ventilate as usual. SAD can be left or removed over the AIC before intubate.

Plan B summary
- Maximum two attempts for SAD placement.
- FOI assisted better technique for intubating via a SAD.
- Always use an uncut tracheal tube when intubating through any SAD.

Plan C: maintain oxygenation and ventilation—wake patient up and postpone surgery
- If plan B unsuccessful the safest option is to wake patient up.
- Face mask ± airway adjuncts: (oropharyngeal/nasopharyngeal airway) or cLMA.
- Reverse muscle relaxant (neostigmine + glycopyrronium, sugammadex).

Plan D: 'can't intubate, can't ventilate' rescue techniques
Help should be present. Adopt plan D immediately if significant hypox-aemia (SpO$_2$ <90%, FiO$_2$ 1.0) or unable to ventilate.

Surgical cricothyroidotomy
Relatively easier to learn with fewer complications than needle techniques. Can be quicker to perform and ventilation is by a standard anaesthetic circuit.
- Equipment—scalpel, small tracheal tube (e.g. 6.0 mm) ± bougie or tracheal hooks and dilators.
- Extend neck and palpate cricothyroid membrane; make horizontal incision with scalpel.
- Dilate with handle, pass bougie or tracheal tube directly then inflate cuff.

Cannula cricothyroidotomy
A variety of kits are available—all require practice before use.
- Wide bore (>4 mm)—ventilate via 15-mm connector with anaesthetic circuit:
  - Melker® (Cook)—Seldinger technique, 5-mm cuffed tube.
  - Quicktrach® (VBM, Germany) V.1 uncuffed and V.2 cuffed. 4-mm tube slides over trochar into trachea. Potential for posterior wall damage.
- Narrow bore (<4 mm)—jet ventilation via cannula relying upon patient's airway for expiration. Avoid 14-G cannula technique as kinks too easily. Short-term solution only, needs urgent surgical airway (ENT).
  - Posterior wall trauma, surgical emphysema and failure possible.
  - Ravussin® cannula (13–16G, VBM, Germany). Pass needle through cricothyroid membrane, aspirate air and advance cannula over needle.
  - Jet ventilate (Manujet 3®, VBM, Germany) until chest rises, taking care to avoid barotrauma.

Rapid sequence induction unanticipated failed intubation
- Follow plan A unless fails; plan C is then the safest option (Fig. 16.2).
- Cricoid pressure may impair intubation—may need to relax briefly for intubation.
- **No** plan B *except* for non-waking patient:
  - pLMA is an alternative because it has a gastric drainage port and improved seal.
  - Time limit for FOI because suxamethonium has a short duration of action.

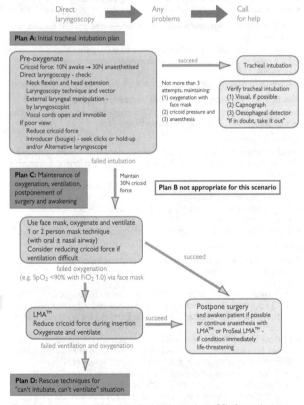

Fig. 16.2 Unanticipated difficult tracheal intubation during RSI of anaesthesia in non-obstetric adult patient. Reproduced with permission from the Difficult Airway Society, Difficult Airway Society Guidelines 2004.

Obstetric failed tracheal intubation

- Must establish maternal risk (see ▣ Chapter 11, p.266).
- Plan A as for unanticipated failed intubation with RSI.
- Mother's life *not* in danger: waking the mother recommended.
- If CICV at any stage: implement plan D immediately.

Further reading

Cook TM, Woodall N, Frerk C. Major complications of airway management in the UK: results of the Fourth National Audit Project of the Royal College of Anaesthetists and the Difficult Airway Society. Part 1: Anaesthesia. *Br J Anaesth* 2011; **106**:617–31.

Cook TM, Woodall N, Harper J, *et al.* Major complications of airway management in the UK: results of the Fourth National Audit Project of the Royal College of Anaesthetists and the Difficult Airway Society. Part 2: intensive care and emergency departments. *Br J Anaesth* 2011; **106**:632–42.

Cook TM, Lee G, Nolan JP. The ProSeal™ laryngeal mask airway: a review of the literature. *Can J Anesth* 2005; **52**:739–60.

Difficult Airway Society Guidelines. Available at: ℘ http://www.das.uk.com

Popat M (ed). *Difficult Airway Management*. Oxford: Oxford University Press, 2009.

Pulmonary aspiration of gastric contents

Key points
- Risk of chemical pneumonitis/pneumonia/atelectasis after pulmonary aspiration.
- Prevention is key, e.g. fasting, tracheal intubation, awake extubation.
- Preoperative antacids may prevent severity of lung injury if aspiration occurs.
- Supportive therapy based on respiratory signs and symptoms.

Background
- Pulmonary aspiration of gastric contents during GA has been estimated at 1:4000 for elective procedures, rising to 1:900 for emergency procedures.
- Morbidity results from lung injury (chemical pneumonitis from gastric acid, pneumonia from upper airway organisms, ARDS) and atelectasis or segmental collapse distal to particulate matter—as well as the immediate threat to life if regurgitated matter causes large airway obstruction.
▶ Anticipation of risk and use of preventative measures is essential.
- Risk factors include a full stomach (e.g. not fasted, intestinal obstruction, delayed gastric emptying due to drugs/trauma/pain), ↓ lower oesophageal sphincter pressure, pregnancy, obesity, pre-existing gastro-oesophageal reflux, hiatus hernia, drugs, difficult airway/difficulty with intubation, delay in securing airway, air inflation of the stomach, ↓ upper airway reflexes, LA to upper airway, emergency, laparoscopic, procedures requiring Trendelenburg or lithotomy position.

Prevention
- Preoperative fasting: minimum 6h for food/milk-containing drinks; 4h for breast milk; 2h for water and clear/non-fizzy fluids.
- Antacids: H_2 receptor antagonists are more effective than proton-pump inhibitors (in healthy test subjects), both at increasing gastric pH and reducing gastric volume. They may have a premedication role in the patient at risk of aspiration, but are not recommended for routine preoperative prescription.
- RSI of anaesthesia in patients at risk of aspiration and cuffed tracheal tube placement.
- Nasogastric tube placement and emptying of gastric contents prior to induction of anaesthesia may be appropriate for patients with intestinal obstruction.
- Extubation of patient sitting up awake and cooperative, or left-lateral head down.

Recognition

- Pulmonary aspiration of gastric contents can occur at any stage of anaesthesia.
- Signs include tachypnoea, ↑ inspiratory pressures, tachycardia, and hypoxaemia.
- Gastric contents may be visible in the oropharynx or airway device.
- Wheeze or crepitations may be heard on auscultation.
- The differential diagnosis includes bronchospasm, ARDS, tracheal tube/circuit obstruction.

Management

- The immediate priority is to prevent further aspiration and lung injury, and ensure adequate oxygenation of the patient.
- The best option will depend on the circumstances. Aspirated matter will need removing from the trachea and airways.
- If a large amount of aspiration, intubate the trachea and suck any solid and particulate matter from the airways before ventilation; this prevents blowing aspirate further into the lungs.
- Consider bronchoscopy to remove solid matter if necessary.
- Cricoid pressure and suctioning the oropharynx rapidly before tracheal intubation may prevent further aspiration.
- Traditional teaching recommends that regurgitation of gastric contents at induction be managed by tilting the patient head-down and positioning in the left lateral position. This can make airway management more difficult and positioning can be difficult to do in large patients.
- If the patient is nearly awake and breathing spontaneously (at start or end of anaesthetic), consider head-down/left-lateral recovery position with high-flow oxygen until fully awake. Monitor patients, because they may need to be resedated and intubated if they develop respiratory distress.
- In the intubated patient PEEP of 5–10 cmH$_2$O may improve oxygenation during positive pressure ventilation and will help reduce atelectasis. Increase FiO$_2$ as necessary, and give bronchodilators for wheeze.
- Decide with the surgical team whether or not to proceed with surgery; this depends on the severity of lung injury and urgency of surgery.
- Insert a nasogastric tube and empty the stomach before extubation.
- If suspicion of larger airways obstruction by solid food (hypoxia not responding to PEEP/high FiO$_2$), consider bronchoscopy to remove debris via the tracheal tube.
- Arrange a chest X-ray. This may be normal or show infiltrates, evidence of lung collapse, and consolidation. Right-sided and dependent lung changes are more common because of the more vertical alignment of the right main stem bronchus.
- Assess the patient's respiratory function—if oxygenation and lung compliance is normal and the patient is stable, extubate. Otherwise keep sedated and intubated and discuss transfer to ICU.

Postoperative

- Patients who can be woken and extubated should be monitored closely for at least 2 h after extubation: if no respiratory symptoms and normal clinical assessment they can be discharged from recovery.
- Consider admission to a critical care unit for those who develop cough or wheeze, are tachycardic or tachypnoeic, have low oxygen saturation on room air, or show new changes on chest X-ray. Patients can develop pneumonitis, ARDS, or pneumonia.
- In ventilated patients with evidence of lung injury, use a protective ventilation strategy, e.g. set tidal volumes <6 mL kg^{-1} (ideal weight derived from height and sex), a plateau pressure <30 cmH$_2$O, and allow gradual hypercarbia if necessary.
- Do not give antibiotics prophylactically, although 20–30% of patients with significant aspiration will develop pneumonia subsequently (treat according to microbiology sensitivities). Often mixed aerobic, anaerobic infections.
- Steroids may limit the inflammatory process but do not reduce mortality and their routine use is not recommended.

Further reading

Bernadini A, Natalini G. Risk of pulmonary aspiration with laryngeal mask airway and tracheal tube: analysis on 65 712 procedures with positive pressure ventilation. *Anaesthesia* 2009; **64**:1289–94.

Clark K, Lam LT, Gibson S, et al. The effect of ranitidine versus proton pump inhibitors on gastric secretions: a meta-analysis of randomised control trials. *Anaesthesia* 2009; **64**:652–7.

Englehardt T, Webster NR. Pulmonary aspiration of gastric contents in anaesthesia. *Br J Anasth* 1999; **83**:453–60.

Ng A, Smith G. Gastroesophageal reflux and aspiration of gastric contents in anesthetic practice. *Anaesth Analg* 2001; **93**:494–513.

World Health Organization. *WHO guidelines for safe surgery.* Geneva: WHO, 2009. Available at: ℬ http://whqlibdoc.who.int/publications/2009/9789241598552_eng.pdf.

Cardiac arrest and peri-arrest arrhythmias

Key points
- Intraoperative cardiac arrest is uncommon.
- Clinical signs and monitoring should enable early diagnosis of cardiac arrest during anaesthesia.
- Ensure high-quality chest compressions with minimal interruption.
- Identify and correct reversible causes during CPR.

Background
- CPR is needed in about 1 in 2000 GAs and 1 in 5000 RAs. Most are related to the patient's presenting problem—e.g. massive trauma, bleeding. About 10% of arrests are directly related to GA (e.g. anaphylaxis, airway problems) and 50% to RA (e.g. high block, respiratory depression, LA toxicity).
- Pulseless electrical activity (PEA) or asystolic cardiac arrest caused by bleeding is the commonest cause of cardiac arrest during anaesthesia. An unexpected primary ventricular fibrillation, pulseless ventricular tachycardia cardiac arrest in individuals with cardiac disease can also occur.
- Survival to discharge after cardiac arrest during anaesthesia is better than for cardiac arrest in other settings (out of hospital, ward).

Management of intraoperative cardiac arrest
Management of cardiac arrest should be according to the advanced life support (ALS) algorithm (Fig. 16.3).

Diagnosis of cardiac arrest during anaesthesia
- Patient monitoring together with clinical signs enables early diagnosis of cardiac arrest. Diagnosis should take <10s.
- Cardiac arrests with reversible causes (e.g. hypovolaemia, hypoxaemia) will have a period of deterioration beforehand.
- A decrease in cardiac output will be associated with a decrease in $ETCO_2$. It is rare in early cardiac arrest to see a flat $ETCO_2$ waveform—if this occurs check tracheal tube/airway placement.
- During hypovolaemia with a tachycardia, the exact moment of PEA cardiac arrest may be difficult to identify. In patients with invasive arterial monitoring this may show a very low blood pressure that responds to fluids and vasopressors. Non-invasive blood pressure monitors cannot measure very low BPs. If other signs indicate cardiac arrest, start CPR.

Starting CPR and modifications for intraoperative cardiac arrest
- Make surgeons and other team members aware that the patient is in cardiac arrest and ask for senior help. Organize the team to ensure everyone knows the plan and that interruptions to chest compressions are minimized.

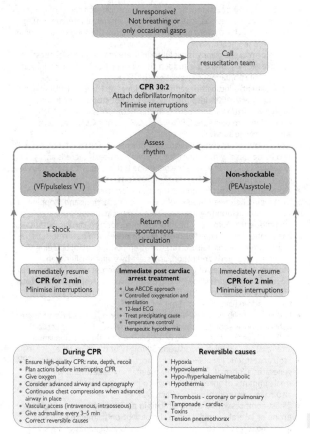

Fig. 16.3 Adult ALS algorithm. Reproduced with the kind permission of the Resuscitation Council (UK).

- Start chest compressions (depth 5–6 cm ensuring full recoil of chest between compressions, rate 100–120 min^{-1}, minimal interruption). If the patient's chest/upper abdomen is open, ask the surgeon to directly compress the heart.
- Waveform capnography is useful to indicate effectiveness of chest compressions. If there is a sudden rise in the ETCO$_2$, this may indicate a return of spontaneous circulation (ROSC).
- If the patient is intubated, ventilate the lungs at 10 min^{-1} (tidal volume 6 mL kg^{-1}) with 100% inspired oxygen. Do not stop compressions to give ventilations. Both pauses in chest compression and a high ventilation rate decrease CPP. A high CPP during CPR is associated with improved survival.
- Continuous chest compressions without pauses for ventilation may also be possible with a supraglottic airway device. If there is an excessive leak, change to a tracheal tube if this is easy to do; otherwise, give two ventilations every 30 compressions.
- If the patient has profound intraoperative bradycardia unresponsive to atropine, followed by asystole, chest compressions and stopping surgical stimulation (e.g. traction on eye muscle, decompressing pneumoperitoneum) may be effective in restoring a cardiac output.
- If the patient has a *non-shockable (PEA/asystole) cardiac arrest*, start chest compressions, ensure surgical attempts to control bleeding continue, give fluids and blood, and start by giving smaller than recommended doses of adrenaline (e.g. 50 micrograms IV increments = 0.5 mL 1:10 000 adrenaline). If the patient has not responded to a total of 1 mg IV adrenaline in the first few minutes of cardiac arrest, give further adrenaline doses of 1 mg for every 3–5 min.
- For *ventricular fibrillation (VF)/tachycardia (VT)* arrest, start CPR and attempt defibrillation as soon as defibrillator is available (see following section). If VF/VT, give first dose of 1 mg IV adrenaline after three defibrillation attempts, and also give amiodarone 300 mg IV at the same time.
- Stop anaesthetic agents—for very short cardiac arrests or where CPR generates a 'normal' BP, consider maintaining anaesthesia with very small amounts of anaesthetic drugs to prevent awareness. They may also have a neuroprotective effect.
- Chest compressions may be difficult in patients who are positioned prone or lateral—rapidly move the patient on to their back if simple initial measures fail to restore circulation. Use of adhesive pads will enable defibrillation in prone patients.
- In some specialist units it may be possible to institute emergency cardiopulmonary bypass during CPR. This will buy time to identify and treat a reversible cause.
- The decision on continuing surgery needs to be made on a case-by-case basis. Continue life-saving surgery (e.g. ruptured aortic aneurysm), stop non-life saving elective procedures where feasible.

Defibrillation

- Minimize interruption to chest compressions for shock delivery.
- Place adhesive pads on patient's chest while chest compressions ongoing. Pause briefly to confirm rhythm. If VF/VT resume chest compressions whilst the defibrillator is charged (use manufacturer's

recommended shock energy or set to highest shock energy). Once defibrillator charged, ensure everyone stands clear. Deliver shock and then resume chest compressions. Complete 2 min of CPR.

- The gap between compressions and shock delivery is called the preshock pause. Even short (e.g. 5 s) increases in preshock pause decrease shock success.
- If the chest is open, adhesive pads can still be used. Alternatively use internal paddles if available. The surgeon should continue compressions with the internal paddles whilst charging (20-J biphasic shock energy) before delivering a shock.
- In patients at high risk of VF/VT arrest, consider placing pads preoperatively. Multifunctional pads with an appropriate defibrillator will enable transcutaneous pacing.

Identification of reversible causes
- During CPR, identify potential reversible causes using the '4 Hs' (hypoxia, hypovolaemia, hypo/hyperkalaemia/metabolic, hypothermia) and '4 Ts' (thrombosis, tamponade, toxins, tension pneumothorax).
- Ultrasound by a skilled operator can be useful to diagnose tamponade and tension pneumothorax during CPR. Ensure interruptions to chest compression are kept to a minimum.

Cardiac arrest due to local anaesthetic toxicity
- Patients with cardiac arrest (or cardiovascular collapse) attributed to LA toxicity may benefit from 20% lipid emulsion IV in addition to CPR and ALS measures.
- Give a 1.5-mL kg^{-1} (about 100 mL in a 70-kg patient) lipid bolus followed by an infusion at 15 mL kg^{-1} h^{-1}. Give up to three bolus doses of lipid at 5-min intervals and continue the infusion (increase the rate to 30 mL kg^{-1} h^{-1} after 5 min) until the patient is stable or has received up to a maximum of 12 mL kg^{-1} of lipid emulsion.

Post cardiac arrest care
- After a short period (e.g. a few minutes) of cardiac arrest, consider waking up the patient if this is feasible. This will enable neurological assessment.
- After prolonged cardiac arrest, once the patient has stabilized, transfer the patient sedated and ventilated to ICU for ongoing care. Patients often develop a systemic inflammatory response (post cardiac arrest syndrome).
- Reversible myocardial dysfunction is common. Patients will require fluids, vasopressors and inotropes. This will require invasive monitoring.
- Consider therapeutic hypothermia (32–34°C) for 24 h. Cool with cold IV fluids (e.g. 2–3 L of cold Hartmann's solution), maintain with surface cooling devices or intravascular cooling, and rewarm slowly at 0.25°C h^{-1}. Most evidence in support of cooling is for VF/VT arrest, but it is also commonly used after PEA/asystolic arrest.
- In patients with a suspected acute coronary syndrome, discuss early coronary angiography and PCI with a cardiologist. Patients with cardiogenic shock may also benefit from insertion of an intra-aortic balloon pump. This may require transfer of the patient to a cardiology centre. The benefits of anticoagulant and antiplatelet drugs need to be balanced against the risks of bleeding in the surgical patient.

- Ensure that an experienced member of the team speaks to the relatives, the incident is investigated and that those involved receive appropriate support from colleagues.

Summary of ALS interventions by age groups
Differences in ALS interventions by age groups are given in Table 16.1.

Table 16.1 ALS interventions by age group

	Adult	Child (1 year–puberty)	Infant (<1 year)	Newborn
C:V Compressions at 100–120 min^{-1}	30:2	15:2	15:2	3:1
Start with:	Compressions first	5 ventilations first		Ventilations first
Landmark	Middle of lower half sternum	1 finger breadth above xiphersternum—lower 1/3 of chest		Just below internipple line—lower 1/3 the chest
Depth	5–6 cm	At least 1/3 AP diameter of chest		
Adrenaline dose	1 mg	10 micrograms kg^{-1}		
Amiodarone dose	300 mg	5 mg kg^{-1}		
Defibrillation dose	According to manufacturer or max. setting	4 J kg^{-1}		

C : V = compression : ventilation ratio; AP = anterior-posterior

Peri-arrest arrhythmias

Algorithms for the treatment of bradycardia and tachycardia are shown in Figs. 16.4 and 16.5.

Further reading

Association of Anaesthetists of Great Britain and Ireland. *Catastrophes in Anaesthetic Practice – dealing with the aftermath*. London: AAGBI, 2005. Available at: ℗ http://www.aagbi.org/ publications.

European Resuscitation Council Guidelines for resuscitation 2010. Available at: ℗ http://www. cprguidelines.eu/2010/.

Resuscitation Council (UK). *Resuscitation Guidelines 2010*. Available at: ℗ http://www.resus.org.uk.

Sprung J, Warner ME, Contreras MG, *et al.* Predictors of survival following cardiac arrest in patients undergoing noncardiac surgery: a study of 518,294 patients at a tertiary referral center. *Anesthesiology* 2003; **99**:259–69.

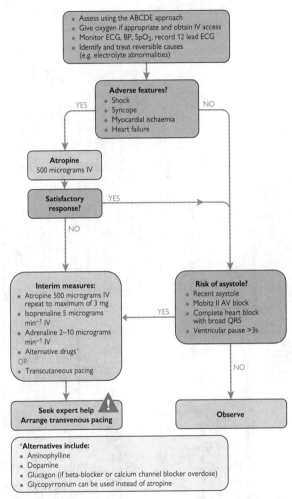

Fig. 16.4 Adult bradycardia algorithm. Reproduced with the kind permission of the Resuscitation Council (UK).

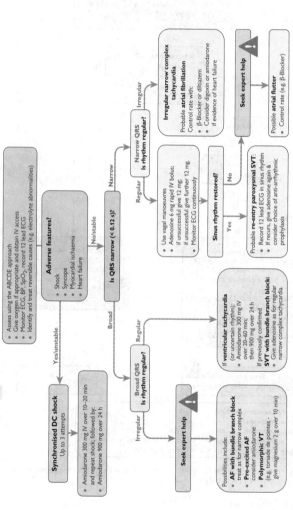

Fig. 16.5 Adult tachycardia algorithm. Reproduced with the kind permission of the Resuscitation Council (UK).

Anaphylaxis

Key points

- Anaphylaxis is a severe, life threatening, generalized or systemic hypersensitivity reaction characterized by life-threatening airway, breathing, or circulation problems, usually associated with skin changes.
- The commonest triggers are: neuromuscular blocking agents (NMBAs) 60%; latex 20%; antibiotics 15%; colloids 4%.
- Use an ABCDE approach to diagnose and treat anaphylaxis.
- Treat anaphylaxis with IV adrenaline early and in small increments (e.g. adults 50-microgram increments, children 1 microgram kg^{-1}).
- Send mast cell tryptase samples for investigation.
- Refer patients with suspected anaphylaxis to a specialist clinic to confirm diagnosis and ensure plan for future anaesthetics in place.

Background

- The incidence of anaphylaxis during anaesthesia has been estimated at between 1 in 10 000–20 000. 10% of reported reactions in the UK are fatal but this is likely to be an overestimate.
- Anaphylaxis can have allergic (2/3 cases, reaction is mediated by an immunological mechanism such as IgE, IgG, or complement activation) and non-allergic (1/3 cases) mechanisms. The term anaphylactoid is no longer used. The underlying mechanism does not affect treatment.
- Females more likely to have reactions to NMBAs and latex. Antibiotic reactions are commoner in smokers.
- NMBAs are the commonest cause (60%) of anaesthetic reactions. Previous exposure is not necessary and all groups of NMBAs have been implicated and cross-sensitivity between different groups can occur. Individuals should therefore be tested for all NMBA groups to identify a safe NMBA to use in the future.
- Latex allergy can be immediate or delayed. ↑ risk in patients with atopy, dermatitis of hands, numerous childhood procedures (spina bifida), healthcare professionals/occupational latex exposure, and those allergic to fruits (banana, avocado, chestnuts).
- Penicillins and cephalosporins (both have a beta-lactam ring) are responsible for 70% of antibiotic reactions. Patients allergic to penicillins have a higher incidence of reactions to 1st-generation cephalosporins (e.g. cefalexin). As there are alternative antibiotic groups available, unless there are compelling microbiological reasons to use a cephalosporin in a penicillin-allergic patient, use something else. A test dose is not useful unless miniscule doses and long periods of observation used—this is not practical.
- LA, opioid, and induction drug reactions are rare and there are no reported reactions to volatile agents.
- Colloid-related reactions tend to be most commonly linked to gelatins and dextrans. Stop a colloid and use a crystalloid if colloid thought to be cause of reaction.

- Numerous other triggers include NSAIDs, chlorhexidine, oxytocin, IV contrast.
- Identify previous reactions during preoperative assessment and avoid trigger agents.
- There is no evidence that pretreatment with antihistamine and steroid reduces risk or severity of anaphylaxis.

Clinical features of anaphylaxis

- Anaphylaxis during anaesthesia usually presents with life-threatening breathing (bronchospasm) or circulation (hypotension due to severe vasodilation and capillary leak, tachycardia, bradycardia (10% cases), cardiac arrest) problems. There are usually skin changes (flushing, urticaria) but these can be absent or subtle.
- Onset is usually rapid (within minutes) after an IV trigger but can be slower after a cutaneous trigger, colloids, antibiotics, or on tourniquet deflation.

Emergency treatment of anaphylaxis during anaesthesia

- Consider anaphylaxis if a patient develops hypotension or bronchospasm.
▶ As the diagnosis is not always immediately obvious, an ABCDE approach to identify and treat problems as they are found is best.
- If cardiac arrest occurs, start CPR according to ALS guidelines (see 🕮 Cardiac arrest and peri-arrest arrhythmias, p.366).
- Stop any potential trigger and call for help early.
- Give 100% inspired oxygen, and ensure trachea intubated, and IV fluids running (large volumes may be needed).
- Give increments of IV adrenaline (adults 50 micrograms, children 1 microgram kg^{-1}). Adrenaline has bronchodilator, vasopressor, and inotropic effects and may decrease mediator release. Titrate to effect—if multiple doses are needed, start an adrenaline infusion.
- If the patient remains hypotensive consider alternative vasopressors (noradrenaline, metaraminol, vasopressin according to experience).
- Consider IV salbutamol, aminophylline, or magnesium for bronchospasm.
- Antihistamines (chlorphenamine—10 mg IV adults) and steroids (hydrocortisone 200 mg IV adults) are 2nd-line drugs and there is time to check doses for children. They will speed up resolution of any skin changes. H_2 blockers are not useful.
- Serum mast cell tryptase (released on mast cell degranulation associated with anaphylaxis) values may help the retrospective diagnosis of anaphylaxis. Values rise and fall rapidly (peak 1 h; half-life 2 h). A normal value does not exclude the diagnosis. Take a sample for mast cell tryptase (5–10 mL clotted bottle) as soon as feasible once resuscitation started, and a 2nd sample at 1–2 h after onset of symptoms. A 3rd sample can be taken at 24 h or at follow-up to measure baseline (some individuals have a high baseline). Ensure samples are labelled and timed and liaise with the hospital laboratory.
- Transfer patient to critical care area for ongoing care. Reactions usually resolve within 2–8 h but some patients may have protracted reactions.

Investigation and follow-up

- Refer patients with suspected anaphylaxis to a specialist clinic (see ℘ http://www.aagbi.org). Ensure accurate details of events, and copy of anaesthetic, recovery, and drug chart provided.
- Skin tests (skin prick test, or intradermal test (more likely to trigger systemic reaction)) should be done only by specialists and should be interpreted with caution. A negative test does not exclude allergy.
- Blood tests for allergen-specific IgE antibodies may give evidence of sensitization but again need specialist interpretation.

Anaesthesia for latex allergy

History and investigations will help classify reaction type:

- Systemic reaction (type 1 hypersensitivity reaction involving specific IgE). This is severe but the least frequent reaction and occurs in genetically predisposed individuals. Blood test for latex specific IgE (75–90% sensitive) or skin prick testing will help identify these high-risk patients.
- Contact dermatitis (delayed type IV hypersensitivity reaction) eczema-like 24–48h after repeated skin or mucosal contact. This is non-life-threatening but can predispose to a severe systemic reaction. Patch testing will help confirm this.
- Irritant dermatitis (non-immune) from irritant effect. This is most common and limited to the contact area.

Avoidance of latex during perioperative period according to local policy is important.

Further reading

Association of Anaesthetists of Great Britain and Ireland. *Suspected anaphylactic reactions associated with anaesthesia*. London: AAGBI, 2009. Available at: ℘ http://www.aagbi.org.

Resuscitation Council (UK). *Emergency treatment of anaphylactic reactions*. London: Resuscitation Council (UK). 2008. Available at: ℘ http://www.resus.org.uk.

Malignant hyperthermia

Malignant hyperthermia

Key points
- Malignant hyperthermia (MH) is a rare, potentially life-threatening condition triggered by all volatile anaesthetic agents and suxamethonium.
- The prognosis is good if MH is recognized and treated early.
- Patients with MH can have had a previous uneventful GA with trigger agents.
- Presentation of MH varies—the onset can be rapid or insidious.
- ▶Supportive treatment, removing trigger, and IV dantrolene are key treatments—know where dantrolene is stored in your hospital.
- Propofol and other IV induction drugs, opioids, non-depolarizing neuromuscular blockers, and nitrous oxide are considered safe.

Background
MH susceptibility shows autosomal dominant inheritance and has a prevalence of 1 in 3000 individuals. Most affected individuals have a mutation of the ryanodine receptor gene (*RYR1*), which encodes the skeletal muscle calcium release channel. MH is estimated to occur in 1 in 10 000–15 000 anaesthetics. Triggering agents in susceptible individuals cause hypermetabolism, sustained skeletal muscle contraction, and muscle breakdown with the release of intracellular contents.

Malignant hyperthermia crisis
Diagnosis
Consider MH if using any volatile agent and/or suxamethonium.

Early signs
- Masseter spasm occurs after giving suxamethonium.
- Unexplained, unexpected increase in $ETCO_2$.
- Unexplained, unexpected increase in O_2 consumption.
- Sweating and mottling of skin.
- Unexplained, unexpected tachycardia.
- Hyperventilation (if spontaneously breathing).
- Cardiovascular instability, arrhythmias, peaked T waves on ECG.
- Generalized muscle rigidity.

Late signs
- Increase in core temperature.
- Hyperkalaemia, ↑ blood creatine phosphokinase, ↑ myoglobin levels, coagulopathy.
- Cardiac arrest.

Differential diagnosis
Insufficient anaesthesia or analgesia, sepsis, anaphylaxis, phaeochromocytoma, thyroid crisis, neuromuscular disorder, malignant neuroleptic syndrome.

Immediate management
- Call for help and use a structured ABCDE approach.
- Stop all trigger agents—remove the vapouriser.
- Maintain anaesthesia with IV propofol.

- Adjust FiO_2 and ventilation to maintain normal oxygen saturation (94-98%), PaO_2, $ETCO_2$, and $PaCO_2$. Use high gas flows and hyperventilate—this will help remove volatile agent from patient and anaesthetic circuit.
- Conclude surgery as soon as is safely possible (ensure senior surgeon present).
- Give dantrolene $2–3\,mg\,kg^{-1}$ IV, then $1\,mg\,kg^{-1}$ up to a total dose of $10\,mg\,kg^{-1}$. May need to exceed maximum recommended dose—give until cardiorespiratory stability. Dissolve dantrolene in sterile water (not saline). Request extra assistance to prepare.
- Switch to a new machine and circuit only when the situation has stabilized. Changing the machine during the acute phase will waste time and resources.

Early management
- Start invasive BP and CVP, core (e.g. oesophageal) and peripheral temperature, and urine output monitoring.
- Check ABG, K^+, platelets, clotting, and haematocrit.
- Treat hyperthermia with cold IV fluids ($2–3\,L$ of 0.9% NaCl at $4°C$), cooling blankets, ice to groins and axillae. Use other cooling devices if available and aim for temperature $<38.5°C$.
- If hyperkalaemia consider IV calcium (chloride has more Ca^{2+} than gluconate and repeated doses may be needed) to protect the heart (especially if ECG changes). Infuse glucose ($50\,mL$ of 50% glucose) with 10 units insulin, and salbutamol (nebulized or IV) to shift K^+ into cells (see ⌨ Electrolytes, p.30). Bicarbonate may also be helpful.
- Cardiac arrhythmias (may resolve with treatment of hyperkalaemia): consider magnesium, amiodarone, or beta-blockers (calcium channel blockers interact with dantrolene).
- Maintain urine output—optimize fluid resuscitation and consider furosemide ($0.5–1\,mg\,kg^{-1}$ IV) or mannitol $1\,g\,kg^{-1}$ IV. Consider forced alkaline diuresis (aim for urine output $>3\,mL\,kg^{-1}$, urine pH >7.0) if there is myoglobinaemia.
- DIC: seek advice from haematologist, give FFP, cryoprecipitate, platelets.

Intensive care management
- Continue invasive monitoring and supportive treatments.
- Further doses of dantrolene may be necessary for up to 24h.
- Watch out for development of renal failure, DIC, and compartment syndrome.
- Check creatine phosphokinase (peaks at 12–24h), urinary pH, and myoglobin.
- Consider alternative diagnosis if no response to dantrolene (e.g. sepsis, thyrotoxic storm, phaeochromocytoma, other myopathies).

Late management

- Ensure alert placed on patient notes.
- Counsel patient and family regarding implications of MH.
- Patients suspected of being MH-susceptible should undergo diagnostic testing using *in vitro* contracture testing (IVCT) and if needed genetic testing at a designated MH-laboratory* (see Ⓢ http://www.emhg.org).
- Ensure plans in place for future anaesthetics and patient is aware of this.

*UK MH Investigation Unit, Academic Unit of Anaesthesia, Clinical Sciences Building, St. James's University Hospital Trust, Leeds LS9 7TF, UK. Direct line: 0113 2065274. Emergency hotline: 07947 609601.

Safe anaesthesia for malignant hyperthermia-susceptible patients

- Avoid trigger agents.
- Consider RA—LAs safe.
- IV anaesthesia safe.
- Safe drugs include: propofol, thiopental, ketamine, benzodiazepines, non-depolarizing neuromuscular blockers, opioids, neostigmine, atropine, glycopyrronium.

Further reading

Glahn KPE, Ellis FR Halsall PJ, *et al*. Recognizing and managing a malignant hyperthermia crisis: guidelines from the European Malignant Hyperthermia Group. *Br J Anaesth* 2010; **105**:417–20.

The Association of Anaesthetists of Great Britain & Ireland. Guidelines for the management of a Malignant Hyperthermia Crisis. London: AAGBI, 2007. Available at: Ⓢ http://www.aagbi.org.

Suxamethonium apnoea

Key points
- Prolonged neuromuscular blockade with suxamethonium caused by reduced level/activity of plasma cholinesterase.
- It is not life threatening but if identified early, anaesthesia can continue until effects of suxamethonium wear off.
- Most common in young people having emergency surgery.
- Prolonged neuromuscular block can also occur with mivacurium.
- May identify from family or anaesthetic history.

Background
The incidence of significant suxamethonium apnoea is 1:2800.

Inherited
- Genes encoding plasma cholinesterase have autosomal inheritance.
- There are several variations of the normal enzyme E1u.
- Three main variants:
  - E1a (atypical/dibucaine resistant) 0.03% population.
  - E1s (silent) 0.001%.
  - E1f (fluoride resistant) 0.003%.
- Heterozygotes (E1u/E1a) have ↑ recovery time (~30 min).
- Homozygotes (E1a/E1a) can take about 3 h to recover.

Acquired
- Normal plasma cholinesterase but with reduced activity/level.
- Delayed recovery in minutes as opposed to hours.
- Causes include:
  - Disease—hypothyroid, anaemia, malnutrition, collagen disorders, carcinomatosis, liver disease, tetanus.
  - Drugs—tetracaine, combined oral contraceptive pill, ketamine, propranolol, ecothiopate eye drops, chlorpromazine, cyclophosphamide, organophosphate insecticides/weedkiller ingestion, pancuronium, neostigmine, monoamine oxidase inhibitors.
  - Physiological—last trimester pregnancy, newborn.
  - Miscellaneous—radiotherapy, plasmapheresis, burns, extracorporeal circulation.

Perioperative
Recognition
- Usually apparent at the end of a GA when suxamethonium (or mivacurium) has been used.
- Routine use of a nerve stimulator will indicate continued paralysis.
- Should waking be attempted (removal of the anaesthetic), the patient will remain paralysed and exhibit signs of awareness (tachycardia, hypertension, sweating, dilated pupils, lacrimation).

Treatment

- If waking was attempted, re-anaesthetize immediately.
- Maintain anaesthesia in a place of safety (operating room/ICU).
- Keep the patient warm and monitor temperature.
- Monitor neuromuscular transmission with a nerve stimulator—the patient should regain four twitches with no fade on train-of-four (TOF) testing.
- If no nerve stimulator is available then maintain anaesthesia until breathing spontaneously.
- Infusion of FFP (contains plasma cholinesterase) will speed up metabolism of suxamethonium. This is not routinely recommended because of the risks associated with infusing a blood product and because it will not gain much time.
- Extubate awake when breathing spontaneously, obeying commands and able to lift their head off the pillow (10 s).
- Reassure the family who may be very anxious.
- Document events.

Follow-up

- The patient may have experienced awareness—explain fully, and offer any support needed.
- Take blood samples at follow-up to measure plasma cholinesterase, dibucaine number and fluoride number (results take 2–3 weeks). Contact laboratory for further information.
- Dibucaine inhibits plasma cholinesterase—a low dibucaine number (above 70 normal) indicates ↓ plasma cholinesterase activity.
- Do not take samples during apnoea or within 24 h of giving suxamethonium. If FFP or plasma cholinesterase preparations have been given wait 6 weeks before taking sample.
- If the tests show an inherited form, family members should also be referred for testing.
- Inform the patient, patient's general practitioner, and ensure clearly documented in notes.

Air/gas embolism

Key points

- Air/gas embolism is usually iatrogenic and prevention is the key.
- A low venous pressure and an open vein cause air/gas entrainment.
- It may cause a sudden fall in $ETCO_2$ and arterial oxygen concentration, followed by cardiovascular collapse.
- Treat with 100% oxygen, raise the venous pressure (e.g. fluids, vasopressors, head-down), start resuscitation, stop further air/gas entrainment, and consider aspirating air/gas from right atrium via a central line.

Background

- Air/gas in the right ventricle/pulmonary artery will cause obstruction to blood flow, right heart strain, and cardiovascular collapse. Air/gas in the pulmonary vasculature also causes an inflammatory response.
- Venous air embolism can occur in presence of open veins, and negative venous pressure, most commonly when the surgical site is above the heart (e.g. neuro-, ENT, orthopaedic, spinal, thoracic surgery, CVC insertion). It can also occur with extracorporeal circuits (e.g. bypass, haemofiltration), IV fluid infusions (especially if pressurized), and from trauma/blast injuries. Air can also be accidentally injected or infused into the venous circulation.
- Carbon dioxide can accidentally enter the venous circulation during laparoscopic surgery. CO_2 embolism is less dangerous than air as it is more rapidly absorbed.
- Outcome depends on the rate/volume of gas entrainment, use of nitrous oxide (will make air bubbles larger—so avoid/stop), patient status, and the presence of a patent foramen ovale (potentially in up to 10% adults; will permit systemic gas and CNS effects). The closer the vein of entrainment to the right heart, the smaller the lethal gas volume (as little as 20 mL can be harmful, 0.5 mL in a coronary artery can cause VF).

Recognition

- Presents with a sudden fall in $ETCO_2$ and fall in SpO_2, followed by cardiovascular collapse or even cardiac arrest. The ECG will show right heart strain, arrhythmias, and ST changes. A rise in ET nitrogen is also seen.
- The surgeon may notice air/gas entrainment/sucking into vein.
- Transthoracic or oesophageal Doppler or ultrasound will show gas bubbles passing through right heart and into pulmonary circulation. Classically a 'mill-wheel murmur' is heard with a stethoscope.
- Ensure other causes are also excluded (e.g. hypovolaemia, anaphylaxis).

Treatment

- Stop further air/gas entrainment—inform the surgeon. Interventions include flooding wound with saline and occluding blood vessels, stopping gas insufflation/decompression of the pneumoperitoneum for laparoscopy, applying bone wax to open bone sinuses, ensuring vascular lines are flushed and closed to air, removing air from extracorporeal circuits.

- Use an ABCDE approach, give 100% inspired oxygen, and stop nitrous oxide.
- Increase CVP—give fluids, vasopressors, put patient head-down, occlude neck veins for cranial surgery.
- Head-down, left-lateral position may prevent gas entering pulmonary circulation—this may, however, hinder resuscitation efforts.
- If a CVC present—aspirate gas from right atrium.
- If cardiac arrest occurs, start CPR according to standard guidelines (see 📖 Cardiac arrest and peri-arrest arrhythmias, p.366).
- Hyperbaric oxygen therapy (if available) speeds up resolution of air bubbles.

Further reading

Mirski MA, Lele AV, Fitzsimmons L, *et al.* Diagnosis and treatment of vascular air embolism. *Anesthesiology* 2007; **106**:164–77.

Equipment failure

Key points
- Human error can contribute to equipment failure.
- Breathing system leaks or disconnections are a common problem.
- Familiarity with equipment and a systematic approach to dealing with problems is essential.
- Maintaining patient safety, rather than precise identification of the fault, is the first priority with anaesthetic equipment failure.
- Improved equipment design, back-up systems, robust checking procedures, and training in crisis management can minimize risks to patients.

Background
- Human error causes >80% of anaesthetic adverse incidents. Equipment failure is the cause in 0.2–2.1%; human error is a contributing factor in 1/4 of these. The incidence of actual or potential harm from equipment failure is 2–11%.
- Early recognition of equipment failure and a systematic approach to finding and dealing with the cause is essential. Familiarity with equipment, an understanding of appropriate preoperative checks, an awareness of risk factors for equipment failure, and maintaining vigilance are key to early identification and subsequent management of equipment-related incidents.
▶ Patient safety (i.e. maintenance of oxygenation, adequate depth of anaesthesia, and cardiovascular stability) must be prioritized above the search for the equipment fault.

Specific equipment problems

Breathing system leak or disconnection
Almost half of anaesthetic machine problems are due to leakage/misconnection of the breathing system.

Risk factors
- Inadequate checking of breathing system.
- Damaged or infrequently changed breathing system.
- Moving the patient or operating table whilst connected.
- Shared airway.
- Changing components of breathing system, e.g. CO_2 absorber, sampling lines, refilling vaporizer.
- Using fresh gas outlet for oxygen without reconnecting breathing system.
- Too small an uncuffed paediatric tracheal tube.

Presentation
Spontaneous ventilation:
- Reservoir bag empties.
- Loss/change $ETCO_2$ waveform.
- Fall in FiO_2/volatile concentration leading to hypoxaemia or light anaesthesia.

IPPV:
- Ventilator bellows empties.
- No chest movements.
- Smell of volatile.
- Audible gas leak/change in ventilator sounds.
- Ventilator alarms—apnoea, low airway pressure, low tidal volume (VT)/minute ventilation (MV).

Management

Increase the fresh gas flow (FGF), close the APL valve and manually ventilate with 100% oxygen, checking chest expansion and capnograph:
- Ventilation possible:
  - Check for leaks around the airway device and breathing circuit.
- Unable to ventilate/inadequate:
  - Discard breathing system and use separate Mapleson C system or self-inflating reservoir bag.
  - Still a problem: (a) check airway/tracheal tube displacement/cuff leak; (b) remove airway device and facemask ventilate if necessary
- Maintain IV anaesthesia.

Methodical check of all the breathing system and connections:
- Side-stream sampling ports; filters; condensers; humidifiers; pressure sensor; flowmeter; oxygen analyser; PEEP valve; CO_2 absorber; reservoir bag; and inspiratory/expiratory limb.

Also consider:
- Placement of nasogastric tube in trachea.
- Tracheo-bronchial leak.
- APL valve unintentionally open/stuck open when ventilating with a Bain system.
- Leaking or incorrectly seated CO_2 absorber housing.
- Active gas scavenging system ports occluded, causing negative pressure in breathing system.
- Ventilator/breathing system pressure relief valve set too low or stuck open.
- Fresh gas flow too low, not switched on, or supply failure.
- Ventilator failure or not switched on.

Further detail

Spontaneous ventilation:
- Change in capnograph trace depends on disconnection site:
  - If the sampling port is in a section of circuit disconnected from exhaled gas, there will be complete loss of the waveform.
  - If it remains connected, it will detect a variable amount of re-breathing of carbon dioxide.
  - If air is entrained, there may be a fall in inspired/expired oxygen, inhalational agent or a rise in inspired/expired nitrogen.

Positive-pressure ventilated:
- Bag-in-bottle ventilator: ascending bellows will collapse (bag generates 2–4 cmH$_2$O PEEP); descending bellows will fall to fully expanded position and may not reveal disconnection.
- Minute volume dividers continue to function if disconnection is distal.
- Many ventilators do not have a visible reservoir, e.g. Penlon Nuffield 200®.

Ventilator failure

Risk factors
- Unfamiliarity with ventilator.
- Inadequate machine check.
- Interruption of power supply.
- Power surge and disruption of ventilator programming.
- Recent anaesthetic machine service or poor maintenance.
- Brand new equipment.
- Old or poorly maintained equipment.

Presentation
- Bellows stop moving (but may not empty).
- Ventilator cycling stops (may be audible).
- Absent chest movements and breath sounds.
- Loss of normal breathing system pressure trace.
- Loss of normal capnograph waveform.
- Apnoea, low tidal/minute volume alarms sound.
- Switching to manual ventilation restores the status quo.
- Falling oxygen saturation is normally a later presentation.

Management
- Check ventilator is switched on and ensure manual/ventilator selector switch is set correctly.
- Switch to manual ventilation with a simple breathing system and manually ventilate patient.
- Consider allowing return of spontaneous ventilation if appropriate, or call for another ventilator.
- Maintain adequate minute ventilation and anaesthesia until another ventilator is available.
- If the reservoir bag will not fill or empties quickly consider:
  - Possible inadequate fresh gas flow settings.
  - Oxygen pipeline failure (and thus ventilator driving gas failure).
  - Disconnection or large leak in breathing system.
  - Unintentional extubation, displacement of airway device, or cuff leak.
- If the reservoir bag fills, but there is resistance on squeezing consider the causes and management of high airway pressure (see following section)
- Once ventilation is re-established, label clearly and remove any faulty ventilator from use (if integral the whole anaesthetic workstation will need removing), log the critical incident, and inform appropriate personnel.

Also consider:
- Manual/ventilator switch incorrectly set or faulty.
- Improper assembly or failure of ventilator, breathing system, pressure sensors, or pressure relief valves.

- Ventilator, anaesthetic workstation, or general power failure (see following section).
- Inappropriate ventilator settings causing pressure relief valve to open.
- Excessive tidal volume for inspiratory time; excessive inspiratory flow.
- Pressure relief threshold too low.
- Bellows or ventilator mechanism stuck.
- Failure of secondary driving gas to some anaesthetic workstation ventilators.
- High airway pressures (see following section), large leaks, or inadequate fresh gas flow.

High airway pressure (P_{insp} >30 cmH$_2$O)
Risk factors

- Inadequate breathing system check; re-use of single-use equipment.
- Cleaning or re-assembly of the circle system.
- Presence of small objects (e.g. IV cannula caps) around anaesthetic station.
- Airway pressure is appropriate for clinical situation: obesity; severe restrictive lung or chest wall disease; patient position, e.g. steep headdown; small diameter microlaryngoscopy tube; raised intra-abdominal pressure, e.g. pneumoperitoneum, ileus.

Presentation

- High measured airway pressure; high airway pressure alarm; sound of ventilator pressure relief valve; low tidal volume and minute volume alarm.
- Audible leaks; abnormal cycling sounds from ventilator.
- Poor chest expansion; ↑ or ↓ ETCO$_2$—depending on the cause.
- Diminished cardiac output secondary to raised intrathoracic pressure.

Management

- Switch to manual ventilation with 100% oxygen; squeeze the reservoir bag and verify difficult ventilation.
- Scan the breathing system, heat and moisture exchanger (HME), and the airway device/tracheal tube for obvious obstructions or signs of reflux.
- Look for signs of light anaesthesia (laryngospasm/coughing/straining/biting with occlusion of the airway device) and deepen anaesthesia intravenously accordingly.
- If ventilation is inadequate, discard breathing circuit and HME to exclude breathing system obstruction and assess ventilation with an alternative system (e.g. self-inflating reservoir bag) connected directly to the airway device.
- If ventilation remains difficult, the problem lies in the airway device or the patient. Check the airway device/tracheal tube is in the right position and patent (an appropriately sized suction catheter or a gum-elastic bougie should pass easily through the whole length of the airway device); replace airway device if necessary.
- If airway device is patent and correctly positioned:
  - Lift drapes and look for skin flushing, urticaria, and subcutaneous emphysema.
  - Examine chest movement, neck veins, tracheal position, and auscultate lungs.

- Examine for evidence of bronchospasm; endobronchial intubation; pulmonary aspiration of gastric contents; pneumothorax; lung/lobar collapse; anatomical/pathological obstruction of the airway or trachea; acute pulmonary oedema; consider CXR, ABG, bronchoscopy.

Also consider:
- Occult obstruction of circuit/airway device (e.g. kink, foreign body, sputum, clot).
- Soaked or clogged filter/HME (e.g. gastric contents, pulmonary oedema).
- Surgical team applying retractors or leaning on the patient.
- Opioid-induced chest wall rigidity.
- Airway pressure alarm malfunction or inappropriately set.
- Ventilator settings inappropriate: excessive tidal volume or inspiratory flow; excessively short I:E ratio; long I:E ratio with gas-trapping.
- Ventilator/manual selector in the wrong position; APL valve stuck or unintentionally closed (especially after switching from mechanical ventilation).
- Ventilator malfunction—expiratory/PEEP valve malfunction.
- Malfunction of scavenging system.
- Oxygen flush depressed inadvertently or stuck open.
- Failure of flow restrictors or machine regulators allowing gas under high pressure to enter breathing system.

Pipeline oxygen supply failure
Risk factors
- No machine check performed; failure to reconnect pipeline after machine check; unfamiliar pipeline connections.
- Anaesthetic workstation not plugged in or unintentionally switched off.
- Recent machine or pipeline maintenance, repair, or replacement.
- Fault during refilling of central oxygen source.
- Exhausted hospital central oxygen source.

Presentation
- Oxygen failure alarm sounds and pressure gauge falls.
- Oxygen and linked flowmeters fall; emergency oxygen flush fails.
- Pipeline oxygen-driven ventilators stop.
- Audible escape of gas if pipeline connection leaking.

Management
- Turn on the reserve oxygen cylinder and check that the pressure gauge indicates an adequately filled cylinder; check oxygen analyser confirms return of oxygen flow.
- Verify pressure failure on the pipeline pressure gauge.
- Check for disconnection between the pipeline and wall and re-attach it if possible
- Preserve cylinder oxygen: use low oxygen flows; in circle system—close the APL valve; switch to manual ventilation if oxygen driven ventilator.
- Inform the surgeon of the event and make a plan to expedite surgery.

Once established on cylinder oxygen:

- Disconnect the pipeline supply if failure has occurred upstream from wall outlet. Re-establishment of pipeline may result in a temporary flow of gas that is contaminated, or the wrong gas may be reconnected at source.
- Inform other hospital areas where pipeline oxygen is used.
- Find out when the oxygen supply is likely to be reliably restored and arrange for an appropriate number of oxygen cylinders to safely complete the surgery.
- If the cylinder oxygen supply runs out, as a last resort, allow the patient to breathe room air or ventilate using a self-inflating reservoir bag whilst maintaining anaesthesia intravenously.

Operating room or anaesthetic station power failure
Risk factors

- Lack of room uninterruptible back-up power supply/emergency generator.
- Lack of back-up batteries or inadequate battery maintenance in vital equipment.
- Injudicious unplugging of room equipment—lack of charge in back-up batteries.
- Running power cables along the floor between equipment and power sockets.
- Emergency generator tests, hospital construction work, or natural disaster.

Presentation

- AC power failure alarms sound on devices with charged back-up batteries
- Devices without charged back-up batteries stop working: anaesthetic workstations (potentially stopping fresh gas flow); monitors; electronically managed ventilators; infusion devices; warming devices; essential surgical instruments (e.g. diathermy); electrically powered operating tables and beds; cardiopulmonary bypass machines.
- Lights may go out; operating room air-conditioning and laminar flow systems fail.

Management

- Call for help and light if necessary (daylight, torches, pen-torches, mobile phone displays, laryngoscopes).
- Check flow meters if visible (e.g. if fluorescent, back-lit, or electronic display with battery back-up).
- If flow meters not visible, listen and feel for fresh gas flow at the common gas outlet.
- If fresh gas flow has stopped, either continue low-flow spontaneously breathing anaesthesia temporarily with a closed circle system if equilibrated, or use a self-inflating reservoir bag with cylinder O_2 and maintain anaesthesia intravenously.
- Check ventilator is still functioning and switch to manual ventilation if necessary.
- Maintain clinical monitoring as far as possible:
  - Visual—chest rise/fall, cyanosis, pupil size, movement, sweating.
  - Tactile—pulses (peripheral or at surgical site), capillary refill time.
  - Auditory—stethoscope, sphygmomanometer.

- Obtain battery-powered monitors: portable pulse oximeters; defibrillator ECG; transport monitors.
- Call for help and information about duration of operating room power failure.
- If necessary, continue with a pneumatic anaesthetic machine and ventilator if pipeline gas supplies or cylinders allow.
- Under difficult circumstances it may be safer to establish spontaneous ventilation.
- Be aware of limited battery life—especially infusion pumps.
- If infusions need to be titrated and electric pumps fail, use volumetric burettes and measure drop rates.
- Ask surgical team to finish as quickly as possible or abandon operation.
- Reallocate personnel and resources to areas where they are needed.
- A hospital disaster plan may have to be initiated.

Further reading

Aitkenhead AR. Injuries associated with anaesthesia. A global perspective. *Br J Anaesth* 2005; **95**:95–109.

Anderson WR, Brock-Utne JG. Oxygen pipeline supply failure. A coping strategy. *J Clin Monit* 1991; **7**:39–41.

Carter JA. Checking anaesthetic equipment and the Expert Group on Blocked Anaesthetic Tubing (EGBAT). *Anaesthesia* 2004; **59**:105–7.

Cooper JB, Newbower RS, Kitz RJ. An analysis of major errors and equipment failures in anaesthesia management. Considerations for prevention and detection. *Anesthesiology* 1984; **60**:34–42.

Fasting S, Gisvold SE. Equipment problems during anaesthesia – are they a quality problem? *Br J Anaesth* 2002; **89**:825–31.

Keith RL, Pierson DJ. Complications of mechanical ventilation. A bedside approach. *Clin Chest Med* 1996; **17**:439–51.

Raphael DT, Weller RS, Doran DJ. A response algorithm for the low-pressure alarm condition. *Anesth Analg* 1988; **67**:876–83.

Robinson H, Crean P, Chisakuta, A. *Risks associated with your anaesthetic. Information for patients. Section 13: Equipment failure.* London: The Royal College of Anaesthetists, 2010. Available at: ℅ http://www.rcoa.ac.uk.

Runciman WB, Kluger MT, Morris RW, *et al.* Crisis management during anaesthesia: the development of an anaesthetic crisis management manual. *Qual Saf Health Care* 2005; **14**:e1.

Index